Drug Injecting and HIV Infection

Social Aspects of AIDS

Series Editor: Peter Aggleton

Institute of Education, University of London

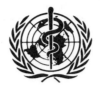

WORLD HEALTH ORGANIZATION

Drug Injecting and HIV Infection: Global Dimensions and Local Responses

Edited by

Gerry V. Stimson, Don C. Des Jarlais
and Andrew L. Ball

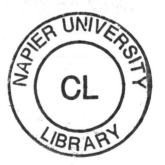

UCL PRESS
Taylor & Francis Group

© World Health Organization, 1998

First published in 1998 by UCL Press

UCL Press Limited
1 Gunpowder Square
London EC4A 3DE
UK

and

1900 Frost Road, Suite 101
Bristol
Pennsylvania 19007-1598
USA

The name University College London (UCL) is a registered trade mark used by
UCL Press with the consent of the owner.

British Library Cataloguing-in-Publication Data
A catalogue record for this book is available from the British Library.

Library of Congress Cataloging-in-Publication Data are available

ISBNs: 1–85728–824–6 HB
1–85728–825–4 PB

Typeset by Wilmaset Ltd, Birkenhead, UK.
Printed by TJ International Ltd, Padstow, Cornwall

Contents

Contents

List of Figures

List of Tables

Foreword

In 1989 the World Health Organization initiated a comparative study of drug injecting behaviour and HIV infection which has involved 12 cities (Athens, Bangkok, Berlin, Glasgow, London, Madrid, New York, Rome, Rio de Janeiro, Santos, Sydney and Toronto). Recruitment of 6390 current drug injectors took place between October 1989 and March 1992, with most being recruited from outside of drug treatment settings.

The study was launched against a background of the rapid spread of HIV infection in a number of cities around the world. It was apparent that the HIV epidemics amongst drug injectors were unfolding in different ways, but there was a lack of comparable information between cities. This study represents the largest international project of its kind, using a standardized methodology and instrument for the collection of data.

The decision to embark on the study showed considerable foresight. Apart from the wealth of data collected in each of the participating cities, the study has contributed much to the development of research methods and has established international collaborative networks. Over 150 scientific publications have been published, along with a World Health Organization report of the study (WHO, 1994).

Most significantly, the study has played an important role in informing national policies, and in placing drug injecting, HIV and related health and policy issues on the international agenda.

A key finding is that there is now substantial evidence from this and other studies that injecting drug users do change their behaviour in response to information about HIV/AIDS and with access to the means of behaviour change. In turn, this behaviour change has helped prevent epidemics in some cities. Nonetheless many policy makers may still believe the stereotype that drug injectors do not change their behaviour, and then use this as a rationale for not implementing AIDS prevention programmes.

This book was inspired by the study. It uses data gathered from the collaborating sites. Considerable further information has been added from other studies, thus presenting a comprehensive overview of what is currently known about drug injecting, HIV infection, epidemic dynamics, and possibilities for prevention.

Examining the context of drug injecting has helped to inform our understanding of factors which influence the spread of HIV infection among this population. In work developing from this study, it has been shown that HIV epidemics among injectors have been contained in communities which responded quickly to the threat. There is now a considerable weight of evidence indicating the importance of interventions at early stages in HIV epidemics, or even where prevalence is negligible. Specifically, prevention efforts in cities where epidemics have been contained included the widespread legal availability of sterile needles and syringes, and the provision of outreach services to drug injectors which disseminated information and which built trust between injecting drug users and health workers. Such outreach often incorporates the efforts of informal and formal drug user organizations. Other strategies found to be associated with low seroprevalence rates among injectors in some cities have included the distribution of bleach and the expansion of drug treatments, such as increasing access to methadone programmes, counselling and in-patient detoxification and rehabilitation services.

The study was conceived in 1986/7 before there was much awareness of the problem of HIV infection among drug injectors in developing countries. Bangkok, Rio de Janeiro and Santos were the only centres that participated from developing countries. In the time since the study commenced, there is now considerable evidence about further diffusion of drug injecting practices, particularly in developing countries. Considering the dynamic changes in injecting behaviour and the rapid spread of HIV infection among drug injectors in many developing countries, and the emergence of new routes for drug transit, sites in Africa, Eastern Europe, Central and South America, the Caribbean and parts of Asia should be included in future studies. There is also an urgent need to develop appropriate interventions in such areas. Since the limited resources and expertise available in some developing countries often preclude the use of large studies, particular consideration should therefore be given to the development and the implementation of simple rapid assessment methods which can inform cost-effective and culturally appropriate interventions.

As the broader HIV epidemic unfolds, it is evident that HIV transmission among and from drug injectors plays a critical role. Transmission occurs through both drug injecting and sexual practices. Drug injectors are often the population affected at the early stage of HIV epidemics. The control of HIV infection in such populations is therefore crucial to the control of HIV epidemics in the wider population.

Ten years ago many countries were faced with what appeared to be an imminent public health disaster. Indeed for many, during the first year of antibody testing in 1985, HIV prevalence rates were at such high levels that the preventive task seemed to be insuperable. We now know that rapid spread of infection is not inevitable. Pessimism has been replaced by cautious optimism.

This book is testimony to the importance of linking research to intervention and policy making. It indicates the major benefits to be derived from comparative international studies. We now know a considerable amount about the successful public health response to drug injecting and HIV infection. Although the precise nature of preventive projects might vary from place to place, in broad terms, the kinds of strategic interventions that are required have been identified. The main problem is in convincing governments that intervention is necessary, can be successful and is cost-effective.

Gerry V. Stimson
Don C. Des Jarlais
Andrew L. Ball

On behalf of all those who have collaborated in the World Health Organization Multi-City Study and related research.
Vancouver, 1996.

Reference

WHO (1994) World Health Organization International Collaborative Group, *Multi-City Study on Drug Injecting and Risk of HIV Infection* (WHO/PSA/94.4), Geneva: World Health Organization.

Series Editor's Preface

The sharing of needles and syringes is one of the principal means by which HIV is transmitted. Information is needed therefore to document the forms that injecting drug use takes in different parts of the world, and the risks involved. This book offers the most comprehensive analysis of drug injecting behaviour and HIV infection yet prepared. With funding and support from the World Health Organization, the multi-site studies described here provide insights from a wide range of different countries. They identify the health and social consequences of drug injecting, sexual risk, issues of mobility and migration, the risks associated with special environments such as prisons, and future priorities for prevention. Certain to become a standard reference text, and invaluable for all those working in the field, *Drug Injecting and HIV Infection* offers a state of the art appreciation of key issues pertaining to injecting drug use and HIV-related risks worldwide.

Peter Aggleton

Acknowledgments

We would like to express our thanks to the numerous researchers, collaborators, interviewees and funders from all the cities participating in the study. We would also like to express thanks to the WHO Programme of Substance Abuse, WHO Global Programme on AIDS, and the United Nations International Drug Control Programme, for financial support. We are grateful to Jo Hooper for editorial assistance on the manuscript.

Chapter 1

Global Perspectives on Drug Injecting

Gerry V. Stimson and Kachit Choopanya

The self-injection of drugs is a problem of global dimensions, with major significance for the spread of HIV-1 infection and other blood-borne diseases. The injection of drugs occurs in all global sectors. It is found in countries with a relatively long 'tradition' of self-injection, as in North America, Western Europe, and Australasia; and it is now found in many developing countries where self-injection is a somewhat 'new' phenomenon. It occurs even in countries which were formerly thought to provide their populations with some resistance to drug injecting because of their cultural heritage, their religious or spiritual history, their traditional patterns of drug use or their political or economic conditions. To the contrary, as Figure 1.1 shows, drug injecting is found in countries of all religious persuasions, all stages of economic development and all political systems.

One of the less optimistic features arising from collaboration in the World Health Organization Multi-City Study on Drug Injecting and Risk of HIV Infection, has been the growing awareness of the global extent of drug injecting, and the fact that the diffusion of injecting and the recruitment of new injectors has been occurring since international agencies, political leaders and government officials first became aware of HIV-1 and AIDS.

That the rapid spread of injecting drug use has been occurring and continues worldwide has major repercussions for global public health (see Chapter 3). For example, Myanmar (formerly Burma) in south-east Asia, Yunnan in south-west China, and Manipur in north-east India, saw the spread of injecting followed shortly after by the spread of HIV-1 infection. HIV-1 among injecting drug users appeared in Thailand by 1987, spread north to Myanmar and Yunnan in 1989, and to Manipur by 1990. In this sub-region, rates of HIV infection among drug injectors — peaking in some areas at over 80 per cent — are the highest that have been reported in the world (Stimson, 1994).

By 1992 drug injection had been reported in over 80 countries worldwide (Stimson, 1993). By 1995, reports of injecting had been received from 121 countries. The increase from 1992 probably reflects to some extent new reports of existing problems. However, the evidence is that these reports mainly reflect *new* problems: none of the studies that have been carried out in those countries reporting injecting drug use for the first time suggest that injection has been around for long periods of time and is only now being reported.

1

The list of countries in Figure 1.1 can do little more than give a general overview. A simple count of countries indicates the existence of injecting, but detailed information about the nature and extent of an illicit activity which is engaged in by a largely hidden population, is difficult to determine. In some of the countries listed there may have been no more than isolated reports of injecting, while in others injection may be a preferred mode of administration for widespread use of drugs such as heroin and cocaine. While it is extremely difficult to assess the scale of injecting, Jonathan Mann and colleagues in their book *AIDS in the World* (1992) estimate that there may be 5 million persons throughout the world who inject illicit drugs. This is probably an underestimate.

Albania	Guatemala	Oman
Argentina*	Haiti	Pakistan*
Australia*	Honduras*	Panama*
Austria*	Hong Kong*	Paraguay*
Azerbaijan	Hungary*	Philippines*
Bahamas*	Iceland*	Poland*
Bahrein*	India*	Portugal*
Bangladesh	Indonesia*	Puerto Rico*
Belarus*	Iran	Romania
Belgium*	Iraq	Russia*
Bermuda	Ireland*	San Marino*
Bolivia	Israel*	Saudi Arabia
Boznia-Herzegovina	Italy*	Senegal
Brazil*	Jamaica	Singapore*
Brunei*	Japan*	Slovak Republic
Bulgaria*	Jordan	Slovenia*
Cambodia*	Kazakhstan	South Africa
Canada*	Kirgystan	Spain*
Chile*	Korea	Sri Lanka*
China*	Kuwait	Sudan
Colombia*	Laos*	Surinam
Costa Rica*	Latvia*	Sweden*
Côte d'Ivoire	Lithuania	Switzerland*
Croatia*	Luxembourg*	Syria*
Czech Republic*	Macao*	Tanzania
Denmark*	Macedonia	Thailand*
Dominican Republic*	Malaysia*	Tunisia*
Ecuador*	Malta*	Turkey*
Egypt*	Mauritius*	Turkmenistan
El Salvador*	Mexico*	Uganda
Estonia	Moldova	Ukraine*
Fiji*	Monaco*	United Kingdom*
Finland*	Morocco*	Uruguay*
France*	Myanmar*	United States of America*
French Polynesia*	Nepal*	Venezuela*
Gabon	Netherlands*	Vietnam*
Georgia	New Caledonia*	Yugoslavia*
Germany*	New Zealand*	Zambia
Ghana	Nicaragua*	
Greece*	Nigeria	
Guam*	Norway*	

* = *Those countries reporting IDU with HIV infection*

Figure 1.1 Countries and territories with injecting drug use and HIV infection among IDUs, by July 1996
Source: The Centre for Research on Drugs and Health Behaviour

In some of the countries listed in Figure 1.1 drug injection has been established over many years and may be found in many groups of the population, albeit with a higher prevalence in certain sectors. In other countries drug injecting may still be very much a minority activity and may be found only in particular social groups. The recent diffusion of drug injecting in developing countries, and the rapidity with which this may occur, are indicated by its existence in rural as well as in urban populations, among rich and poor people in large cities as well as among tribal peoples in remote areas.

Reasons for the spread of injecting drug use are complex and multiple. At the individual level, injecting offers several advantages to the drug user: the technology of use is more straightforward than some other means of ingestion; there are economic advantages in that more of the drug is consumed; heroin injecting may be easier to conceal than, for example, opium smoking; and the effects may be preferred over other routes of use. But there are factors that may be operating at other levels that facilitate the spread of injecting. These include the patterns of communication within and between areas that allow transfer of knowledge about techniques of administration, and the influence of drug production and trafficking on the local availability of injectable preparations. For example, the local adoption of drug injecting in south-east Asia has been influenced by the development of opiate production in that region. The trafficking of heroin through parts of West Africa and in Mauritius has led to the local use of heroin. The potential is there for injecting to be adopted, as the case of Mauritius shows.

The uptake of new patterns of drug use is also influenced by the social, economic and political changes that are taking place in many parts of the world, for example in the Newly Independent States and the countries of Central and Eastern Europe. In some of these countries (with a few notable exceptions) the spread of drug use and injecting has happened mainly from 1990, in parallel with the major changes in these societies.

The complex interweaving of factors may have ramifications for drug use in many locations and among different populations. This is well illustrated by the Vietnamese war. That war was associated with American servicemen smoking and injecting heroin in Vietnam (many of whom stopped on being returned to the USA) (Robins *et al.*, 1974). 'Rest and recreation' visits of American servicemen during the war helped to establish the Kings Cross district of Sydney, Australia, as an illicit drug use and dealing centre, particularly with regard to heroin injecting. Anti-Communist insurgents and tribal groups in several parts of South-east Asia — who were often also engaged in opiate production and trafficking — were supported by the USA. Drug production and trafficking routes and infrastructures were established, and drug trafficking routes were often associated with arms trafficking (and later gem and sex workers trafficking). These events had major implications for the development of heroin production in Myanmar and the later adoption of heroin smoking and injection there. The lack of analgesics in North Vietnam during the war resulted in the use of parenteral opium, and possibly heroin, to treat wounded North Vietnamese soldiers and civilians, some developing chronic dependence (McCoy, 1972, 1991). Many Vietnamese refugees in Hong Kong were introduced to heroin use through criminal networks there, where they have been used for cheap labour, drug trafficking and dealing.

It is not possible, given the current state of knowledge, to fully describe, let alone explain, the dynamics of the diffusion of injecting on a global basis. The rest of this chapter attempts an overview of the current situation. It draws on reports from the World Health Organization Regional Offices and the United Nations International Drug Control Programme, a review of published and unpublished literature, and information from researchers, doctors and prevention workers around the world.

North America

The United States of America has one of the longest histories of self-injection of drugs, starting long before drugs such as heroin and cocaine were illicit (Musto, 1987). The invention of the hypodermic syringe in the early part of the nineteenth century, and the synthesis of morphine, contributed to the widespread use of morphine injections in self-treatment, particularly among injured military survivors of the Civil War. Self-injection of morphine was known as the 'army disease' (Terry and Pellens, 1970). Heroin was first introduced as a cough suppressant in 1898, and its use both for self-medication and for pleasure rapidly spread. Its rising popularity between 1905 and 1915 led Terry and Pellens, writing in 1928, to describe it as 'the very remarkable history of the rapid increase of the use of this drug' (p. 86), a comment that is applicable to the later experience of many other countries.

Between 1910 and 1920 the sniffing of heroin was well established, but was mainly concentrated in New York and other north-eastern cities (Terry and Pellens, 1970). Sometime between 1915 and 1925, there was a shift to subcutaneous injection and a little later, by the early 1920s, heroin users discovered the effects of heroin injected directly into a vein (O'Donnell and Jones, 1968). The popularity of heroin might have been influenced by the ban on the import of smokable opium in 1909, and controls over cocaine importation soon after. In 1920, heroin sniffing was largely confined to New York and nearby cities, with morphine users mostly located elsewhere. The diffusion of heroin use and injection radiated out from New York, so that by 1932 heroin injection had spread to most US cities. By 1940, heroin was the drug of choice in nearly every large city and the 'heroin mainliner' had emerged as the 'dominant underworld type' (Courtwright, 1982). One of the earliest reported epidemics of a syringe-transmitted blood-borne disease was an outbreak of estivo-autumnal malaria reported among drug injectors in New York City in 1932 (Helpern, 1934). In the period before the Second World War about 40 per cent of opiate users seeking treatment were injecting, and this number had risen to between 70 and 90 per cent by 1950 (O'Donnell and Jones, 1970).

After 1945 heroin use spread among minority youth in New York, and in other urban settings. The US heroin supply came mainly from Turkey's opium production in the 1940s, 1950s and 1960s, and into the early 1970s through the 'French Connection'. There occurred a further spread of heroin use in American cities (for example Washington and Chicago) between 1969 and 1972. When Turkish opium production was reduced to a small legal crop in the early 1970s, Mexican production began to fill this vacuum, followed later by heroin from South-east Asia (DuPont and Greene, 1973; Hughes, Senay and Parker, 1992; Hunt, 1974).

The US experience therefore illustrates both that the diffusion of injecting can be rapid and that the periodic diffusion of injecting (rapid incidence) may be followed by relative plateaux, only to be followed later by further diffusion (Crider, 1985; O'Donnell and Jones, 1970; Helpern and Rho, 1967; Gibson Hunt and Chambers, 1976).

The National Institute on Drug Abuse has invested substantial sums in the development of household and other surveys to estimate the prevalence of drug use in the USA. It estimates that over 700 000 people in the USA (about half of 1 per cent) injected drugs in 1990, and that over 3.33 million have injected at some time in their lives (National Institute on Drug Abuse, 1991). The data are considered to be a marked underestimate, and the current estimate of drug injectors is approximately 1.3 million (Des Jarlais, personal communication). New York has been viewed as the drugs capital of the world: it is believed that there are 200 000 injectors, most of whom use heroin and cocaine. In localities marked by high social deprivation, prevalence of injecting can be extremely high: in the Bronx in New York City, it is estimated that 17 per cent of all males aged between 25 and 44 years are drug injectors (Drucker and Vermund, 1989).

As a close neighbour of the United States, sharing a long and unguarded border, Canada has shared in the US drug problem. Montreal was for a long time an important trans-shipment point for drugs going to New York. Vancouver has also had a long history of narcotic use, with injection as the dominant route of administration (Michael Rekert, personal communication).

In Canada, until the early part of the twentieth century, patent medicines, including many containing opiates or cocaine, flourished (Blackwell, 1988). As in the United States, opium smoking was introduced to Canada by Chinese labourers who came to work primarily in the western part of the country. The first attempt to outlaw opiates, including opium smoking itself, occurred in 1908. Until that year, cocaine too was legal and could be readily purchased without a prescription. As was the pattern in the United States, introduction of drug legislation was followed by a sharp increase in the price of opium, and its gradual replacement by morphine and then by heroin, which were easier to smuggle and conceal. Along with this shift to more potent drugs, injecting began to replace sniffing or smoking as a more efficient mode of administration. The numbers of users are likely to have been relatively small, however, with very little illegal opioid use during and immediately following the Second World War. During the 1950s, British Columbia was believed to have over half of Canada's estimated

2000 heroin users. Most of these were reported to be white males who had grown up in circumstances which were economically marginal but not severely impoverished.

During the 1960s, there developed in Canada, as in the United States, a phenomenon of injection of large doses of amphetamines among young polydrug users who were known as 'speeders'. Their numbers peeked at an estimated 2000 to 3000 in 1970, after which use of this drug declined rapidly. In the early 1970s there were estimated to be about 15 000 Canadian regular heroin users, mainly injectors. Heroin injection has continued to be an important issue in large Canadian cities such as Montreal, Toronto and Vancouver, and more recently there has been an upsurge in the use of cocaine, both by injection and in smokable form ('crack'). Generally speaking, problems with injecting drug use have tended to parallel those of the United States, but here rates of use have tended to be lower, and have not followed the same racial patterns, with the majority of drug injectors being white. In recent years, increasing concern has developed about involvement of First Nations persons (native Indians) as injecting drug users, particularly in western cities such as Edmonton and Vancouver. This problem is closely related to severe impoverishment and social disruption experienced by many young persons from First Nations moving to these large cities from reserves (Peggy Millson, personal communication).

It is estimated that there are now aout 50 000 to 100 000 drug injectors in Canada, of which about 8000 to 10 000 are located in Toronto. It is estimated that 1 per cent of adults and between 1 and 2 per cent of students have used heroin at some time in their lives.

Western Europe

Like the USA, Western Europe also has a long experience with drug injecting. The more recent experience — from the 1960s — illustrates that the diffusion of drug use patterns is a subregional phenomenon, rather than just a unique experience of particular cities and countries.

In many parts of Western Europe some recreational drug injecting occurred within specific social groups in the first two decades of the twentieth century. In particular, it was found in those 'pleasure classes' (Stimson, 1995) characterized by a lifestyle which provided the income and the opportunity to indulge in recreational drug use: in cultural, artistic and bohemian circles, among the aristocracy and the upper classes, and among the criminal underworld and sex workers.

There was some evidence of the spread of injection in some cities in the late 1940s and 1950s, but it tended to be confined to relatively small social networks. For example, in Stockholm intravenous use of amphetamine emerged in the late 1940s, but was rare until the late 1950s when it increased in artistic, bohemian and criminal groups. London saw morphine and heroin injection spread from the mid-1950s.

But the main diffusion of drug injecting happened in Europe from the early 1960s onwards. In Sweden, by the 1960s drug injecting in Stockholm (mainly of amphetamine) was substantially established with peak incidence (to 1970) occurring between 1963 and 1968 (Bejerot, 1977). In West Berlin, heroin injecting developed in the late 1960s and spread in the 1970s. By 1979 the number of heroin users in that city was estimated to be 6000, increasing to 8800 by 1990. About 75 per cent of these were injectors. Around 1971–2 heroin became widely available in the Netherlands, by 1972–5 it had spread to Surinamese residents, and by 1975 to 'blue-collar' (working class) adolescents. At the end of the 1970s a second wave of heroin users emerged (Grund, 1993).

In Scotland, drug injecting was introduced to Glasgow in the late 1970s and early 1980s, but did not escalate to significant levels until 1983. By 1985 it was estimated that there were 5000 injectors in Glasgow, and approximately 8500 by 1990 (Frischer, 1992). The main drugs injected were heroin, benzodiazepines and buprenorphine. In Greece, injecting appears to have started to spread in Athens around the mid-1970s, when there was a major increase in the use of illicit drugs in younger age groups. There are now estimated to be 80 000 opioid users, of which 50 per cent are injectors (Ball *et al.*, 1994). In Spain, drug use and injection spread later, around 1977–9, and involved the injection of manufactured opioids, sedatives and stimulants. In Italy, injecting was initially limited to the young middle class in specific urban areas. The prevalence of injecting increased significantly in the 1980s, and spread across all socio-economic classes.

Increases in the use and injection of heroin were seen across European cities in different stages and waves in the early 1970s, and again in the early 1980s. In much of Western Europe injecting was initially adopted by a few individuals in minority creative groups (such as jazz musicians, bohemians and students), but it rapidly spread to new social groups in the 1970s with an illicit heroin market served by heroin from South-east Asia (Stimson and Oppenheimer, 1982). Political upheavals in Iran in 1979 led to a further flow of heroin to Europe, with the expansion of both heroin smoking and injecting in the early 1980s. From then on, injection became associated with poorer and disadvantaged social groups.

Europe illustrates how diffusion may involve various social groups at different stages: the pattern of the diffusion of drug injecting from upper- and middle-class innovators to poorer groups has also occurred in other parts of the world.

The history of drug injecting in Western Europe shows that trends in the spread of drug use often transcend state boundaries. Subregional diffusion of injecting was probably linked to the cultural homogenization that occurred within Europe in the period following the Second World War. Significant were the increasing opportunities for mobility and migration, proliferation of, and lessening state control over, media sources, and the rise of youth subcultures distinguished by fashion and style (including choice of drugs).

Eastern Europe

The earlier spread of injecting in Western Europe had not, for the most part, been echoed in Eastern Europe. Injecting has until recently been relatively uncommon, although in Poland *Kompot* (a home-made opiate from poppies) has been used extensively (Boyes, 1984). Oral histories of drug users who emigrated to New York indicate that narcotic injection occurred in a minor way in the Soviet Union during the Brezhnev era (Des Jarlais, personal communication). But in the more recent period, diffusion appears to be associated with social, economic and political changes in Eastern Europe: these are facilitating the adoption of new drug use patterns in those countries where drug injecting was formerly uncommon, mostly since about 1990.

In East Berlin there appears to have been no significant drug scene until 1990. Heroin is the most commonly injected drug, but cocaine use has also increased. Heroin use has spread in Lithuania since 1990, and in the Ukraine there was a major spread of injecting, identified during 1994 and 1995. In the Czech Republic, relatively small-scale patterns of drug use developed in the 1970s, fed mainly by domestic products, but drug consumption here has increased dramatically since 1990 with a major growth in 1992–5. Up to 70 per cent of drug agencies' clients in Prague are injectors (Country Report for the Czech Republic, 1994). This followed the loosening of restrictions on movement, and the use of Czech territory for trans-shipment of illicit drugs, compounded by the war in former Yugoslavia which cut the traditional transit route to Western Europe. In Slovenia in former Yugoslavia, injection is recent and there are now thought to be between 4000 and 8000 injectors. Macedonia has had a growing problem with heroin use since 1990 and there are thought to be between 3000 and 5000 heroin users in a population of about 3 million, but injection is still relatively rare.

North Africa, the Eastern Mediterranean and the Middle East

Egypt has had a history of injecting drug use since the 1920s (Biggam, 1929). The syringe-transmitted epidemic of malaria among drug injectors in Egypt is probably the first report of blood-borne transmission on record, occurring in 1928 and preceding the report of the outbreak in New York City in 1932. In more recent years it would appear that heroin injecting has been present since at least the beginning of the 1980s, with an estimated 40 000 heroin users of whom an estimated one-third inject. There are also reports of the injection of amphetamine and cocaine.

The Bekaa valley in Lebanon (controlled by Syria) is considered to be a major opium growing and heroin producing area. Drug injecting has been reported from Israel since at least 1986 and is on a sufficient scale to warrant the introduction of methadone maintenance treatment (Dan *et al.*, 1989, 1992).

Elsewhere in the area there have been only a few published reports of drug injection, for example in Bahrain (Fulayfil and Baig, 1991) and Saudi Arabia (Bari *et al.*, 1993).

Sub-Saharan Africa

The injection of illicit drugs has been relatively uncommon in many African countries, even though the use of injections in folk and regular medical treatment may be relatively common. There is considerable evidence of the development of drug use in many countries in sub-Saharan Africa. A number of African cities are trafficking routes for a variety of psychoactive drugs including cannabis, methaqualone, heroin and cocaine. The contemporary experience of West Africa illustrates the impact of drug trafficking routes on the diffusion of new drug use practices and the potential spread of illicit drug injection.

Most of the — still few — reports of injection come from West Africa. Here there had been no traditional use of opioid drugs or cocaine but, from the beginning of the 1980s, this area became an important trafficking route for cocaine from South America and heroin from South-east Asia *en route* for Europe and North America. Initially this involved Nigeria, then Côte d'Ivoire, Mali, Ghana and Senegal. Law enforcement in some countries of West Africa has led to the diversion of distribution routes to adjacent countries. Local drug trans-shipment has had a spillover effect and heroin and cocaine use has been on the increase in almost all countries on the continent, and particularly among those which were major trafficking and transit zones such as Nigeria, Liberia, Côte d'Ivoire, Senegal, Chad, Ghana, Kenya, South Africa and Mauritius (Stimson, Adelekan and Rhodes, 1996; Adelekan and Stimson, 1996).

In Nigeria, from the early 1980s, heroin appeared on the local market, and was soon followed by cocaine. Treatment data indicate increasing use of heroin and cocaine since the mid-1980s. Although smoking and inhalation have been the modes of use most commonly reported by 'area boys and girls' (groups of young, mainly unemployed men and women) in Lagos, there have been recent anecdotal reports of injection. Initially the use of cocaine and heroin was limited to the upper middle classes, but it has now broadened to other groups. The price of one gram of heroin or cocaine has fallen from about N1000 in 1992 to N20 and N25 in Lagos in 1995 (Olukoya, 1995).

Some injection has also now been reported from Gabon, Ghana, Mauritius, Senegal, South Africa, Tanzania, Uganda and Zambia. The risk of heroin injecting spreading is illustrated by the experience in the island of Mauritius, where, as a consequence of being a drug trafficking country, first heroin smoking, and latterly injecting, have spread. In the 1980s brown sugar heroin was introduced into the country and its use rapidly acquired epidemic dimensions. This was controlled in 1987 and 1988 following the adoption of new legislation and firmer enforcement. There followed a temporary reduction in the supply of heroin, but an increase in the consumption of alcohol and licit psychoactive drugs such as codeine, ephedrine and benzodiazepines. Since 1991 heroin use has again increased, with a switch to injecting which is now the predominant mode of use.

With the current situation of prevalence of HIV-1 and AIDS in Africa, the introduction of drug injecting may bring further enormous public health costs. Of significance is the fact that groups currently vulnerable to HIV-1 infection in Africa, such as truck drivers, unemployed youths, the military, street youth and sex workers, are also the ones which may be the most vulnerable to the spread of drug injection.

Caribbean and Central America

Some injecting, although on a relatively small scale, has been reported from Central America and the Caribbean, including the Dominican Republic and Honduras. Puerto Rico has higher levels of injection, associated with the link between Puerto Rican and New York populations (Drucker, 1990). Puerto Rico has become a major trans-shipment point for cocaine, with a substantial local consumption.

South America

In South America, at least two patterns of drug use may be detected. In the southern cone (Argentina, Chile, Paraguay and Uruguay) and in Brazil the use and injection of cocaine is common. However, little was known about the prevalence of cocaine injection prior to the emergence of AIDS. About a quarter of all AIDS cases in these parts of South America are thought to be due to drug injecting, and some HIV-1 infection associated with injecting was reported as early as 1986 in Brazil and 1987 in Argentina (Libonatti *et al.*, 1993). Later reviews of AIDS case reporting by the AIDS Reference Centre of São Paulo dated the first AIDS case in a drug injector as occurring in 1983. Within Brazil, there are marked variations in the geographical distribution of drug injecting, most of it being concentrated in the south and south-east. The diffusion of injection of cocaine appears to mirror cocaine distribution routes (see Chapter 10). In Brazil, in addition to transmission of hepatitis B and C, HIV-1 and HTLV-I/II, transmission of malaria has also been associated with shared injecting among cocaine users.

In the Andean region, and especially in Colombia, while there is extensive consumption of coca, cocaine and other coca products such as basuco, administration is almost entirely by chewing, inhalation and smoking. Cocaine users in Colombia seem to have had no preference for, and possibly an antipathy towards, injecting. At the end of the 1980s, some of the cocaine cartels in Colombia introduced poppy growing in order to produce heroin there. This shift was aided with the help of refining experts from South-east Asia. The production of heroin for export has in turn led to an increase in its local availability, with by 1994 some reports of heroin injecting among cocaine and basuco users in Bogota and Cali (Tim Rhodes, personal communication). Some of these users, having injected heroin, have moved to this means of administration with cocaine. There are indications, therefore, that Colombia may be verging on the transition to drug injecting. There are also recent anecdotal reports of cocaine injection, particularly among students, in Bolivia.

Indian Subcontinent

Within the Indian subcontinent, there is a major heroin-producing and transit area in Pakistan, and the north-east Indian states of Manipur and Nagaland which share borders with the opiate producer country of Myanmar. The pattern of heroin use and injection is quite varied, with pockets of high use in some places and few reports of use in others. In Pakistan there was only a handful of heroin users at the beginning of 1980. After the end of the Afghan war, there was an increase in the availability of heroin. By 1990 it was estimated that there might be 1 million heroin users, but there had until now been few reports of the injection of heroin (Gossop, 1995). Indeed it was thought that most heroin users smoked the drug. Recent evidence from Karachi suggests that about 20 to 25 per cent of heroin users practise injection (McCormick, 1995).

A shift to injecting also appears to be occurring in several cities in India. For example, in Madras, the smoking of brown sugar heroin imported from Pakistan began in 1983 among students and middle-class youth. By 1986 it had spread to slum areas. The first reports of injecting occurred in 1987. At first this had appeared to be confined to Sri Lankan Tamils and people from north-east Indian states such as Manipur, but there were a number of factors that are thought to have encouraged a shift to injection in Madras. The first of these was that after the assassination of Rajiv Ghandi there was a police crackdown on Sri Lankan militants, who were also trading brown sugar heroin. The second was that some local doctors began to sell injections of buprenorphine (known under the brand name Tidigesic), purportedly as a cure for dependence. The third was the long-standing migration of young people and students from Manipur to Madras. This facilitated the importation of injectable heroin from South-east Asia. By 1990 injecting, though still relatively rare, was found in many sectors of Madras. By 1996, there had been an increase in the availability of brown sugar heroin from Pakistan. In Madras there are now heroin injectors, buprenorphine injectors and those who inject cocktails of buprenorphine, diazepam and diphenhydramine. Buprenorphine injection has also been reported in other areas of India since the 1990s, for example in Chandigarth (Basu *et al.*, 1994).

The state of Manipur in north-east India has a border with Myanmar, and is on a major drug distribution route to other parts of India and to Nepal. It is a further example of the impact of drug trafficking on the development of local drug problems. It appears that at the beginning of the 1980s there was little preference for heroin in Manipur, but that heroin smoking and then injecting spread in the mid-1980s, so that by the end of the decade it was estimated on the basis of local surveys that there were about 15 000 heroin injectors. The geographical distribution of new drug use patterns is well reflected by the incidence of heroin use along the main highway leading from Myanmar (Sarkar *et al.*, 1991). Most of the heroin users are found along Highway 39, a heroin trans-shipment route starting at the Myanmar border and running through Manipur and north to Nagaland.

Japan

The 'epidemic' of amphetamine injection in post-war Japan was preceded by large stocks of oral methamphetamine released onto the market and widely advertised as pep pills. The first stimulant-dependent person was admitted to hospital in Tokyo in 1946, and soon afterwards all prefectures in Japan had reported cases of amphetamine dependence. Injectable amphetamine was initially limited to cultural élites and occupational groups such as drivers, students and night workers. However, use by injection spread quickly to economically deprived and displaced youths in cities. By 1951 all classes and areas in Japan were affected. When amphetamine use peaked in 1954 it was estimated that 2 million people were using amphetamines and 55 000 people were arrested that year for drug offences. It is not clear what proportion of the 2 million were injecting the drug. By 1956 there was a dramatic decrease in use, apparently following massive public education campaigns (Brill and Hirose, 1969; Kato, 1990; Tamura, 1989). The spread of amphetamine injection and its later reversal indicate the importance of understanding mechanisms that might influence the transition away from injecting to other modes of administration.

Australasia

In Sydney, injecting drug use was relatively rare until the late 1960s. Its spread was facilitated by visits from US servicemen during the Vietnam war. Due to their proximity to air and seaports, eastern parts of Sydney have generally had a concentration of injectors. Heroin is the most commonly injected drug, but the injection of amphetamine increased in popularity in Australia during the 1980s. It is estimated that there are between 12 000 and 15 000 injectors in New South Wales, of which about 8000 to 10 000 would be in Sydney.

South-east Asia and China[1]

Much of South-east Asia has a relatively recent experience with drug injecting, with older patterns of drug use being replaced by the diffusion of injection mainly as a consequence of local heroin production and distribution (Stimson, 1996).

The region includes the Golden Triangle, which is the world's largest opium producing area and encompasses parts of Laos, Myanmar and Thailand.

Until the 1960s opium was produced for export and refined elsewhere, and local consumption was confined to opium. Heroin was unavailable locally unless imported (for example the first case of heroin addiction in Thailand involved heroin brought in from Hong Kong). The late 1960s onwards saw the expansion of the refining of opium to heroin in this area. This new development taking place in refineries in or close to the growing areas was influenced by the prospect of lower production costs, the growth of the world markets, successful law enforcement against production in Mediterranean countries and later in Mexico, and local political conditions — control of opium and heroin being significant in local political control and in the financing of insurgent activity. In 1991 this area accounted for 70 per cent of global opium production. The refining and distribution of heroin — originally intended for export — in turn facilitated the local availability of heroin and thus the emergence of new markets for heroin.

Much of the heroin for world export went in transit through Bangkok, but with enforcement and government activity against dissident groups in Myanmar, the cost of local 'taxes' on transport (that is, corruption) and the development of new transport networks, there was a shift in overland export routes through Shan state to Yunnan in China and on to Hong Kong. In the mid-1980s, an overland route north-east of Myanmar through Manipur and north-east India also developed. In the early 1990s, the first major seizure of heroin at Ho Chi Minh City airport in Vietnam was reported, suggesting a new transit route.

Patterns of local drug consumption and modes of administration underwent marked transformations. In Thailand local heroin use paralleled the trade in heroin for American service people based in Vietnam and the growth of world heroin markets. In a period of 20 years starting in the late 1950s, Thailand saw the gradual transition from opium smoking to heroin smoking, and then to heroin injection (Vichai Poshyachinda, 1992). A second heroin 'epidemic' in Thailand extended well into the 1980s. Drug injecting is now found in all the major cities of Thailand as well as in rural areas. Injecting drug use is commonly reported by more than 60 per cent of clients in treatment services in Thailand, and 80 per cent in Bangkok. In Bangkok it is estimated that there are 36 600 opiate users of which 90 per cent are injectors. Within a period of 25 years or less the pattern of drug dependence in Thailand has thus shifted from mainly opium smoking to a more complex one involving mainly heroin, but also other drugs such as amphetamines and inhalants.

Myanmar (Burma) is the world's largest producer of heroin, with an estimated 200 tonnes produced each year. It has major opium poppy growing and heroin refining areas, mainly in the eastern part of the country in Shan State. As in Thailand, the expansion of poppy growing and heroin refining occurred at the time of the war in Vietnam. Myanmar itself became a major consumer of heroin from the mid-1970s onwards, and heroin injection began to take over from heroin smoking as the main problematic form of drug use. Within a few years injection was reported by those in treatment in many of its major cities. Injection is also found in the mining areas, and among fishermen (employed on Thai boats in the southern part of the country). These are mainly socio-economic groups with above average income because, although heroin is produced in the country, its cost is relatively high. Problems of drug dependence and heroin injection are found among the tribal groups and insurgent armies that are involved in the heroin trade, such as the Wa in Shan State, and the Kachins in northern Myanmar.

Drug injection was probably reintroduced into Yunnan in southern China from Myanmar, from about 1990 onwards. Yunnan is on a heroin trade route from Myanmar, and many tribal population groups straddle the China/Myanmar border, including the Wa and the Kokang. Drug use in China appears to be concentrated in the south-west (Yunnan, Guizhou, and Sichuan provinces), the south (Guangdong and Guangxi) and the north-west (Sha'anxi, Gansu and Inner Mongolia); in most of these provinces injecting is relatively rare except in Yunnan and Guangxi (Zheng *et al.*, 1995). The main drug injected is heroin. Outside of Yunnan, most drug users (over 80 per cent in one survey) had begun injecting since 1990, and the earliest report of injecting was in 1988. In 1992 the Chinese government estimated that there were 250 000 drug users in China, with 30 per cent in Yunnan. Geographic variation in the proportion of those injecting drugs is thought to be related to variation in the availability of injectable grade heroin. Heroin was the most common drug reported in Guangxi, Guangdong and Sichuan provinces, which, with Yunnan, are heroin smuggling routes from the Golden Triangle region of Myanmar, Laos and Thailand. Less injectable drugs such as 'yellow crust' (heroin and opium) and opium were more common in regions remote from the drug trade routes (Zheng *et al.*, 1995). The 1994 estimate for China is 380 000 known users: this is an underestimate of the total number, but it does represent a fivefold increase over the 1990 estimate of 70 000 (Des Jarlais, personal communication).

In Vietnam the situation is rather unusual. There was major consumption of heroin, mainly by smoking but also by injection, among American military personnel during the war. There was also almost certainly some injection of heroin by Vietnamese people at that time. However, after the end of the war there were few reports of heroin injection. Injection of opium solution was identified at the beginning of the 1990s, illustrating the diffusion of the injecting technique before the diffusion of heroin use, and heroin injection re-emerged in both Hanoi and Ho Chi Minh City around 1993, and also in provincial cities such as Nha Trang.

It is estimated that up to 95 per cent of addicts in contact with treatment services in Myanmar and Thailand prefer to inject drugs (Vichai Poshyachinda, 1994). In Ruili, in the border area of Yunnan and Myanmar the prevalence of injectors among treated addicts rose from 24 per cent in 1990 to 36 per cent by 1992 (Zheng *et al.*, 1994). In Vietnam, it appears that most opium users (97 per cent) inject, boiling raw opium or the residue of smoked opium and injecting the liquid.

In other parts of South-east Asia, some injecting has recently been reported from Laos. It appears to have been rare but on the increase in Bangladesh (Ahmed and Begum, 1994) and there have been a few anecdotal reports of injecting from Cambodia.

Implications of the Diffusion of Drug Injecting

Some important features of the diffusion of injection can be noted.

First, is the fact that human beings often find psychoactive drugs reinforcing — they 'like' to take drugs. This applies to 'legal' drugs such as alcohol and nicotine, as well as to 'illegal' drugs.

Second, both the legal and illegal drug industries have undergone globalization over the last two decades. With heroin, this is typified by the shift of refining to opium growing areas, a technology transfer that takes advantage of improved communications and transport, and the reduction of production and transport costs by moving production to areas of cheap labour. International improvements in transport facilitate the movement and marketing of drugs using well co-ordinated production and distribution networks.

Third, is the availability and characteristics of the drugs. In some parts of the world the available drug preparations are more suitable for injection that for smoking.

Fourth, laws against drugs tend to raise the price and risks to the consumer (and the potential profits to the producers who avoid law enforcement) (Des Jarlais, personal communication). The illegal status of heroin and cocaine provides an incentive for consumers to inject. Injecting is more cost-efficient in that most of the drug is delivered to the brain — rather than going up in smoke. The injectable forms of drugs are usually more compact than the non-injectable ones (heroin is less bulky than opium, and so is cocaine hydrochloride compared to cocaine paste) and therefore easier to smuggle. Injection is also easier than opium smoking, requiring less time for preparation and consumption. These economic considerations should not be taken as arguments for legalization of currently illegal drugs, but as an indication that there are economic incentives for injection as a route of administration.

Fifth, is that diffusion of injection can be rapid. In many parts of the world it took only a few years to happen. This means that countries presently without injecting need to be able to identify the potential for its spread. Rapid incidence may be followed by relative plateaux, only to be followed later by further diffusion.

Sixth, is that certain groups are more likely to encounter opportunities to use and inject drugs than others. Initial adoption is followed by more general dispersion. The spread of drug use and specific practices (such as injecting) may perhaps be understood in a similar fashion to the diffusion and adoption of other innovations.

Seventh, is the significance of networks of communication. Information about drugs permeates through a wide variety of communication channels, and drug use practices are passed from one person to another through social networks. At an extreme, mixing and mobility and consequent diffusion of drug use practices may be witnessed in multinational drug scenes that occur in many inner-city areas in Europe. London, Amsterdam, Barcelona and Berlin are all examples of cities where drug tourism has been significant. The spread of injecting in Madras is in part influenced by links with Manipur. In Italy, most drug injectors from North African countries started to inject after they arrived in Italy. It may be important therefore to understand the cultural, communicative, migration and social links between population groups (see also Chapter 7). Networks of communication are important for understanding the spread of both the behaviour — drug injecting — and the infection — HIV-1 and other blood-borne diseases. They are both passed from person to person, both are *communicable*. The diffusion of injecting and the transmission of infection occur through the networks created by drug injectors. As they communicate and interact with one another, their behaviours may lead them to risk of infection, or indeed away from risk of infection. Therefore, crucial to prevention activities is an understanding that the networks through which both injecting and HIV-1 infection may spread, are also the networks through which prevention messages may be communicated.

Eighth, are the legal, cultural, economic and political conditions under which new patterns of drug use are likely to occur. Rapid social changes, changes in political institutions, changes in legislation and reductions in barriers to communication, may all be important considerations for understanding the diffusion of injecting. Linked to this is the necessity of seeing diffusion as a subregional phenomenon, rather than something that can only be understood at the city or country level.

Ninth, is that the spread of drug injecting is connected with the geopolitics of drug production and distribution: drug producer and transit countries eventually develop indigenous drug problems. This has implications for international and national law enforcement.

Tenth, is the issue of whether the diffusion of injecting is reversible. This is little documented, but there is historical evidence in the case of the decline of the Japanese amphetamine injecting 'epidemic', and more recent indications from cities as diverse as São Paulo (Brazil), Edinburgh (Scotland), New York (USA) and Yangon (Myanmar) that there is a shift away from injection towards other modes of administration.

Drug Injecting and HIV-1 Infection

The diffusion of injecting provides the backdrop for consideration of health risks for drug injectors, particularly HIV-1 infection. HIV-1 infection in drug injectors has now been reported in 83 different countries worldwide (Figure 1.1). This is a substantial increase over the 52 countries known to have HIV-1 infection among drug injectors in 1993. Some countries have experienced rapid spread of HIV-1 infection. Hepatitis B and C are also major problems (see also Chapter 3).

South-east Asia provides an illustration of both the rapid dissemination of HIV infection and how that spread can follow soon after the introduction of drug injecting. This region saw perhaps the most rapid diffusion of HIV infection among injecting drug users found anywhere in the world. Many areas reached a prevalence of 40 per cent or more among injectors within approximately 12 months. In Bangkok, HIV rates of zero or 1 per cent among drug injectors were found in various surveys from 1985 through to 1987 (Weniger *et al.*, 1991). These climbed rapidly from the beginning of 1988 to reach between 32 and 43 per cent by August and September of 1988. Extremely high seroconversion rates were found in Bangkok: 20 per cent of drug injectors who were negative in February 1988 had seroconverted by September of that year. In Chiang Rai in northern Thailand, prevalence was 1 per cent in 1988 and rose to 61 per cent in 1989. *Ad hoc* surveys revealed similarly high rates among drug injectors in remote hill-tribe areas. In south-west China, in the town of Ruili, 13 per cent of injecting drug users were positive at the end of 1989, increasing to 58 per cent by 1990 (Zheng *et al.*, 1994). In Manipur, the first seropositive drug injector was not detected until October 1989; within three months 9 per cent were positive, and in the next three months, the prevalence rate had increased to 56 per cent — a rise from zero to 56 per cent within six months (Sarkar *et al.*, 1994). In Myanmar, no HIV positive drug injectors were found in the years up to 1988. High levels of HIV infection were discovered among drug injectors from 1989 onwards in geographically distant parts of the country, with rates ranging from 73 to 96 per cent (Department of Health, Union of Myanmar, 1993).

Preventing the Spread of HIV-1 Infection and Discouraging the Spread of Injection

Many national leaders and élites invoke 'national immunity myths' (Stimson and Adelekan, 1996) to affirm their belief that they will not suffer the problems of injecting and HIV-1 infection that have been experienced elsewhere, and that they have some protective factor by which their population is immune from the spread of injecting and its consequences. However, the evidence is that since the WHO Multi-City Study was launched, the number of countries with drug injecting and with associated HIV-1 infection has continued to grow. Further, the new 'epidemics' of injecting are occurring in countries where injecting is an additional health and social burden, overlain on a multitude of existing burdens and lack of resources for dealing with them.

Starting from the mid-1980s, major attention has been given to the problem of preventing the spread of HIV-1 infection among current injectors, and the problem of secondary transmission to sexual partners. There is now a wealth of experience, from both developing and developed countries, in the design and

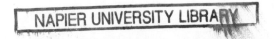

implementation of prevention programmes that can help injectors change their behaviour and reduce their risk of HIV-1 infection. Other chapters in this book point to substantial evidence that the course of epidemics may be changed by public health interventions. There is evidence that HIV-1 prevention programmes have helped current injectors to make large reductions in their injecting (and to a lesser extent in their sexual) risk behaviour, and that this is associated with lower HIV-1 incidence. There have been some notable successes for public health programmes in this field.

Public health interventions also need to focus on the process itself of the spread of injecting. The global urgency of this task is underlined by demographic trends: drug use and injecting are predominantly (though not exclusively) engaged in by younger urban people. There is the growing urbanization of the global population — by the year 2000 the majority of births in the world will be in urban settings. And the proportion of young people is increasing — almost 30 per cent of the total world population is aged between 10 and 24, and between 1960 and 1990 the total youth population (aged 15 to 24) increased by 99 per cent (World Health Organization, 1995).

There has been little experience with programmes to discourage the spread of injecting. The challenge for policy makers, prevention experts and researchers is to develop appropriate research methods, local and regional competence, and low-cost models for the prevention of injection and its consequences. At the same time, this must be done without marginalizing and repressing current injectors. Programmes might target individuals to help them avoid the transition from the smoking and sniffing of drugs to injection, or at a community level, aim to discourage the broader diffusion of injecting to new social groups.

The spread of drug injecting has been insufficiently documented so far; the mechanisms for spread remain under-researched and poorly conceptualized and the reasons poorly understood. In many parts of the world these 'epidemics' remain hidden or are inadequately reported. An understanding of the process of diffusion of new drug-using practices may lead to indications about how they may be curtailed or reversed by social interventions.

Note

1 Parts of this section first appeared in Stimson (1996).

References

ADELEKAN, M. and STIMSON, G.V. (1996) 'Problems and prospects of implementing harm reduction for HIV and injecting drug use in high risk sub-Saharan African countries', *Journal of Drug Issues*, **27** (1), pp. 97–116.

AHMED, S.K. and BEGUM, K. (1994) 'Patterns and trends of drug abuse in Dhaka, Bangladesh', in NAVARATNAM, V., FOONG KIN and TAN BEE LENG (Eds) *Report of the Asian Multi-City Epidemiology Work Group*, Malaysia: Centre for Drug Research.

BALL, A., DES JARLAIS, D.C., DONOGHOE, M.C., FRIEDMAN, S.R., GOLDBERG, D., HUNTER, G.M., STIMSON, G.V. and WODAK, A. (1994) *Multi-City Study on Drug Injecting and Risk of HIV Infection*, Geneva: World Health Organization.

BARI, N., SBEIH, F. and KHAN, M.Y. (1993) 'Tetanus: A complication of parenteral drug abuse', *Saudi Medical Journal*, **14**, 1, pp. 76–7.

BASU, D., MATTOO, S.K., ARORA, A., MALHOTRA, A. and VARMA, V.K. (1994) 'Pseudoaneurysm in injecting drug abusers: Cases from India', *Addiction*, **89**, pp. 1697–9.

BEJEROT, N. (1977) 'Drug abuse and drug policy: An epidemiological and methodological study of drug abuse of intravenous type in the Stockholm Police arrest population 1965–1970 in relation to changes in drug policy', *Supplementum 256*, pp. 1–277, Stockholm: Department of Social Medicine, Karolinska Institute.

BIGGAM, A.G. (1929) 'Malignant malaria associated with the administration of heroin intravenously', *Transactions of The Royal Society of Tropical Hygiene and Hygiene*, **23**, 2, pp. 147–53.

BLACKWELL, J. (1988) 'An overview of Canadian illicit drug use epidemiology', in BLACKWELL, J. and ERIKSON, P. (Eds) *Illicit Drugs in Canada: A Risky Business*, Ontario: Nelson.

BOYES, R. (1984) 'Poland grows its own drug problem', *The Times*, 19 June 1984.

BRILL, H. and HIROSE, T. (1969) 'The rise and fall of a methamphetamine epidemic: Japan 1945–55', *Seminars in Psychiatry*, **1**, 2, pp. 179–94.

COUNTRY REPORT FOR THE CZECH REPUBLIC (1994) Czech Republic: National Drug Commission.

COURTWRIGHT, D.T. (1982) *Dark Paradise: Opiate Addiction in America Before 1940*, London: Harvard University Press.

CRIDER, R.A. (1985) 'Heroin incidence: a trend comparison between national household survey data and indicator data', in ROUSE, B.A., KOZEL, N.J. and RICHARDS, L.G. (Eds) *Self-Report Methods of Estimating Drug Use*, pp. 125–40, Washington: US Department of Health and Human Services.

DAN, M., ROCK, M. and BAR-SHANY, S. (1989) 'Prevalence of antibodies to human immunodeficiency virus among intravenous drug users in Israel — association with travel abroad', *International Journal of Epidemiology*, **18**, 1, pp. 239–41.

DAN, M., CAHANA, A., FINTSI, Y. and BAR-SHANY, S. (1992) 'Human immunodeficiency virus infection among intravenous drug addicts in Israel: Stable low prevalence over 34 months', *International Journal of Epidemiology*, **21**, 3, pp. 561–3.

DEPARTMENT OF HEALTH, UNION OF MYANMAR (1993), AIDS Prevention and Control Programme, Sentinel Surveillance Data, March.

DRUCKER, E. (1990) 'Epidemic in the war zone: AIDS and community survival in New York City', *International Journal of Health Services*, **20**, 4, pp. 601–15.

DRUCKER, E. and VERMUND, S.H. (1989) 'Estimating population prevalence of human immunodeficiency virus infection in urban areas with high rates of intravenous drug use: A model of the Bronx in 1988', *American Journal of Epidemiology*, **130**, 1, pp. 133–42.

DUPONT, R.L. GREENE, M.H. (1973) 'The dyanamics of a heroin addiction epidemic', *Science*, **181**, pp. 716–22.

FRISCHER, M. (1992) 'Estimated prevalence of injecting drug use in Glasgow', *British Journal of Addiction*, **87**, pp. 235–43.

FULAYFIL, R. and BAIG, Z.H.B. (1991) 'Prevalence of HIV antibodies in high risk groups, Bahrain', M.D.4161, June, VII International Conference on AIDS, Florence.

GIBSON HUNT, L. and CHAMBERS, C.D. (1976) *The Heroin Epidemics*, New York: Spectrum Publications.

GOSSOP, M. (1995) 'Counting the costs as well as the benefits of drug control laws', *Addiction*, **90**, 1, pp. 16–17.

GRUND, J.C. (1993) *Drug use as a social ritual: Functionality, symbolism and determinants of self-regulation*, Rotterdam: IVO Addiction Research Institute.

HELPERN, M. (1934) 'Epidemic of fatal estivo-autumnal malaria', *American Journal of Surgery*, **XXVI**, 1, pp. 111–23.

HELPERN, M. and RHO, Y. (1967) 'Deaths from narcotism in New York City', *The International Journal of the Addictions*, **2**, 1, pp. 53–84.

HUGHES, P.H., SENAY, E.C. and PARKER, R. (1992) 'The medical management of a heroin epidemic', *Archives of General Psychiatry*, **27**, pp. 585–91.

HUNT, L.G. (1974) 'Recent spread of heroin use in the United States', *American Journal of Public Health*, **64** (suppl.), pp. 16–23.

KATO, M. (1990) 'Brief history of control, prevention and treatment of drug dependence in Japan', *Drug and Alcohol Dependence*, **25**, pp. 213–14.

LIBONATTI, O., LIMA, E., PERUGA, A., GONZALEZ, R., ŽACARIAS, F. and WEISSENBACHER, M. (1993) 'Role of drug injection in the spread of HIV in Argentina and Brazil', *International Journal of STD and AIDS*, **4**, pp. 135–41.

MCCORMICK, J. (1995) 'WHO drug injecting study: Phase II planning meeting', unpublished report.

MCCOY, A.W. (1991) *The Politics of Heroin: CIA complicity in the global drug trade*, Chicago: Lawrence Hill Books.

MCCOY, A.W. (1972) *The Politics of Heroin in South East Asia*, New York: Harper and Row.

MANN, J.M., TARANTOLA, O.J.M. and NETTER, T.W. (Eds) (1992) *AIDS in the World*, Cambridge: Harvard University Press.

MUSTO, D.F. (1987) *American Disease: Origins of Narcotic Control*, Oxford: Oxford University Press.

NATIONAL INSTITUTE ON DRUG ABUSE (1991) *National Household Survey on Drug Abuse: Population Estimates 1990*, Washington: US Department of Health and Human Services.

O'DONNELL, J.A. and JONES, J.P. (1968) 'Diffusion of the intravenous technique among narcotic addicts in the United States', *Journal of Health and Social Behaviour*, pp. 120–30.

O'DONNELL, J.A. and JONES, J.P. (1970) 'Diffusion of the intravenous technique among narcotic addicts', in BALL, J.C. and CHAMBERS, C.D. (Eds) *The Epidemiology of Opiate Addiction in the United States*, pp. 147–64, Springfield: Charles C. Thomas.

OLUKOYA, S. (1995) 'A worrisome development: Hard drug consumption is gaining ground in Nigeria', *Newswatch*, 13 March, pp. 21–2.

ROBINS, L.N., *et al.* (1974) 'Drug use by U.S. Army enlisted men in Vietnam', *American Journal of Epidemiology*, **99**, p. iv.

SARKAR, S., MOOKERJEE, P. and ROY, A.E. (1991) 'Descriptive epidemiology of intravenous heroin users: A new risk group for transmission of HIV in India', *Journal of Infection*, **23**, 2, pp. 201–7.

SARKAR, S., DAS, N., PANDA, S. *et al.* (1994) 'Rapid spread of HIV among injecting drug users in north-eastern states of India', *Bulletin on Narcotics*, **XLV**, pp. 91–105.

STIMSON, G.V. (1993) 'The global diffusion of injecting drug use: Implications for human immunodeficiency virus infection', *Bulletin on Narcotics*, **XLV**, 1, pp. 3–17.

STIMSON, G.V. (1994) 'Reconstruction of subregional diffusion of HIV infection among injecting drug users in south-east Asia: Implications for early intervention', *AIDS*, **8**, 11, pp. 1630–2.

STIMSON, G.V. (1995) 'Preventing HIV-1 infection among drug injectors in Europe, the challenge for social and behavioural scientists', in GEORGAS, J., MANTHOULI, M., BESEVEGIS, E. and KOKKEVI, A. (Eds) *Contemporary Psychology in Europe*, Gottingen, Germany: Hogrefe and Huber.

STIMSON, G.V. (1996) 'Drug injecting and the spread of HIV infection in south-east Asia', in SHERR, L., CATALAN, J. and HEDGE, B. (Eds) *The Impacts of AIDS: Psychological and Social Aspects of HIV Infection*, Reading: Harwood Academic Publishers.

STIMSON, G.V., ADELEKAN, M. and RHODES, T. (1996) 'The diffusion of drug injecting in developing countries', *International Journal of Drug Policy*, **7** (4), pp. 245–55.

STIMSON, G.V. and OPPENHEIMER, E. (1982) *Heroin Addiction: Treatment and Control in Britain*, London: Tavistock.

TAMURA, M. (1989) 'Japan: Stimulant epidemics past and present', *Bulletin on Narcotics*, **XLI**, 1 and 2, pp. 83–93.

TERRY, C.E. and PELLENS, M. (1970) *The Opium Problem*, New Jersey: Patterson Smith.

VICHAI POSHYACHINDA (1992) 'Drugs and AIDS in south-east Asia', *Forensic Science International*, **62**, pp. 15–28.

VICHAI POSHYACHINDA (1994) 'Drug injecting and HIV infection among the population of drug abusers in Asia', *Bulletin on Narcotics*, **XLV**, pp. 77–90.

WENIGER, B.G., KHANCHIT, L., KUMNUAN, U. *et al.* (1991) 'The epidemiology of HIV infection and AIDS in Thailand', *AIDS*, **5** (2), S71–S85.

WORLD HEALTH ORGANIZATION (1995) *A Picture of Health: A Review and Annotated Bibliography of the Health of Young People in Developing Countries*, WHO/FHE/ADH/95.14, Geneva: World Health Organization.

ZHENG, X., TIAN, C., ZHANG, J., CHENG, M., YANG, X. *et al.* (1994) 'Injecting drug use and HIV infection in south-west China', *AIDS*, **8**, pp. 1141–7.

ZHENG, X., TIAN, C., ZHANG, J., LI, D., LIU, X., HU, D.J., WENIGER, B.G. and DONDERO, T.J. (1995) 'IV risk behaviors but absence of infection among drug users in detoxification centers outside Yunnan province, China, 1993', *AIDS*, **9**, pp. 959–63.

Chapter 2

The Social Context of Injectors' Risk Behaviour

Neil McKeganey, Samuel R. Friedman and Fabio Mesquita

There is a popular view that the reason why injecting drug users share each other's injecting equipment is that they are unconcerned with their health and the health of others. There is now sufficient evidence from studies carried out in many countries worldwide that injectors *are* concerned with their own and others' health. Studies of drug injectors from both developed (Celentano *et al.*, 1994) and developing countries (Bueno *et al.*, 1996; Des Jarlais *et al.*, 1994) have shown that where they are given information and resources, injectors have made significant reductions in their HIV-related risk behaviour. Much the most impressive reductions have occurred in relation to the sharing of injecting equipment; however, recent research has shown that injecting drug users are also able to reduce their sexual risk behaviour (Friedman *et al.*, 1994; Vanichseni *et al.*, 1993).

The HIV-related risk behaviour of injecting drug users does not occur within a vacuum but within a social context which exerts a powerful influence on the nature and extent of that behaviour. Contextual factors influence the overall level of sharing between injectors, who shares with whom, and the use or non-use of condoms. In this chapter we look at the range of factors which have been cited as having an influence on risk behaviour. Our focus is on the behaviour of those individuals injecting drugs on a 'non-therapeutic basis'; we do not consider influences on the behaviour of those providing and receiving therapeutic injections — an activity which occurs within a number of developing countries and which, depending upon the availability of sterile injecting equipment and the scope for sterilization of injecting equipment, can carry a risk of HIV transmission.

Most of the research which we examine in this chapter has been carried out in developed countries. This reflects the balance of research carried out to date; however, there is a clear need to conduct more work on contextual influences, and on risk behaviour within developing countries. In describing the contextual influences, this chapter is not confined to research carried out as part of the WHO Multi-City Study on Drug Injection and Risk of HIV Infection.

In the absence of an effective vaccine against HIV the major prospect of limiting the spread of the epidemic is through reducing the occurrence of those behaviours known to transmit infection. In order to alter behaviour, we need to understand the various ways in which it may be influenced by both psychological factors and social context. Interventions aimed at reducing HIV-related risk behaviour need to operate at both the individual and the contextual levels if they are to be effective. Understanding the contextual influences on risk behaviour is therefore an essential component in the design of such interventions.

The Availability and Accessibility of Injecting Equipment

The single greatest factor influencing the sharing of injecting equipment among injectors is the availability and accessibility of sterile equipment. Put crudely, where injecting equipment is widely available and accessible to injectors, sharing tends to be low; conversely where availability and accessibility are poor, sharing tends to be high.

There is no evidence that drug injecting itself is diminished by shortages in the availability of injecting equipment. The clearest evidence for this has come from studies of injecting drug use within prisons. In virtually every prison study which has collected data on drug use over the last few years, injecting and the sharing of injecting equipment have been identified (Covell *et al.*, 1993; Turnbull, Dolan and Stimson, 1990; Carvell and Hart, 1990; Magura *et al.*, 1993; Muller *et al.*, 1995). In reporting on the first documented outbreak of HIV within a Scottish prison population, Taylor *et al.* (1995) found that in 1993, 43 per cent of inmates reported injecting within the prison – and all but one of these individuals had shared injecting equipment with other prisoners. Similar findings have been reported from a prison study carried out in Brazil (Rozman *et al.*, forthcoming) (see also Chapter 11). Beyond such settings as prisons there is no evidence that obstacles to the availability of injecting equipment reduce the incidence and prevalence of injecting. In most of the United States the possession of injecting equipment by drug users has been outlawed, yet there are an estimated 200 000 injectors living within New York City alone.

That politics can influence the availability of injecting equipment is beyond doubt. That the politics of needle and syringe provision can in turn influence the level of sharing has been documented on the basis of research comparing the situation in different cities and countries. Des Jarlais (1994), for example, contrasted the situation of those areas where HIV infection among injectors has remained low for a number of years (Glasgow, Sydney, Lund, and Tacoma) with those where there has been a rapid expansion of HIV-1 infection levels among injectors (Manipur, Bangkok, India). What the low prevalence areas had in common, and what distinguished them from the high prevalence areas, was the speedy implementation of a policy of needle and syringe provision combined with outreach services to injectors (see also Chapter 12). On the basis of this comparison Des Jarlais points out that:

> Given the evidence that it is possible to prevent epidemics of HIV among IDUs a failure to do so should be considered primarily a local political failure rather than a failure of scientific knowledge or the technological means for behaviour change. (Des Jarlais, 1994, p. 389)

The exception to this, as Des Jarlais recognizes, are those developing countries where there simply are not the resources to supply sterile injecting equipment for medical purposes, let alone for the purpose of illicit drug use.

Equally as important as the matter of the availability of injecting equipment is the issue of accessibility. By and large the worlds of health care provision and injecting drug use exist within different social and economic space and time. As a result there is a need not only to make injecting equipment available within clinic-type settings but to ensure that it is accessible within the actual situations in which drugs are used. The importance of the accessibility of injecting equipment was demonstrated by recent research in Glasgow, Scotland, a city with an extensive network of needle exchanges. Injectors were asked to say how they thought they might act in a range of situations in which they had drugs to inject but no access to sterile injecting equipment. Although one option was to leave the situation and acquire sterile injecting equipment, 68 per cent of the respondents stated that they would rather borrow someone else's injecting equipment than leave the situation or postpone their drug use (McKeganey *et al.*, 1995). This highlights the importance of not only making injecting equipment available within medical or clinic settings but of gaining access to the actual situations where drugs are used, through, for example, outreach services that take injecting equipment to injectors (Broadhead and Fox, 1990; Rhodes and Hartnoll, 1996). In Salvador, Brazil, the first needle exchange programme was established in a health centre in 1995. Although the number of syringes distributed by this centre was small (less than 200 per month), its very existence served as an example of what could be done and a more successful project organized by a non-governmental organization (IEPAS) has now been set up to distribute needles and syringes on an outreach basis. In many locations in Australia and the Netherlands, the provision of needles and syringes to injecting drug users has been made easier by funding drug users' own organizations ('junky unions') to provide syringe exchange outreach services at times and places which are convenient to drug users themselves (Friedman, de Jong and Wodak, 1993).

The Cultural Dimensions of Sharing

In Howard and Borges's classic study 'Needle sharing in the Haight' (1970), it was recognized that the sharing of needles and syringes had an important function in symbolizing the relationship between injectors. Before looking at the cultural dimensions of sharing it is worth discounting what might appear to be a conflict between explanations of sharing in terms of availability and accessibility, and explanations couched in terms of the social and symbolic significance of sharing. While shortages in the availability of injecting equipment can be seen as the context within which sharing occurs, this does not necessarily mean that the sharing itself will be devoid of social meaning or symbolic significance. To understand the sharing of injecting equipment one needs to recognize the importance of the cultural context within which it occurs, as well as its social meaning for the individuals involved.

In his book *The Gift*, Marcel Mauss (1925) provided an elegant analysis of the importance of gift giving and reciprocity in human social relationships. Such an analysis is important in reminding us that although in the era of AIDS it may be difficult to think of the sharing of injecting equipment in any terms other than as a risk behaviour, in fact it may also be seen as part and parcel of a wider culture of sharing within communities. In ethnographic work carried out on a working-class community in Glasgow, the sharing of injecting equipment was part of a wider culture of sharing among local people generally. All manner of items including clothing, food and cigarettes were shared on an everyday basis among local people, whether they were were injecting or not (McKeganey and Barnard, 1992). Similar anthropological research looking at the cultural dimension of syringe sharing has also been carried out in Brazil (Fernandez, 1994). Within the Netherlands, Grund, Kaplan and Adriaans (1991) and Grund *et al.* (1992) have looked at the cultural meaning of sharing among Dutch drug users:

> Addicts share many valued things such as housing, food, money, clothing and childcare. Often they help one another with daily problems associated with the addict life where sharing fits the broader context of coping with craving, needs for human contact and the hardships of life on the margins of society. In this context the sharing of drugs serves as a strong symbolic binding force. (Grund *et al.*, 1992, p. 383)

On the basis of his ethnographic work Grund noted that Dutch injectors would sometimes use the barrels of possibly contaminated syringes for dividing drugs prior to their use among friends. Such practice (known as 'frontloading' or 'backloading') has been described in numerous other cities including London (Hunter *et al.*, 1995), New York (Jose *et al.*, 1993; Grund *et al.*, in press) and Glasgow (Green *et al.*, 1993), and is likely to constitute a significant further risk of HIV infection (Jose *et al.*, 1993) and HTLV-11 infection among drug injectors (Vlahov *et al.*, 1995).

The impact of cultural expectations of reciprocity among injectors is also apparent in the passing on of previously used injecting equipment. In an ethnographic study carried out in Glasgow, the majority of injectors interviewed stated that they would be prepared to help out someone who had drugs to inject but no access to injecting equipment by passing on their own equipment if asked to do so, although they generally added that they would not accept back injecting equipment lent in this way. While being aware of the risks to themselves, the injectors in this study also recognized the importance of helping out a fellow injector in need (McKeganey, Barnard and Watson, 1989). The passing on of previously used injecting equipment can be seen both as part of a local culture among people generally and as a specific set of obligations shared among injectors.

Who Shares with Whom: The Importance of Social Relations

While the availability and accessibility of injecting equipment influence the overall level of sharing, they do not altogether determine who shares with whom; this is an issue which is heavily determined by the relationship between injectors. Information on who shares with whom is crucial in understanding and predicting HIV spread among injectors. The extent and nature of HIV spread is likely to be different depending upon whether most sharing occurs within relatively closed social networks of injectors, between sexual partners or between injectors who are socially distant from each other.

The clearest evidence for this has been the data on drug injecting venues (such as 'shooting galleries'). Shooting galleries have been identified in some of the areas where very rapid spread of HIV has occurred among injectors (New York, Edinburgh). The characteristic feature of shooting galleries, which explains their important role in HIV spread, is the fact that they enable sharing to occur between individuals who are socially distant from each other. A similar process may also explain the rapid spread of HIV in parts of Asia where it has been reported that injectors are often given the location of a hidden set of injecting equipment, which they use and then replace for others to use; or where injection with used needles is performed by a professional injector and drug seller on customers as they come *seriatim*. Such serial anonymous sharing, as in the case of shooting galleries, facilitates the sharing of injecting equipment among injectors who are socially distant from each other.

The impact of social networks in shaping the social pattern of sharing and thus of HIV spread has been studied in some detail in the US by Friedman, Neaigus and colleagues. Friedman, for example, contrasted the level of sharing and HIV positivity among new and experienced injectors. While the former were sharing at a relatively high level, only about 20 per cent of them, as opposed to 50 per cent of old injectors, were HIV positive. One explanation for this apparent paradox may be the fact that although the new injectors were sharing injecting equipment, their sharing partners tended to be other individuals who had similarly only recently begun injecting and who therefore may have had only a limited exposure to HIV. Over time, as the social networks of new injectors expand to encompass individuals who have been injecting for longer periods, their risk of being exposed to HIV increases and the prevalence of HIV among those individuals may begin to rise (Friedman *et al.*, 1989).

Analysis of social and risk-taking networks has been developed further by

Neaigus and colleagues (1994) who found that in New York such networks were homogeneous in certain respects, for example race, and socially diverse in others, for example they cross-cut gender and lengths of time individuals had been injecting. By analyzing the composition of these networks the researchers were able to provide information relevant to understanding the social pattern of HIV spread within a given area. They were able to show that although a given network may appear closed in terms of the sharing practices of most of its members, nevertheless networks with very different risk profiles may overlap as a result of the activities of a small number of injectors who may simultaneously participate in multiple networks:

> Although drug injectors' direct risk networks commonly involve social ties between network members, their risk networks can also be mediated and anonymous. Thus infected syringes particularly those which are centred in shooting galleries, can circulate among injectors who have no direct social ties to one another. (Neaigus *et al.*, 1994, p. 75).

Neaigus *et al.* (1994) have also shown that syringe sharing is more likely among pairs of drug injectors who have closer social ties, and among those who see their peers' norms as supportive of sharing (Friedman *et al.*, in press). Curtis *et al.* (in press, a and b) have shown that drug injectors at the core of large social networks are more likely to share syringes than more peripheral injectors. Analysis of the composition of social and risk-taking networks may be of value in developing peer education and support interventions which can involve both the injecting and non-injecting members of injectors' social networks in facilitating and maintaining their behaviour change (Friedman *et al.*, 1992).

Although the pattern of sharing that has evolved within such high prevalence areas as New York may serve to link individuals who are otherwise socially distant from each other, within many of the low prevalence areas most of the sharing that takes place is between sexual partners or good friends. Sharing between sexual partners or among close friends is likely to be influenced by cultural perceptions of risk, social distance, and trust — individuals who are socially distant may be perceived as representing a greater risk than individuals who are socially close (Neaigus *et al.*, 1994). Furthermore, between sexual partners or good friends there may be an assumption that one's sharing partner would not share with anyone else outside the particular relationship.

Gender

A number of studies have pointed to the significance of gender upon injectors' sharing practices and have suggested that women may be at increased risk of sharing. There are likely to be various reasons for this. First, injecting drug use carries greater stigma for females than for males, especially if the females are mothers (Taylor, 1993). In an ethnographic study, female injectors reported being unwilling to reveal their drug injecting to agency staff not only because of the stigma, but in the case of young mothers, because their drug use may lead to concerns being expressed by agency staff as to their competence to care for their children. There appeared to be no similar fears among the male injectors (Barnard, 1993). As a result, female injectors may be less likely than their male counterparts to attend services providing sterile injecting equipment. Research carried out in needle exchanges within the UK has consistently shown fewer women than men (relative to the estimated female-to-male ratio of injecting drug users) attending such services (Stimson, 1989; Hart *et al.*, 1989); however, in New York, men and women were equally likely to report having used syringe exchanges (Tortu, in press).

The second area where gender may have an influence on risk behaviour is in the finding that male injectors are more likely to have non-injecting female sexual partners compared to female injectors, who mostly have male partners who are also injectors (Klee *et al.*, 1990; Donoghoe, 1992; Freeman, Rodriquez and French, 1994). In their study of 769 injectors from Patterson, New Jersey, Freeman and colleagues found that although females were less likely than males to attend shooting galleries, they were significantly more likely to inject with a sex partner:

> nearly half the females shot up at least some of the time with a sex partner, while only 21.5 per cent of the males reported doing so. Males are significantly more likely than females to inject at least some of the time with a person they identify as a running partner (injecting partner). Almost 28 per ent of the females, compared to 16 per cent of the males reported that they had never shot drugs alone in the previous six months. (Freeman, Rodriquez and French, 1994)

The authors of this report noted, for example, that the female injectors in their study

> were often injected by their male drug shooting partner after he had injected himself, a sequence that clearly places the woman at elevated risk of acquiring the virus in the absence of consistent and thorough needle cleaning.

Among injecting couples it is likely that the two risk practices of sharing injecting equipment and having unprotected sex reinforce each other. In Glasgow, for example, many of the female injectors who were sharing with their male sex partner described their reason for continuing to do so precisely in terms of the fact of their having unprotected sex with their partner; within such a situation, they explained, there was little point in not sharing injecting equipment (Barnard, 1993).

Racial and Ethnic Differences in Injecting Behaviours

In some countries such as the United States, race/ethnicity is a major element of social stratification. HIV seroprevalence data among injecting drug users in many areas — but not all — of the United States indicate that African-Americans and those of Latino or Puerto Rican origin or descent are more likely to be seropositive than whites (Chitwood *et al.*, 1993; Friedman *et al.*, 1987; Friedman, Sufian and Des Jarlais, 1990; Hahn *et al.*, 1989; Koblin *et al.*, 1990; LaBrie *et al.*, 1993; Marmor *et al.*, 1987; Nwanyanwu *et al.*, 1993). High risk injecting behaviours vary by race/ethnicity in the United States, but this variation is extremely complex. The race/ethnicity of drug injectors is mediated by the racial/ethnic composition of the city in which they live (Friedman *et al.*, 1992). Among African-American drug injectors there is some evidence that two contradictory processes may be operating: first, an 'inequality' theme which suggests that deprivation of access to resources and services which African-Americans face may engender a degree of higher-risk behaviour among them; and second, a 'culture of resistance' theme which suggests that their long-term experience of survival and struggle has made them particularly capable of adapting their norms and behaviours in ways that have led to a greater degree of deliberate reduction of HIV-risk behaviours among them.

The Salience of Risk in the Drug-using Lifestyle

In their article 'Taking care of business — the heroin users' life on the streets', Preble and Casey (1969) describe the everyday activity of maintaining a drug habit; this involves the near continuous activity of obtaining money, locating drugs, buying drugs, avoiding the police, using the drugs, experiencing the effects of the drugs, and then beginning the cycle anew. This cycle is likely to be repeated several times a day. It is also a cycle within which there are multiple risks: of being arrested, of not locating drugs, of not having sufficient money to buy drugs or of being sold fake drugs (Power *et al.*, 1995). Since risk is a highly salient feature of the addict's lifestyle it cannot be assumed that HIV will be recognized by addicts as the pre-eminent risk they face. If they appear to pay less attention to HIV within certain situations than health educationalists might desire, this may not be because they are unconcerned with the risks of infection but because other risks are more immediately pressing.

Drug Use

A number of studies have attempted to identify whether particular drugs may be associated with higher levels of injecting or sexual risk taking. Within parts of the US the combined use of heroin and cocaine ('speedball') or the use of cocaine alone appears to be associated with increased risk of HIV transmission. This could be partly due to differences in the frequency of drug injecting — users who combine heroin with cocaine, or who inject cocaine alone, often report more frequent injecting than do users of heroin alone. In addition, the drugs used may affect certain features of drug preparation that may be associated with higher levels of HIV infection. Greenfield, Bigelow and Brooner (1992), for example, found that more than two to three times the amount of blood was involved when cocaine and heroin were injected together than when heroin alone was injected. 'Blood booting' (drawing blood back into the syringe to mix it with the drug) among those reporting needle sharing, was significantly more likely during cocaine use than heroin use. In other countries the risk of HIV transmission is associated with the practice of mixing drugs in a common pot, from which individual injection amounts are withdrawn. Such a practice has been reported as occurring within countries as diverse as Poland and Vietnam.

The likelihood of needle and syringe sharing has also been demonstrated to be associated with the level of drug dependency. Gossop and colleagues (1993a) found that the more severely dependent injectors were more likely to have shared injecting equipment. In Madrid, both frequency of injection and use of cocaine were independent significant predictors of syringe sharing (Rodriguez *et al.*, in press). The possible effects of drug use on sharing practices is not confined to injected drugs. Saxon and Calsyn (1992) found that those injectors who reported using alcohol were also more likely to report needle and syringe sharing compared to injectors who did not report using alcohol. Similarly, Latkin *et al.* (1994a) found that among the male injectors in Baltimore, heavy drinking was significantly associated with having multiple sex partners and exchanging sex for money or drugs. The authors recommend that services focus particular attention on injecting drug users reporting heavy use of alcohol.

Drug Use Settings

The influence of the setting on drug users' activities has had a long-standing place in drug use research (Zinberg, 1984). Despite this, the effect of drug setting on HIV-related risk behaviour has received rather less attention than one might have anticipated. It seems likely that such factors as whether injecting is occurring within a derelict tenement block without an adequate clean water supply or in an individual's own home, will have a significant impact on injectors' risk behaviours. Latkin *et al.* (1994b) paid particular attention to the significance of drug use setting in their Baltimore study. They note that:

> Frequency of injecting with others was significantly associated with these three risk behaviours (frequency of sharing, always using cleaned equipment and slipping, i.e. using a needle after someone else without cleaning it). Frequency of sharing needles in the prior six months was significantly associated with reports of injection at friends' residences, shooting galleries and semi-public areas. Moreover recent slipping was

also significantly associated with reported injecting at friends' residences, shooting galleries and semi-public areas. (Latkin *et al.*, 1994b)

Attention has also been directed at the way in which changes in the social structure of drug markets can have an impact on risk behaviour. Curtis *et al.* (in press, a) have looked at the way in which drug-related activities may, through a variety of social processes including policing, be concentrated within certain areas with the result that what is created is a kind of drug supermarket. Analysis of risk behaviour within those areas revealed that both the sharing of injecting equipment and the sharing of drugs (via 'backloading') was more likely to occur. Newcomers to the area were more likely to buy drugs through association with a sponsor with whom an agreement may be made to share the drugs, resulting in an increased likelihood that injecting equipment may also be shared. In addition, the hyperactivity of such areas may lead to more frequent injecting (particularly with cocaine or drug mixing with crack smoking), resulting in more sharing.

Curtis *et al.* (in press, b) also suggest that changes in residential patterns in some areas of a city can lead to extreme overcrowding within these. The reduction in the space available may have simultaneously led to a reduction in the number of local shooting galleries within certain areas, with a corresponding increase of activity in others. Such changes may also lead to an increased likelihood of injecting occurring within semi-public settings where the pressure to inject quickly before attracting the attention of the police may result in less attention being given to the preparation and cleaning of injecting equipment.

The association between homelessness and the sharing of injecting equipment has been noted by a number of researchers (Beardsley *et al.*, 1992). As well as influencing the setting where injecting occurs, homelessness may also be indicative of a level of chaos within an individual's life in which maintaining a clear sense of the ownership of injecting equipment may be more difficult. In an ethnographic study (McKeganey and Barnard, 1992), some of the drug injectors described their own sharing as resulting from confusion over the ownership of equipment. Such confusion may be more likely to occur within the more chaotic life circumstances of an individual who is homeless.

Sexual Risk Behaviour and Injecting Drug Users

Despite the focus of attention being upon equipment sharing practices, most injectors are also at risk of contracting and, if infected, of spreading HIV through sexual contact (Abdul-Quader *et al.*, 1990). In their study in England, Klee *et al.* (1990) report that 88 per cent of drug injectors were sexually active; 82 per cent of attendees at syringe exchange schemes in England were found to be sexually active (Donoghoe, Dolan and Stimson, 1990); and Magura and colleagues (1990) found 73 per cent of injectors enrolled in methadone maintenance clinics in New York to have been sexually active in the previous month.

Contrary to popular beliefs about drug injectors being deviant in every respect, many studies have shown some injectors to be sexually conservative — often being involved in long-term relationships with one partner (Kane, 1991). Although the levels of condom use among injectors are low, in fact condoms are not widely used by the majority of other people involved in long-term relationships. Therefore one needs to be cautious and avoid making easy assumptions that the reasons underpinning injectors' use or non-use of condoms will be different from those of most other people.

Studies carried out by, among others, Nutbeam (1989), MacDonald and Smith (1990), Donoghoe *et al.* (1989) and Klee *et al.* (1990) have all stressed that individuals, injectors and non-injectors, remain unconvinced that they are personally at risk from the sexual transmission of HIV. Similarly, in studies of male and female heterosexual behaviour it has been noted that condoms, where they are used at all, tend to be used at the beginning of relationships. Once it is recognized that the relationship will continue there is often a move to non-barrier methods of contraception (Holland *et al.*, 1990). Condoms tend to be seen as a temporary measure more associated with 'one-off' or occasional sexual contacts than with long-term relationships. Since many injectors are involved in long-term relationships, the suggestion that they should use condoms may be taken by the individuals as signalling a lack of trust in their partner's fidelity.

In the majority of studies which have collected data on the sexual behaviour of injectors, fairly low levels of condom use have been identified. Rhodes *et al.* (1993a) report that 70 per cent of the London injectors and 75 per cent of the Glasgow injectors studied were not using condoms with their primary partners; similarly 34 per cent of the London injectors and 52 per cent of the Glasgow injectors never used condoms with their casual partners. This finding is very much in accord with studies conducted elsewhere; for example in the US, Watkins *et al.* (1993) report 66 per cent of injectors in their study not using a condom on their last sexual encounter.

There are exceptions to this, however; Hando and Hall (1994) report that 32 per cent of their sample of Australian amphetamine users were always using condoms with their regular sexual partners. Somewhat higher levels of condom use have also been recorded in those areas where HIV has been high over a number of years. Friedman *et al.* (1994) found that 38 per cent of injectors reported using a condom on the last occasion of having sex with a primary partner and 59 per cent on the last occasion of having sex with a casual partner. Drug injectors attending syringe exchanges were also significantly more likely than non-exchange attenders to report having used condoms in their last sexual encounter with a primary partner as well as on the last occasion of sex with a casual partner. In New York, Friedman *et al.* (1994) looked at the consistent use of condoms over the last 30 days. They found that condoms were consistently used in only 22 per cent of relationships where both parties were injectors, but in 44 per cent of the relationships where only one of the couple was an injector. Consistent condom use was particularly high (68 per cent) in relationships between seropositive drug injectors and non-injectors. Consistent condom use was also greater in relationships where peer norms were perceived to be supportive of condom use. These data indicate that drug injectors in New York have developed norms favourable to protecting others through condom use.

It is not only in New York, however, that an altruistic dimension of injectors' behaviour has become apparent. A survey in Spain, for example, found that seropositive injectors were more likely to stop sharing and to change their sexual habits than their HIV negative counterparts (Delgado-Rodriguez *et al.*, 1994). In London, injectors who knew they were HIV positive were more likely to use condoms and less likely to share injecting equipment than injectors who were unaware of being HIV positive (Rhodes *et al.*, 1993b). In Glasgow, McKeganey (1990) also found evidence of HIV positive injectors employing a number of means to protect the health of others, including: never sharing injecting equipment, always using condoms, always telling a prospective partner about their HIV status, or remaining celibate. Such measures were often enacted at great personal cost to the individual concerned; however, they reflected a widespread feeling among injectors that the last thing they wanted to do was to pass HIV on to others. Such findings illustrate clearly injectors' willingness not only to be concerned with reducing their own health risks but also to take steps to protect the health of others.

Race and Sexual Risk Behaviours

Attention has been directed at the possible influence of race and ethnicity on sexual behaviour. Anal sex has been reported to be more common among white injecting drug users than among black injectors (Lewis and Watters, 1991) and more common among Latino injectors than either white or black injectors in New York (Friedman *et al.*, 1993b). White injectors have been reported as having fewer non-injecting partners than black injectors (Lewis and Watters, 1991). Identifying the possible impact of race or ethnicity on injectors' sexual behaviour is a very difficult task. Race is not a single variable, but a composite of commonalities in experience, history of social struggle, cultural beliefs, religion, patterns of sociality, education, employment and so on. It is far from clear which, if any, of these things, may exert an influence on sexual behaviour.

Although there have been calls to target sexual risk reduction measures on specific population groups, most notably black injectors, there is a need to avoid the suggestion that it is only the behaviour of certain racial or ethnic groups which needs to be targeted. In their comparison of 19 cities, Friedman *et al.* (1993b) found that sexual risk was common across all racial/ethnic groups. They argue that:

> The self-reported sexual behaviours . . . of all racial/ethnic groups studied — including those of Mexican origin and white drug injectors — place them at high risk of infection . . . Thus contrary to arguments made by others . . . prevention resources should be allocated to

result of HIV, it could be that some relapse from safer injection arises out of a feeling of despair or exhaustion.

Finally, in terms of theoretical developments we need to develop more sophisticated models of explanation that enable us to combine, for example, personality and contextual factors and which avoid the assumption that behaviour derives unproblematically from knowledge and beliefs (the health belief model) or is overly determined by contextual factors.

References

ABDUL-QUADER, A.S., TROSS, S., FRIEDMAN, S.R. *et al.* (1990) 'Street-recruited intravenous drug users and sexual risk reduction in New York City', *AIDS*, **3**, pp. 1075–9.

BARNARD, M. (1993) 'Needle sharing in context: patterns of sharing amongst men and women injectors and HIV risks', *British Journal of Addiction*, **88**, pp. 805–12.

BEARDSLEY, M., CLATTS, M.C., DEREN, S. *et al.* (1992) 'Homelessness and HIV-risk behaviours in a sample of New York City drug injectors', *AIDS and Public Policy Journal*, **7**, pp. 129–52.

BROADHEAD, R.S. and FOX, K.J. (1990) ' "Taking it to the streets": AIDS outreach as ethnography', *Journal of Contemporary Ethnography*, **19**, pp. 332–48.

BUENO, R., LURIE, P., MESQUITA, F., TURIENZO, G. *et al.* (1996) 'A successful outreach project developed in Brazil among IDUs', paper presented at VIII International Conference On the Reduction of Drug-Related Harm, Australia.

CARVELL, A.L.M. and HART, G.L. (1990) 'Risk behaviours for HIV infection among drug users in prison', *British Medical Journal*, **300**, pp. 1383–4.

CELENTANO, D.D., MUNOZ, A., COHN, S. *et al.* (1994) 'Drug-related behaviour change for HIV transmission among American injecting drug users', *Addiction*, **89**, pp. 1309–17.

CHITWOOD, D.D., RIVERS, J.R., COMERFORD, M. and McBRIDE, D.C. (1993) 'A comparison of HIV-related risk behaviours of street-recruited and treatment program-recruited injecting drug users', in FISHER, D.G. and NEEDLE, R.H. (Eds), *AIDS and Community-Based Drug Intervention Programs: Evaluation and Outreach*, Binghampton, NY: Harrington Park Press.

COLON, H.M., ROBLES, R.R., SAHAI, H. and MATOS, T. (1992) 'Changes in HIV risk behaviours among intravenous drug users in San Juan, Puerto Rico', *British Journal of Addiction*, **87**, pp. 585–90.

COVELL, R.G., FRISCHER, M., TAYLOR, A. *et al.* (1993) 'Prison experience of injecting drug users in Glasgow', *Drug and Alcohol Dependence*, **32**, pp. 9–14.

CURTIS, R., FRIEDMAN, S.R., NEAIGUS, A. *et al.* (in press, a) 'Street-level drug market change and its impact on risk-taking behaviours by injecting drug users', *Journal of Contemporary Ethnography*.

CURTIS, R., FRIEDMAN, S.R., NEAIGUS, A. *et al.* (in press, b) 'Street-level drug market structure and HIV risk', *Social Networks*.

DELGADO-RODRIGUEZ, M., DE LA FUENTE, L., BRAVO, M. *et al.* (1994) 'IV drug users: changes in risk behaviour according to HIV status in a national survey in Spain', *Journal of Epidemiology and Community Health*, **48**, pp. 459–63.

DES JARLAIS, D.C. (1994) 'Cross-national studies of AIDS among injecting drug users', *Addiction*, **89**, pp. 383–92.

DES JARLAIS, D.C., CHOOPANYA, K., VANICHSENI, S. *et al.* (1994) 'AIDS risk reduction and reduced HIV seroconversion among drug users in Bangkok', *American Journal of Public Health*, **84**, pp. 425–55.

DONOGHOE, M.C. (1992) 'Sex, HIV and the injecting drug user', *British Journal of Addiction*, **87**, pp. 405–16.

DONOGHOE, M., DOLAN, K. and STIMSON, G.V. (1990) *National syringe exchange monitoring study: interim report*, London: Centre for Research on Drugs and Health Behaviour.

DONOGHOE, M., STIMSON, G.V., DOLAN, K. and ALLDRITT, L. (1989) 'Changes in HIV risk behaviour in clients of syringe exchange schemes in England and Scotland', *AIDS*, **3**, pp. 267–72.

EDLIN, B.R., IRWIN, K., FARUQUE, S. *et al.* (1994) 'Intersecting epidemics — crack use and HIV infection among inner-city young adults', *New England Journal of Medicine*, **331**, pp. 1422–7.

FERNANDEZ, O. (1994) 'The practice of drug injection, the community of sharing syringes and harm reduction related to HIV', in FERNANDEZ, O. (Ed.), *AIDS in Brazil*, Rio de Janeiro: Relume-Dumará.

FREEMAN, R.C., RODRIGUEZ, G.M. and FRENCH, J.F. (1994) 'A comparison of male and female intravenous drug users' risk behaviours for HIV infection', *American Journal of Drug and Alcohol Abuse*, **20**, pp. 129–57.

FRIEDMAN, S.R., DE JONG, W. and WODAK, A. (1993) 'Community development as a response to HIV among drug injectors', *AIDS*, 92/93 (suppl. 1), S263–S269.

FRIEDMAN, S.R., DES JARLAIS, D.C. and STERK, C.E. (1990) 'AIDS and the social relations of intravenous drug users', *The Millbank Quarterly*, **68**, pp. 85–109.

FRIEDMAN, S.R., DES JARLAIS, D.C. and WARD, T.P. (1994) 'Social models for changing health-relevant behaviour', in DI CLEMENTE, R. and PETERSON, J. (Eds) *Preventing AIDS*, pp. 95–116, New York: Plenum Press.

FRIEDMAN, S.R., SUFIAN, M. and DES JARLAIS, D.C. (1990) 'The AIDS epidemic among Latino intravenous drug users', in GLICK, R. and MOORE, J. (Eds) *Drug Abuse in Hispanic Communities*, pp. 45–54, New Brunswick, NJ: Rutgers University Press.

FRIEDMAN, S.R., SOTHERAN, J.L., ABDUL-QUADER, A. *et al.* (1987) 'The AIDS epidemic among Blacks and Hispanics', *The Millbank Quarterly*, **65** (suppl. 2), pp. 455–99.

FRIEDMAN, S.R., DES JARLAIS, D.C., NEAIGUS, A. *et al.* (1989) 'AIDS and the new drug injector', *Nature*, **339**, pp. 333–4.

FRIEDMAN, S.R., NEAIGUS, A., DES JARLAIS, D.C. *et al.* (1992) 'Social intervention against AIDS among injecting drug users', *British Journal of Addiction*, **87**, pp. 393–404.

FRIEDMAN, S.R., JOSE, B., NEAIGUS, A. *et al.* (1993a) 'Female injecting drug users get infected with HIV sooner than males' Session 3137, 121st Annual Meeting of the American Public Health Association, San Francisco, CA.

FRIEDMAN, S.R., YOUNG, P.A., SNYDER, F.R., SHORTY, V., JONES, A., ESTRADA, A.L. and the NADR Consortium (1993b) 'Racial differences in sexual behaviours related to AIDS in a nineteen-city sample of street-recruited drug injectors', *AIDS Education and Prevention*, **5**, pp. 196–211.

FRIEDMAN, S.R., JOSE, B., NEAIGUS, A. *et al.* (1994) 'Consistent condom use in relationships between seropositive injecting drug users and sex partners who do not inject drugs', *AIDS*, **8**, pp. 357–61.

FRIEDMAN, S.R., NEAIGUS, A., JOSE, B. *et al.* (in press) 'Network and socio-historical approaches to the HIV epidemic among drug injectors', in CATALÁN, J., HEDGE, B. and SHERR, L. (Eds) [title under negotiation], Chur, Switzerland: Harwood.

GOSSOP, M., GRIFFITHS, P., POWIS, B. and SRANG, J. (1993a) 'Severity of heroin dependence and HIV risk. I. Sexual behaviour', *AIDS Care — Psychological and Socio-Medical Aspects of AIDS/HIV*, **5**, pp. 149–57.

GOSSOP, M., GRIFFITHS, P., POWIS, B. and STRANG, J. (1993b) 'Severity of heroin dependence and HIV risk. II. Sharing injecting equipment', *AIDS Care*, 5, pp. 159–68.

GREEN, S.T., TAYLOR, A., FRISCHER, M. and GOLDBERG, D.J. (1993) 'Frontloading ("halfing") among Glasgow drug injectors as a continuing risk behaviour for HIV transmission' (1), *Addiction*, **88**, pp. 1581–2.

GREENFIELD, L., BIGELOW, G.E. and BROONER, R.K. (1992) 'HIV risk behaviour in drug users: Increased blood "booting" during cocaine injection', *AIDS Education and Prevention*, **4**, pp. 95–107.

GRUND, J-P.C., KAPLAN, C.D. and ADRIAANS, N.F.P. (1991) 'Needle sharing in the Netherlands: An ethnographic analysis', *American Journal of Public Health*, **81**, pp. 1602–7.

GRUND, J-P.C., STERN, L.S., KAPLAN, C.D. *et al.* (1992) 'Drug use contexts and HIV-consequences: The effect of drug policy on patterns of everyday drug use in Rotterdam and the Bronx', *British Journal of Addiction*, **87**, pp. 381–92.

GRUND, J-P.C., FRIEDMAN, S.R., STERN, L.S. *et al.* (in press) 'Syringe-mediated drug sharing among injecting drug users', *Social Science & Medicine*.

HAHN, R.A., ONORATO, I.M., JONES, T.S. and DOUGHERTY, J. (1989) 'Prevalence of HIV injection among intravenous drug users in the United States', *Journal of American Medical Association*, **261**, pp. 2677–84.

HANDO, J. and HALL, W. (1994) 'HIV risk-taking behaviour among amphetamine users in Sydney, Australia', *Addiction*, **89**, pp. 79–85.

HART, G., CARVELL, A., WOODWARD, N. *et al.* (1989) 'Evaluation of needle exchange in central London', *AIDS*, **3**, pp. 261–5.

HOLLAND, J., RAMAZANOGLU, C., SCOTT, S., *et al.* (1990) 'Sex, gender and power: Young women's sexuality in the shadow of AIDS', *Sociology of Health and Illness*, **12**, pp. 336–50.

HOWARD, J. and BORGES, P. (1970) 'Needle sharing in the Haight: Some social and psychological functions', *Journal of Health and Social Behaviour*, **11**, pp. 220–30.

HUNTER, G.M., DONOGHOE, M.C., STIMSON, G.V. *et al.* (1995) 'Changes in the injecting risk behaviour of injecting drug users in London, 1990–1993', *AIDS*, **9**, pp. 493–501.

INCIARDI, J.A., LOCKWOOD, D. and POTTIEGER, A.E. (1993) *Women and crack cocaine*, University of Delaware, New York: Macmillan.

JOSE, B., FRIEDMAN, S.R., NEAIGUS, A. *et al.* (1993) 'Syringe-mediated drug-sharing ("backloading"): A new risk factor for HIV among injecting drug users', *AIDS*, **7**, pp. 1653–60.

KANE, S. (1991) 'HIV, heroin and heterosexual relations', *Social Science and Medicine*, **32**, pp. 1037–50.

KLEE, H. (1993) 'HIV risks for women drug injectors heroin and amphetamine users compared', *Addiction*, **88**, pp. 1055–62.

KLEE, H., FAUGIER, J., HAYES, C. *et al.* (1990) 'Sexual partners of injecting drug users: The risk of HIV infection', *British Journal of Addiction*, **85**, pp. 413–18.

KOBLIN, B.A., MCCLUSKER, J., LEWIS, B.F. and SULLIVAN, J.L. (1990) 'Racial/ethnic differences in HIV-1 seroprevalence and risky behaviours among intravenous drug users in a multisite study', *American Journal of Epidemiology*, **132**, pp. 837–46.

LABRIE, R.A., MCAULIFFE, W.E., NEMETH-COSLETT, R. and WILDERSCHIED, L. (1993) 'The prevalence of HIV infection in a national sample of injecting drug users', in

BROWN, B.S. and BESCHNER, G.M. (Eds) *Handbook on Risk of AIDS*, pp. 16–37, Westport, CT: Greenwood Press.

LATKIN, C., MANDELL, W., OZIEMKOWSKA, M. *et al.* (1994a) 'The relationships between sexual behaviour, alcohol use, and personal network characteristics among injecting drug users in Baltimore, Maryland', *Sexually Transmitted Diseases*, **21**, pp. 161–7.

LATKIN, C., MANDELL, W.D., VLAHOV, D. *et al.* (1994b) 'My place, your place and noplace: behaviour settings as a risk factor for HIV-related injection practices of drug users in Baltimore, Maryland', *American Journal of Community Psychology*, **22**, 3, pp. 415–31.

LEWIS, D.K. and WATTERS, J.K. (1991) 'Sexual risk behaviour among heterosexual intravenous drug users: Ethnic and gender variations', *AIDS*, **5**, pp. 77–83.

McCoY, H.V. and INCIARDI, J.A. (1993) 'Women and AIDS: social determinants of sex–related activities', *Women and Health*, **20**, pp. 69–86.

MacDONALD, G. and SMITH, C. (1990) 'Complacency, risk perception and the problem of HIV education', *AIDS Care*, **2**, pp. 63–8.

McKEGANEY, N. and (1990) 'Being positive: drug injectors' experience of HIV', *British Journal of Addiction*, **85**, pp. 1113–24.

McKEGANEY, N.P. and BARNARD, M. (1992) *AIDS, Drugs and Sexual Risk: Lives in the Balance*, Buckingham: Open University Press.

McKEGANEY, N., BARNARD, M. and WATSON, H. (1989) 'HIV-related risk behaviour among a non-clinic sample of injecting drug users', *British Journal of Addiction*, **84**, pp. 1481–90.

McKEGANEY, N., ABEL, M., TAYLOR, A. *et al.* (1995) 'The preparedness to share injecting equipment: An analysis using vignettes', *Addiction*, **90**, pp. 1259–66.

MAGURA, S., SHAPIRO, J., SIDDIQUI, Q. and LIPTON, D. (1990) 'Variables influencing condom use among intravenous drug users', *American Journal of Public Health*, **80**, pp. 82–4.

MAGURA, S., KANG, S., SHAPIRO, J. and ODAY, J. (1993) 'HIV risk among women injecting drug users who are in jail', *Addiction*, **88**, pp. 1351–60.

MARMOR, M., DES JARLAIS, D.C., COHEN, H. *et al.* (1987) 'Risk factors and infection with human immunodeficiency virus among intravenous drug abusers in New York City', *AIDS*, **1**, pp. 39–44.

MAUSS, M. (1925) *The Gift: forms and functions of exchange in archaic societies*, New York: Norton Publishing.

MULLER, R., STARK, K., GUGGENMOOS, J. *et al.* (1995) 'Imprisonment: a risk factor for HIV infection counteracting education and prevention programmes for intravenous drug users', *AIDS*, **9**, pp. 183–90.

NEAIGUS, A., FRIEDMAN, S.R., CURTIS, R. *et al.* (1994) 'The relevance of drug injectors' social and risk networks for understanding and preventing HIV infection', *Social Science and Medicine*, **38**, pp. 67–78.

NUTBEAM, D. (1989) 'Public knowledge and attitudes to AIDS', *Journal of Public Health*, **103**, pp. 205–11.

NWANYANWU, O.C., CHU, S.Y., GREEN, T.A. *et al.* (1993) 'Acquired immunodeficiency syndrome in the United States associated with injecting drug use, 1981–1991', *American Journal of Drug and Alcohol Abuse*, **19**, pp. 399–408.

PLANT, M. (1990) 'Alcohol, sex and AIDS', *Alcohol and Alcoholism*, **25**, pp. 293–301.

POWER, R., JONES, S., KEARNS, G. *et al.* (1995) *Coping with illicit drug use*, London: The Tufnell Press.

PREBLE, E. and CASEY, J. (1969) 'Taking care of business: the heroin user's life on the streets', *International Journal of Addiction*, **1**, pp. 1–24.

RHODES, T.J. and HARTNOLL, R. (1996) *AIDS, Drugs and Prevention: Perspectives on Individual and Community Actions*, London: Routledge.

RHODES, T.J., BLOOR, M.J., DONOGHOE, M.C. *et al* (1993a) 'HIV prevalence and HIV risk behaviour among injecting drug users in London and Glasgow', *AIDS Care — Psychological and Socio-Medical Aspects of AIDS/HIV*, **5**, pp. 413–25.

RHODES, T.J., DONOGHOE, M.C., HUNTER, G.M. and STIMSON, G.V. (1993b) 'Continued risk behaviour among HIV positive drug injectors in London: implications for intervention', *Addiction*, **88**, pp. 1553–60.

ROSS, M.W., WODAK, A., GOLD, J. and MILLER, M.E. (1992) 'Differences across sexual orientation on HIV risk behaviours in injecting drug users', *AIDS Care — Psychological and Socio-Medical Aspects of AIDS/HIV*, **4**, pp. 139–48.

ROZMAN, M., MASSAD, E., BURATTININ, M. *et al*. (forthcoming) 'AIDS in a South American Prison', *Journal of AIDS*.

SAXON, A.J. and CALSYN, D.A. (1992) 'Alcohol use and high-risk behaviour by intravenous drug users in an AIDS education paradigm', *Journal of Studies on Alcohol*, **53**, pp. 611–18.

SCHOENBAUM, E., HARTEL, D., SELWYN, P. *et al*. (1989) 'Risk factors for human immunodeficiency virus infection in intravenous drug users', *New England Journal of Medicine*, **321**, pp. 874–9.

SCHOENFISCH, S., ELLENBROCK, T., HARRINGTON, P. *et al*. (1993) 'Risks of HIV infection and behavioural change associated with crack cocaine in pre-natal patients', Abstract PO-C 15 2920, IX International Conference on AIDS, Berlin.

STALL, R., EKSTRAND, M., POLLACK, L. *et al*. (1990) 'Relapse from safer sex: The next challenge for AIDS prevention efforts', *Journal of the Acquired Immune Deficiency Syndromes*, **3**, pp. 1181–7.

STIMSON, G.V. (1989) 'Syringe exchange programmes for injecting drug users', *AIDS*, **3**, pp. 253–60.

TAYLOR, A. (1993) *The career of the female intravenous drug user*, Oxford: Oxford University Press.

TAYLOR, A., FRISCHER, M., McKEGANEY, N. *et al*. (1993) 'HIV risk behaviours among female prostitute drug injectors in Glasgow', *Addiction*, **88**, pp. 1561–64.

TAYLOR, A., GOLDBERG, D., EMSLIE, J. *et al*. (1995) 'Outbreak of HIV infection in a Scottish prison', *British Medical Journal*, **310**, pp. 289–92.

TORTU, S., DEREN, S. and BEARDSLEY, M. (in press) 'Factors associated with needle exchange use in East Harlem', *Journal of Drug Issues*.

TURNBULL, P., DOLAN, K. and STIMSON, G. (1990) 'HIV-related risk behaviour among prisoners', *British Medical Journal*, **85**, pp. 123–35.

VANICHSENI, S., DES JARLAIS, D.C., CHOOPANYA, K. *et al*. (1993) 'Condom use with primary partners among injecting drug users in Bangkok, Thailand and New York City, United States', *AIDS*, **7**, pp. 887–91.

VLAHOV, D., KHABBAZ, R., COHN, S. *et al*. (1995) 'Incidence and risk factors for human T-Lymphotropic virus Type II seroconversion among injecting drug users in Baltimore, Maryland, USA', *Journal of Acquired Immune Deficiency Syndrome and Human Retrovirology*, **9**, pp. 89–96.

WALLACE, M.E., GALANTER, M., LIFSHUTZ, H. and KRASINSKI, K. (1993) 'Women at high risk of HIV infection from drug use', *Journal of Addictive Diseases*, **12**, pp. 77–86.

WATKINS, K.E., METZGER, D., WOODY, G. and McLELLAN, A.T. (1993) 'Determinants of condom use among intravenous drug users', *AIDS*, **7**, pp. 719–23.

WEATHERBURN, P., DAVIES, P., HUNT, A. *et al.* (1992) 'Heterosexual behaviour in a large cohort of homosexually active men in England and Wales', *AIDS Care*, **2**, pp. 319–24.

ZINBERG, N. (1984) *Drug set and setting: the basis for controlled intoxicant use*, New Haven: Yale.

Chapter 3

Health and Social Consequences of Injecting Drug Use

Martin C. Donoghoe and Alex Wodak

While it is generally accepted that drug use can have serious consequences for health and social well being, establishing a causal relationship between substance use and ill-health is problematic. As pointed out with regard to attributing causation between alcohol use and alcohol related problems: 'Causality here is not a matter of Newtonian physics, and uncertainty is part of every equation' (Edwards *et al.*, 1994). The uncertainty in attributing causation is all the greater with substances other than alcohol and tobacco. Users of illicit drugs seldom use only one drug exclusively. Heroin users in some countries, for example, will often use benzodiazepines. In many countries the majority of illicit drug users also use tobacco. Attributing causality to the use of a particular drug is therefore difficult.

Methods commonly used to study the health effects of alcohol and tobacco use, for example large scale general population based longitudinal cohort studies, do not lend themselves well to the study of the health effects of illicit drug use and injecting. Illicit drug users and, in particular, drug injectors are in the first place less accessible than smokers and alcohol drinkers. The stigmatized and often illegal nature of some substance use means that drug use is often a 'hidden' activity. As a result, true random samples of the general drug-using or drug-injecting population will rarely, if ever, be available. Furthermore the overall rates of the use of certain drugs, particularly those which are injected, in the general population are extremely low. Even in very large samples few injectors would be found. The sub-samples become even smaller and less meaningful when stratified for sex and age differences, and type of drug. The low prevalence of use of certain drugs and of drug injecting in the general population may also mean that case control studies are unsuitable for assessing health consequences.

Most studies of the health effects of injecting rely on opportunistic sampling of drug injectors from hospitals, health care agencies, specialist treatment and rehabilitation facilities, and prisons. These are all institutions where drug users will be over-represented. Drug users in these institutions, particularly those in treatment, may have more serious health problems than those not in contact.

Data collected from institutional records may also be biased. Hospital admission data, for example, may underestimate the number of hospitalizations resulting from drug use. Data on drug injecting are rarely collected as a matter of routine from people admitted to hospital, and people may be reluctant to disclose their drug-using behaviour to medical staff.

It is possible to overcome some of these methodological problems. Potential sample bias can be minimized by recruiting 'community-wide' samples of drug injectors, that is in and out of contact with institutions and through multiple site sampling techniques (Donoghoe *et al.*, 1993).

While longitudinal cohort studies are extremely difficult to conduct amongst drug injectors and are resource intensive, they provide ideal methods for studying the health effects and social consequences of drug injecting. Cohort or natural history studies are not new to the study of drug use. One of the earliest cohort studies of opioid users was conducted by Pescor in the early 1940s (Pescor, 1943) and the first documented out-of-treatment follow-up study was conducted by Nurco and Lerner (1971) between 1952 and 1971 with a 91 per cent follow-up rate. Cohorts have also been successfully followed over the longer term by, amongst others, Stimson in the United Kingdom (Stimson and Oppenheimer, 1982), Maddux and Desmond (1981) and Vaillant (1973) in the United States. Such studies cannot be generalized to drug-injecting populations globally or even to different groups of injectors in the same country. However, standardization of definitions and methodologies for collecting health data may allow for improved comparisons within and between countries, in much the same way as the World Health Organization (WHO) Multi-City Study on Drug Injecting and Risk of HIV Infection provided cross-nationally comparable data on drug-injecting behaviour and HIV infection (WHO, 1994).

Health Consequences of Injecting Drug Use

The health consequences of drug injecting will continue to make an increasing contribution to the overall global burden of disease as more people inject in more countries. Estimates suggest that five million people worldwide inject drugs (Mann, Tarantola and Netter, 1992). In Chapter 1 the rapid global diffusion of injecting and globalization of both 'legal' and 'illegal' drug industries was discussed.

Possibly the earliest documented adverse health consequence of illicit drug injection was a case of tetanus in a female morphine injector (Anonymous, 1876). Subsequently, epidemics of malaria in non-tropical areas were attributed to injecting drug use. One of the earliest recorded outbreaks of malaria attributed to the shared use of injecting equipment was in the 1920s in Cairo, Egypt. An outbreak occurred in the 1930s in New York City (Helpern, 1934). In Brazil there have been more recent outbreaks of malaria among drug injectors in areas where malaria had become relatively rare (Barata, Andraguetti and des Matos, 1993). A wide range of infectious complications of injecting drug use have been documented since these early reports (Selwyn, 1993; Cherubin and Sapira,

1993). The addition of HIV infection in the early 1980s has of course had a dramatic impact, and has irrevocably changed the nature of injecting drugs and the way that injecting drug use is perceived.

Human Immunodeficiency Virus

Worldwide around 21 million people are currently living with HIV, over 90 per cent of them in developing countries. Evidence suggests that within 10 years of infection, about 50 per cent of HIV-1 positive people develop an AIDS defining condition and that death often follows within one to three years of the development of AIDS. In developing countries the average survival time for a person with AIDS is six months. Some recent advances in treatment are extending life expectancy for people living with AIDS, but a cure is unlikely.

At a global level the predominant mode of HIV-1 transmission is through sexual contact. However, the shared used of injection equipment has played a critical role in fuelling a number of local, national and regional epidemics. HIV-1 prevalence is high in drug-injecting populations in southern Europe, the north-east of the United States, parts of Asia and parts of South America. Epidemics have more recently been reported in eastern Europe. By 1996 HIV-1 infection among drug injectors had been reported in 83 different countries worldwide, compared with 52 countries in 1993 (Des Jarlais *et al.*, 1996, see also Chapter 1).

HIV can be rapidly spread among drug injectors and such diffusion can follow soon after the introduction of drug injecting. Once established in the injecting population, that population can become important in heterosexual and perinatal transmission (Friedman *et al.*, 1993). Many cities and regions have experienced the rapid spread of HIV both among and from injecting drug users. In some cities and regions (for example Bangkok and Chiang Rai, Thailand; Manipur, north-east India; Ruili, south-west China; in parts of Myanmar; in Edinburgh, Scotland; recently in Sveltogorsk, Belorus; and Odessa, Ukraine) HIV-1 prevalence among drug injectors exceeded 40 per cent within two years of the first reported case.

Questions remain about the relationship between current risk behaviours and the prevalence and incidence of HIV-1 in comparison with other viral infections. It has been suggested (Chapter 12) that changes in injecting risk behaviour have stabilized or lowered rates of HIV-1 in many populations of injectors. However in these same populations, prevalence and incidence of hepatitis C (HCV) remain high or increasing. This may be because HCV is more infectious than HIV and thus more easily transmissable, so that certain behaviours are sufficiently risky for endemic spread of HCV, but not for HIV. Such behaviours may include occasional sharing of equipment or other unsafe practices such as the shared use of water, filters and spoons. The high incidence of hepatitis C can also be attributed in part to the underlying high prevalence of infectious carriers in the population.

Hepatitis

Acute and chronic hepatitis B (HBV) infection are well known and well documented hazards of drug injecting. This virus can also be transmitted horizontally to sexual partners or transmitted vertically from mother to child. Hepatitis B continues to be a common reason for admission of drug injectors to hospital, in the UK for example (Leen *et al.*, 1989), and is also a risk for non-injecting drug users and sexual contacts of drug injectors (Clee and Hunter, 1987). Chronic hepatitis B can result after some years in the development of cirrhosis and liver cancer. The majority of drug injectors who become HBV infected will never have an acute or chronic episode of clinical hepatitis (Blumberg, 1990). It is estimated that only 10 per cent of those who contract HBV infection will develop acute hepatitis, of whom 10 per cent will later develop chronic persistent or chronic active hepatitis which carries an increased risk of cirrhosis or carcinoma of the liver (Strang and Farrell, 1992). Immuno-suppression due to HIV can increase the proportion of chronic carriers. The prevalence of hepatitis B in many populations of injectors is in the range 40 to 60 per cent, though higher rates are not uncommon (Rhodes *et al.*, 1996).

A hepatitis B vaccine is available and is relatively inexpensive, safe and effective, but rarely administered to injecting populations or their sexual partners. Immunization for hepatitis B would also reduce the transmission of hepatitis D since it requires the presence of hepatitis B in order to replicate. Treatment for chronic hepatitis B at present consists of interferon, which is expensive and is only effective in a minority of cases. Epidemics of hepatitis D occur almost exclusively in drug injectors (Turner, Panton and Vandervelde, 1989). Co-infection with hepatitis D is acquired either at the same time as hepatitis B infection or subsequently.

Hepatitis C is prevalent in many populations of drug injectors. Typically 60 to 70 per cent of injectors have antibodies to hepatitis C, although rates of 80 to 100 per cent are not uncommon. Hepatitis C is transmitted by needle sharing (Woodfield *et al.*, 1994), although indirect sharing also carries a high risk of infection. Evidence for sexual transmission is not conclusive. As with hepatitis B, prevalence appears to be directly related to duration of injecting. The incidence of HCV infection may be a more sensitive marker of injecting risk behaviour in cohorts of recent injectors that HBV infection and will not be influenced by hepatitis B vaccination programmes. In Australia, Crofts *et al.* (1993) report an incidence rate of seroconversion of 19 per 100 person years. Similarly high incidence rates are reported for injectors in the United States. In Seattle an incidence rate of 26.9 per 100 person years has been reported (Hagen *et al.*, 1996).

There are few data on long-term outcomes for injectors, but molecular biological approaches indicate that the outcome of chronic HCV infection may be related to the infecting viral strain (Tsubota *et al.*, 1994). Prognosis may vary according to mode of infection and specific subtype. About 20 per cent will develop cirrhosis in 10 to 20 years and a proportion of these will later develop liver failure or cancer. Treatment for chronic hepatitis C at present consists of interferon and ribavirin which are expensive and only effective in a minority of cases. Such treatment also has significant side-effects. No vaccine is available for hepatitis C at present and some argue that the prospects for vaccine development are bleak. Hepatitis C is probably the most prevalent infectious complication in drug injectors worldwide. The social impact of hepatitis C is less dramatic than HIV but the far larger pool of infected injecting drug users and the protracted illness associated with many of the complications of hepatitis C suggest that the health and economic consequences will be considerable in most countries with significant numbers of injecting drug users.

An increased risk of hepatitis A among drug injectors has been reported, but it is likely that this is due to insanitary living conditions rather than drug injection (Boughton and Hawkes, 1980). Hepatitis GB virus C has recently been described and designated (Alter, 1996). This virus has been found in injecting drug users and other groups with blood exposure and appears to have a global distribution.

Sexual Health

Reports of sexually transmittable diseases other than the blood-borne viruses associated with drug injection, including syphilis, gonorrhoea and herpes are not uncommon among drug injectors. This may reflect the fact that some female and male injectors engage in high risk sexual behaviour associated with some patterns and contexts of drug use, for example involvement in sex work. Pelvic inflammatory disease and menstrual irregularities are common in female injecting drug users. Irregular menstrual cycles may suggest to the drug user that pregnancy cannot occur and can lead to unplanned pregnancies.

There is some evidence that drugs, and in particular opioids, may have physiological and psychological effects which impair sexual functioning and lower sexual activity (Mirim *et al.*, 1980). Most research, particularly that related to HIV risk, shows that the majority of drug injectors are sexually active (Donoghoe, 1992). Research has, in the main, focused on: sexual risk behaviour; the potential for heterosexual transmission; condom use; sexual risk and women; commercial sex work; pregnancy; male homosexual activity and drug use; the relationship between drug use and sexual behaviour. Much of this research concerns the assumed disinhibitory effects of drugs on sexual behaviour. Several commentators have highlighted the limitations of this research and conclude that the determinants of the relationship between drug use and sexual behaviour remain unclear (Rhodes and Stimson, 1994). Most evidence suggests that drug injecting risk behaviour has changed to a far greater extent than that related to sexual risk. These issues are discussed in more depth in Chapters 2, 9 and 13.

Overdose

The major cause of death in populations of drug injectors, before HIV, was drug overdose. An overdose is generally understood to be an excessive dose of a drug which results in coma and respiratory failure. Morbidity associated with non-fatal overdose includes anoxic brain damage and organ failure. In injecting populations where HIV-1 has become established, deaths from AIDS often become more common than deaths from overdose.

Drug overdose is poorly understood and there are no clearly established criteria for what constitutes an overdose. Frischer and colleagues (1994) point out that the term itself is misleading since in many cases it is not clearly established that death is a direct consequence of an excessive dose of the drug in question. Respiratory depression is a direct pharmacological action of heroin, other opioids and hypnosedatives. Some deaths from respiratory depression among heroin and other illicit opioid injectors are therefore predictable as the purity of heroin and other illicit drugs sold on the black market is uncertain and varies considerably due to vicissitudes of the market and variations in enforcement activities. However, among decedents of heroin overdose, there is a wide variation in the *post mortem* blood levels of morphine, the major metabolite of heroin, suggesting that other factors are involved. Variable individual tolerance to heroin is likely to be another important and complicating factor. Overdose deaths are more common within days of release from prison or after detoxification when tolerance to heroin has lowered.

The consumption of combinations of depressant drugs at the time of overdose is likely to be an even more important contributory factor. Alcohol is probably the most common other depressant drug consumed at the time of overdose, but benzodiazepines, barbiturates and other pharmaceutical opioids all contribute substantially to deaths from overdose among heroin injectors. In some countries the use of cocaine and heroin combined ('speedballing') is implicated. Occasionally, sudden death may be due to adulterants. Sudden death occurs occasionally among injectors of stimulants, especially cocaine (and more rarely amphetamines). Myocardial ischaemia sometimes occurs in older cocaine users with undiagnosed coronary artery disease. Hypertensive episodes associated with cocaine are rarely complicated by cerebrovascular haemorrhages. Death can also occur from arrhythmias or complications of epileptic seizures.

It is generally accepted that the cause of sudden death following heroin and other drug injection is usually accidental, but a minority of such cases are believed to represent episodes of completed suicide. Suicide has been shown to be a relatively common cause of death among opioid users in some studies (Engstrom *et al.*, 1991). The current International Classification of Diseases (ICD10) allows for the classification of overdoses either as poisoning or acute intoxication (WHO, 1992).

Some commentators suggest that despite commendable efforts to prevent HIV infection little has been done to understand or prevent overdose deaths (Zador, Sunjic and Darke, 1992).

Tuberculosis and Pneumonia

The prevalence of tuberculosis (TB) is increasing worldwide. In 1995 there were three million deaths from tuberculosis. TB is the most common infectious cause of adult deaths worldwide. It is estimated that 50 million people are infected with drug-resistant mycobacterium tuberculosis. TB may be a particular problem for drug users because of their social and material conditions. Rates of infection are highest where people are poorest and where they live in overcrowded conditions. TB is a particular problem for drug injectors because of co-infection with TB and HIV-1. HIV-1 weakens the immune system, allowing for opportunistic infection and, reciprocally, tuberculosis may accelerate the course of HIV-related disease (Whalen et al., 1995). TB is the most common opportunistic infection in the developing world, particularly in poor inner-city areas. In 1992 nearly 4000 cases of TB were recorded in New York City. Furthermore, injecting drug users have been identified as a risk group for non-adherence to preventive therapy and to treatment (Perlman et al., 1995).

Pneumonia is an important cause of hospitalization and death for drug injectors. Whilst pneumonia is a leading cause of death in HIV positive injectors, it is also a significant cause of death and hospitalization in injectors who are HIV negative.

Other Bacterial, Fungal, Parasitic and Viral Infections

Concern about the prevention of HIV infection has highlighted risks to injecting drug users from blood-borne virus infections (Mutchnik, Lee and Peleman, 1991), but has overshadowed the importance of other health risks, such as endocarditis, tuberculosis, pneumonia, abscesses, other local complications of injecting and increased mortality. These typically account for the majority of hospital admissions of injecting drug users (Scheidegger and Zimmerli, 1989), and heavy demands on emergency rooms (Makower, Pennycook and Moulton, 1992) and other health care facilities (Gerada, Orgel and Strang, 1992).

Death following a chronic illness in an injecting drug user is usually due to an infection resulting from use of unsterile injection equipment or contaminated injection materials. This may be due to bacterial, fungal, parasitic, or viral infection. Bacterial infections result in considerable morbidity both from local complications at the injection site, such as abscesses and thrombophlebitis (damage to the veins), as well as distant infections such as lung or brain abscess. Bacterial and fungal endocarditis (infected heart valves) and fungal opthalmitis (eye infection) are also well documented complications of drug injecting. Mortality from infective endocarditis in injecting drug users has been reported to range between 15 per cent and 92 per cent (English et al., 1995). Infective endocarditis is a common cause of death in HIV positive injectors. Anecdotal reports from cities around the world suggest that these conditions have become much less common in areas where vigorous attempts have been made to provide accessible sterile injection equipment and ensure its utilization.

Skin complaints and tissue damage resulting from injection are common. Physical damage from frequent injection includes the characteristic 'track marks' and other scarring. Loss of access to superficial veins may result in using deeper veins which can cause tissue damage. The use of the femoral veins as an injection site may result in damage to the femoral nerve and attendant risk of deep venous thrombosis, pulmonary emboli or venous gangrene. Excessive tissue damage may result from the injection of drugs intended for oral use (for example the various oral formulations of temazepam). Injection into arteries can result in gangrene. Some of these complications result in the need for amputation. Pulmonary fibrosis can result from the injection of insoluble adulterants, such as talc.

Crime, Violence, and Homicide

There is a complex relationship between crime, violence and drug use. Most evidence suggests that the link between drugs and violence is not a direct causal one. Drug use is a complex social phenomenon and its relationship to violence cannot be reduced to one of simple, direct, causation.

Social and family tensions may be exacerbated by the use of drugs and in particular alcohol. These tensions can lead to acts of violence. In these circumstances drugs and alcohol alone are not the cause of the violence, but may contribute to it. Underlying factors such as poverty, lack of education, and other socio-economic deprivations may be as important as alcohol and drug use. The use of certain drugs may create or occur in situations where violence is more likely to occur; however, alcohol and other drug use is not a prerequisite for violent behaviour and often there are other mitigating or confounding factors. Drug use, as with alcohol, may be used as an excuse or justification for aggression, thus negating personal responsibility. This is a phenomenon particularly observed among young males in some societies. Cultural and social norms play an important role in alcohol and drug related violence. Alcohol and drug use is a consideration for public health which goes beyond individualized notions of social behaviour.

Violence itself is a complicated phenomenon that is not easily defined. Aside from physical assaults both within and outside the family, other forms of violence should be considered, such as parental neglect of children, sexual aggression and violence associated with crime and the illegal status of some drugs. Domestic violence associated with other drug use is generally found to be at a lower level than that associated with alcohol. In the United States a study of men involved in domestic violence against women found that between 13 per cent to 20 per cent were under the influence of drugs when violent incidents occurred. Studies of cocaine-dependent mothers show a crude association between maternal use of cocaine during pregnancy and physical or sexual abuse or neglect of young children. Women who use drugs are more likely to be victims of violence than non-drug-using women. This is also the case with drug-using men. This may be associated with the marginalized circumstance that drug users find themselves in and the violence associated with illegal drug markets. Most empirical evidence shows that whilst violence is related to alcohol and drug use the link is not causal. These links need careful study and explanation in order to formulate a response to what is clearly an important social and health issue.

Sudden death from violent causes is common among drug injectors. Incidence rates of 3.8 per 1000 person years among HIV negative injectors in Baltimore and 1.3 in Amsterdam have been reported (van Ameijden *et al.*, 1996). In some countries violence is associated with the use and trade in certain drugs. In the United States violence has been associated with certain drugs such as the crack cocaine trade, with the use of phencylidene (PCP) and increasingly with methamphetamine. This violence is often related to the nature of street distribution networks. Toxicological screening of homicide cases show cocaine to be present in 31 per cent of New York murder victims in the early 1990s.

The lifestyle associated with the acquisition and injection of illegal drugs increases the risk of involvement in crime. Drug injectors generally consume drugs which are classified as illegal. A substantial proportion commit other types of crime before commencing drug use. Following initiation of drug injection, it is generally accepted that crime is often intensified and prolonged by the drug use. Some injectors buy more drugs than they intend to use themselves, selling the residual quantity at a higher price to generate income. Some injectors resort to property crime to generate income to pay for illicit drugs. Violent crime is common in association with drug trafficking. Experience of imprisonment is common among injectors, especially males.

Imprisonment may result in some psychological sequelae and may also be associated with an increased risk of blood-borne viral infections. Studies from many countries show that the majority of drug injectors will be imprisoned at some time in their injecting careers. For some injectors prison is a frequent and recurring event. Studies also show that many injectors continue to inject in prison, where access to sterile equipment is limited. The sharing of injecting equipment in prisons has led to documented outbreaks of HIV and other blood-borne infections. HIV risk behaviours in prisons are discussed in more depth in Chapter 11.

Accidents

Whilst alcohol is clearly a factor in road accidents, the relationship between risk of traffic accidents and use of drugs other than alcohol is more difficult to establish. Studies which have been conducted generally have small samples and results which are not generalizable. Research on the influence of drugs (other than alcohol) in fatal and non-fatal traffic accidents, restricted mainly to developed countries, shows some association. In a small study in New York 18 per cent of drivers killed in traffic accidents tested positive for cocaine metabolites (Skolnick, 1990). Other accidents (or non-intentional injuries) including falls, drowning and other injuries at home or in the workplace may be related to drug use, although evidence is scant.

Mental Health and Social Functioning

Some evidence suggests that certain types of drug use can lead to psychotic states, although generally drug use does not directly cause psychosis. Prolonged use or large dosages of amphetamine, for example, can be followed by mental depression, the so-called 'come down'. Amphetamine use has also been associated with acute paranoid psychosis and toxic delirium. Some studies have associated drug use with schizophrenia (Dixon *et al.*, 1991). Drug users are more likely to have concurrent (or comorbid) psychiatric disorders. Opioid users in the United States have been shown to have higher rates of psychiatric disorders (including depression, anxiety, schizophrenia, anti-social personality disorders) in comparison with the general population (Ward, Mattick and Hall, 1992). Some drug users entering methadone maintenance treatment have high levels of psychiatric disorders. The severity of these disorders can often predict the outcome of the treatment (*ibid.*). Drug problems can exacerbate psychiatric illness and interfere with seeking and adhering to treatment for psychiatric conditions. English and colleagues comment that the poor quality of studies on drug use and psychiatric morbidity does not allow for even a limited causal association (English *et al.*, 1995).

The impact of drug use on social functioning is particularly difficult to assess. Investigators use various measures of social function (for example employment, marriage and parent-hood, involvement in crime, acdemic perfor-mance), but causality is difficult to attribute one way or another. Long-term opioid users have often been characterized as 'socially disabled' with poor employment histories, family and relationship problems, involvement in crime including experience of imprisonment and poor academic achievement (Maddux and Desmond, 1981; Stimson and Oppenheimer, 1982). There is a tendency for the more visible problem drug users to be concentrated in areas of socio-economic deprivation, generally characterized by high levels of unemployment (Pearson and Gilman, 1994). This presents the dilemma of determining the causal factors and the direction of causality with regard to drug use and social functioning.

Mortality — Drug Related Deaths

Substance abuse related mortality (otherwise referred to as drug related deaths) remains poorly documented and poorly understood. In the first place defining what constitutes a drug related death is problematic because of the lack of a common terminology. Second, as discussed at the beginning of this chapter, standard epidemiological techniques cannot easily be adapted to calculate drug related deaths because of the lack of data regarding denominator populations of drug users in the general population. Third, even where mortality data are collected, they are often not comparable across countries, or even within countries, because of the lack of standardization and categorization. In the absence of common definitions for what constitutes a drug related death the World Health Organization recommends a common classification to distinguish direct and indirect drug related causes of death (WHO, 1993). Much of the data available are from developed countries and cause-specific mortality data are rarely available in developing countries.

Frischer and colleagues (1994), in their worldwide review of substance abuse related mortality, report that the number of deaths reported to international agencies have been increasing in recent years. The authors caution, however, that this may partially be a result of improvements in surveillance systems. They estimate that there may be about 200 000 deaths worldwide per year but warn against extrapolation of the available data and generalizing of research findings and epidemiological data across environments.

Studies conducted before HIV began to have an impact on drug injectors show increased mortality rates. The pooled mortality rate of predominately opioid injectors in 12 studies reviewed by Holman and colleagues was 9.6 per 1000 person years. This represents a relative risk of 17.1 compared to non-drug-using age- and sex-matched controls (Holman *et al.*, 1990). Perucci *et al.* (1991), in a retrospective cohort study of drug users enrolled in methadone treatment, calculated a standardized mortality rate of 10.1 per 1000 person years. Rates of 17.1 and 16.0 have been calculated for HIV-1 negative drug injectors in Baltimore (United States) and Amsterdam (Netherlands) (van Ameijden *et al.*, 1996). Excess of mortality in Perucci's study was found for HIV, infectious, circulatory respiratory and digestive diseases; and for violence, overdose and unknown or ill-defined causes. Prior to the advent of HIV, studies indicate that the annual mortality rate among injecting drug users in developed countries was 1 to 2 per cent per annum. Frischer and colleagues (1994) cautiously suggest an estimated all-cause mortality rate for injectors that includes HIV-1 of 3 to 4 per cent per annum.

Studies have demonstrated an increased mortality rate in populations of drug injectors in which HIV has become established even before the onset of AIDS. The increased mortality among HIV infected injectors prior to the development of AIDS has been attributed to opportunistic bacterial infections and tuberculosis. This finding has been observed in both developed and developing countries.

Health Promotion

The health of drug injectors is inexorably linked to the broader social context in which drug injectors lead their lives. The overall health of drug users is not just an issue of individual pathology, but a public health issue which is determined by the wider environment in which drug use and drug injecting occur. Here environment is to be interpreted in its widest sense to include the physical, economic, social, political and cultural environment.

HIV and AIDS led to a major reconceptualization of the nature of drug use and 'addiction' or 'dependence'. This in turn raises questions about the relationship of the concept of 'dependence' to the overall health of drug injectors. Evidence from around the world, some of it presented in Chapters 12 and 13, has shown that drug injectors are capable of making rational decisions about health and are capable of changing their behaviours to remain healthy. This challenges the view of drug 'addiction' which pathologizes drug use as a disease, over which the individual has no control. It also challenges the fatalistic notion of the inevitable decline of the drug user into disease, sickness and early death. It replaces the image of the 'sick junkie' with, for some, an equally disturbing image, that of a more rational, health-conscious drug injector (Stimson and Lart, 1991; Stimson and Donoghoe, 1996).

Stimson and Donoghoe (1996) argue that drug injectors seeking to remain healthy, whilst continuing to inject drugs, demonstrate that they can share common health values with the general non-injecting population. This helps counter the marginalization of drug injectors and opens up opportunities for treatment, care and rehabilitation. This reconceptualization is, in some countries, apparent in the shift away from treating 'addiction' and 'drug dependence' towards preventing health problems resulting from drug use and injection. This, in the age of HIV and other life-threatening conditions, is vitally important because injection and infection can occur among people who are neither addicted nor dependent.

By focusing on the health implications of drug injection, AIDS and HIV have put the overall health of drug injectors onto the agenda. Preoccupations with treating 'addiction' have, in some countries, been replaced with a more pragmatic response of controlling HIV transmission. HIV prevention amongst drug injectors has in turn led to strategies not just to prevent other blood-borne viruses, such as hepatitis B and C, but also towards improvement of the overall health of injectors. Health promotion among drug injectors or the provision of services and information to promote a more health-conscious drug-using and drug-injecting population may not be seen as desirable by someone who confuses health promotion with condoning or advocating drug use and drug injection. Whilst it may be preferable for an individual to abstain from drugs, for many abstinence is neither achievable or sustainable, at least in the short term. In the interest of individual and public health the pursuit of intermediate goals which fall short of abstinence are equally desirable. These intermediate goals are framed by an acceptance that some people will use and inject drugs without condoning or advocating drug use and drug injection. Health promotion for drug injectors signifies a willingness to work with and provide services for drug injectors. This creates possibilities for the wide range of interventions to reduce specific harmful health consequences of drug use and drug injection. Some of these interventions with reference to HIV-1 are described by Ball in Chapter 13. Such interventions are equally applicable for reducing and preventing other harmful health consequences of drug injection.

In spite of the promise shown for health promotion strategies for drug injectors, such strategies are pursued only in a minority of mostly developed countries. Health promotion for drug injectors has often been seen as neither feasible nor desirable for developing countries. It is recognized that poorer, developing countries have different priorities for health, such as the prevention and control of tuberculosis, malaria and diarrhoeal diseases. However, as Ball argues in Chapter 13, in the context of HIV-1, despite competing development priorities there is evidence of growing public health concern about drug injecting in developing countries. These concerns have in some communities been translated into action which seeks to promote general health among drug injectors. Examples include health promotion projects for drug injectors in Nepal and northern Thailand (Gray, 1995). This demonstrates that even amongst the most marginalized and geographically isolated injectors health promotion is possible.

Conclusion

A better understanding of health outcomes for drug injectors, and the role of social and environmental factors in determining those outcomes, is a public health priority. The lessons learned from those countries which, up to now, have averted HIV epidemics among drug injectors need to be carefully considered. However, the speed at which HIV-1 can spread among injectors and into non-injecting populations does not allow for delay. Many countries which reacted quickly and with a range of responses have been able to control HIV-1 in drug injectors. Lessons learned with regard to responding to HIV-1 may be applicable to other health consequences of drug injecting. As with HIV-1 an understanding of the health issues and risk behaviours is essential and mobilization of resources in a swift response must closely follow. Some responses are relatively simple, for example hepatitis B vaccination and educating drug injectors on how to avoid overdose, others, such as changing attitudes towards, and promoting health for, drug injectors, are complicated and may require more time. The experience of HIV has shown that such responses are worthwhile and can make important contributions to public health.

References

ALTER, H. (1996) 'The cloning and clinical implications of HGV and HGBV-C', *New England Journal of Medicine*, **334**, pp. 1536–7.
ANONYMOUS (1876) 'Tetanus after hypodermic injection of morphia', *Lancet*, **2**, p. 873.
BARATA, L.C.B., ANDRAGUETTI, M.T.M. and DES MATOS, M.R. (1993) 'Outbreak of malaria among injectable-drug users', *Revista de Saude Publica*, **27**, pp. 9–14.

BLUMBERG, B.S. (1990) 'Sex-related aspects of hepatitis B and its consequences', in PIOT, P. and ANDRE, F. (Eds) *Hepatitis B: A Sexually Transmitted Disease in Heterosexuals*, Oxford: Excerpta Medica.

BOUGHTON, C.R. and HAWKES, R.A. (1980) 'Viral hepatitis and the drug cult: A brief socio-epidemiological study in Sydney', *Australia and New Zealand Journal of Medicine*, **10**, pp. 157–61.

CHERUBIN, C.E. and SAPIRA, J.O. (1993) 'The medical complications of drug addiction and the medical assessment of the intravenous drug user twenty five years later', *Annals of Internal Medicine*, **119**, 10, pp. 1017–28.

CLEE, W.B. and HUNTER, P.R. (1987) 'Hepatitis B in general practice: Epidemiology, clinical and serological features and control', *British Medical Journal*, **295**, pp. 530–2.

CROFTS, N., HOPPER, J.L., BOWDEN, D.S., BRESCHKIN, A.M., MILNER, R. and LOCARNINI, S.A. (1993) 'Hepatitis C virus infection among a corhort of Victorian injecting drug users', *Medical Journal of Australia*, **159**, pp. 237–41.

DES JARLAIS, D.C., STIMSON, G.V., HAGAN, H., PERLMAN, D., CHOOPANYA, K., BAASTOS, F.I. and FRIEDMAN, S. (1996) 'Emerging HIV infectious diseases and the injection of illicit psychoactive drugs', *Current Issues in Public Health*, **2**, pp. 130–7.

DIXON, L., HAAS, G., WEDIEN, P.J., SWEENEY, J. and FRANCES, A.J. (1991) 'Drug abuse in schizophrenic patients: Clinical correlates and reasons for use', *American Journal of Psychiatry*, **148**, pp. 224–30.

DONOGHOE, M.C. (1992) 'Sex, HIV and the injecting drug user', *British Journal of Addiction*, **87**, pp. 405–16.

DONOGHOE, M.C., RHODES, T.J., HUNTER, G.M. and STIMSON, G.V. (1993) 'HIV testing and unreported HIV positivity among injecting drug users in London', *AIDS*, **7**, pp. 1105–11.

EDWARDS, G., ANDERSON, P., BARBOR, T.F. *et al.* (1994) *Alcohol Policy and the Public Good*, Oxford: Oxford University Press.

ENGLISH, D.R., HOLMAN, C.D.J., MILNE, E. *et al.* (1995) *The Quantification of Drug Caused Morbidity and Mortality in Australia*, Canberra: Commonwealth Department of Human Services and Health.

ENGSTROM, A., ADAMSSON, C., ALLEBECK, P. and RYDBERG, U. (1991) 'Mortality in patients with substance abuse: A follow-up in Stockholm County, 1973–1984', *International Journal of Addiction*, **26**, pp. 91–106.

FRIEDMAN, S.R., DES JARLAIS, D.C., WARD, T.P., JOSE, B., NEAIGUS, A., GOLDSTEIN, M.F. (1993) 'Drug injectors and heterosexual AIDS', in SHERR, L. (Ed.) *AIDS and the Heterosexual Population*, London: Harwood Academic Publishers.

FRISCHER, M., GREEN, S.T. and GOLDBERG, D. (1994) *Substance Abuse Related Mortality: A Worldwide Review*, Austria: United Nations International Drug Control Programme.

GERADA, C., ORGEL, M. and STRANG, J. (1992) 'Health clinics for problem drug misusers', *Health Trends*, **24**, pp. 68–9.

GRAY, J. (1995) 'Operating syringe exchange programs in the hills of Thailand', *AIDS Care*, **7**, pp. 489–99.

HAGEN, H., McGOUGH, J.P., HANSEN, G.R., YU, T., FIELDS, J. and RUSSELL, ALEXANDER E. (1996) 'Incidence of blood-borne viruses in a cohort of Seattle IDUs', paper presented at the Seventh International Conference on the Reduction of Drug Related Harm, Hobart, Australia.

HELPERN, M. (1934) 'Epidemic of fatal estivo-autumnal malaria', *American Journal of Surgery*, **XXVI**, 1, pp. 111–23.

HOLMAN, C.D.J., ARMSTRONG, B.K., ARIAS, L.N. *et al.* (1990) *The Quantification of Drug*

Caused Morbidity and Mortality in Australia, 1988, parts 1 & 2, Canberra: Commonwealth Department of Community Services and Health.

LEEN, C.L.S., DAVIDSON, S.M., FLEGG, P.J. and MADAL, B.K. (1989) 'Seven years experience of acute hepatitis B in a regional department of infectious diseases and tropical medicine', *Journal of Infection*, **18**, pp. 257–63.

MADDUX, J.F. and DESMOND, D.P. (1981) *Careers of Opioid Users*, New York: Praeger.

MAKOWER, R.M., PENNYCOOK, A.G. and MOULTON, C. (1992) 'Intravenous drug abusers attending an inner city accident and emergency department', *Archives of Emergency Medicine*, **9**, pp. 32–9.

MANN, J., TARANTOLA, J. and NETTER, T. (1992) *AIDS in the World*, Cambridge, Mass.: Harvard University.

MIRIM, S.M., MEYER, R.E., MENDLESON, J. and ELLINGBOE, J. (1980) 'Opiate use and sexual dysfunction', *American Journal of Psychiatry*, **137**, pp. 909–15.

MUTCHNICK, M.G., LEE, H.H. and PELEMAN, R.R. (1991) 'Liver disease associated with intravenous drug abuse', in LEVINE, D.P. and SOBEL, J.D. (Eds) *Infections in Intravenous Drug Abusers*, Oxford: Oxford University Press.

NURCO, D.N. and LERNER, M. (1971) 'The feasibility of locating addicts in the community', *International Journal of the Addictions*, **6**, pp. 51–62.

O'DONNELL, J.A. (1969) *Narcotic Addicts in Kentucky*, US Government Printing Office.

PEARSON, G. and GILMAN, M. (1994) 'Local and regional variations in drug misuse: The British heroin epidemic of the 1980s', in STRANG, J. and GOSSOP M. (Eds) *Heroin Addiction and Drug Policy: The British System*, Oxford: Oxford University Press.

PERLMAN, D.C., SALOMON, N., PERKINS, M.P., YANCOVITZ, S., PAONE, D. and DES JARLAIS, D.C. (1995) 'Tuberculosis in drug users', *Clinical Infectious Diseases*, **21**, pp. 1253–64.

PERUCCI, C.A., DAVOLI, M., RAPITI, E., ABENI, D.D. and FORASTIERI, F. (1991) 'Mortality of intravenous drug users in Rome: A cohort study', *American Journal of Public Health*, **81**, pp. 1307–10.

PRESCOR, M.J. (1943) 'Follow-up study of treated narcotic addicts', *Public Health Report*, Supplement No. 170.

RHODES, T. and STIMSON, G.V. (1994) 'What is the relationship between drug taking and sexual risk, social relations and social research', *Sociology of Health and Illness*, **16**, 2, pp. 209–29.

RHODES, T., HUNTER, G.M., STIMSON, G.V., DONOGHOE, M.C., NOBLE, A., PARRY J. and CHALMERS, C. (1996) 'Prevalence of markers for hepatitis B virus and HIV-1 among drug injectors in London: Injecting careers, positivity and risk behaviour', *Addiction*, **91**, 10, pp. 1457–67.

SCHEIDEGGER, C. and ZIMMERLI, W. (1989) 'Infectious complications in drug addicts: Seven year review of 269 hospitalised narcotics abusers in Switzerland', *Reviews of Infectious Diseases*, **11**, pp. 486–93.

SELWYN, P.A. (1993) 'Illicit drug use revisited: What a long, strange trip it's been', *Annals of Internal Medicine*, **119**, 10, pp. 1044–6.

SKOLNICK, A. (1990) 'Illicit drugs take another toll — death or injury from vehicle associated trauma', *Journal of the American Medical Association*, **263**, 23, pp. 3122–5.

STIMSON, G.V. and DONOGHOE, M.C. (1996) 'Health promotion and the facilitation of individual change: The case of syringe distribution and exchange', in RHODES, T. and HARTNOL, R. (Eds) *AIDS, Drugs and Prevention: Perspectives on Individual and Community Action*, London: Routledge.

STIMSON, G.V. and LART, R. (1991) 'HIV, drugs and public health in England: New words, old tunes', *International Journal of the Addictions*, **26**, 12, pp. 1263–77.

STIMSON, G.V. and OPPENHEIMER, E. (1982) *Heroin Addiction: Treatment and Control in Britain*, London: Tavistock.

STRANG, J. and FARREL, M. (1992) *Hepatitis B: what you always ought to have known but didn't know to ask*, London: ISDD.

TSUBOTA, A., CHAYAMA, K., IKEDA, K. *et al.* (1994) 'Factors predictive of response to interferon alpha on therapy in hepatitis C virus infection', *Hepatology*, **19**, pp. 1088–94.

TURNER, G.C., PANTON, N. and VANDERVELDE, E.M. (1989) 'Delta infection and drug abuse in Merseyside', *Journal of Infection*, **19**, pp. 113–18.

VAILLANT, G.E. (1973) 'A twenty year follow-up of New York narcotic addicts', *Archives of General Psychiatry*, **29**, pp. 237–41.

VAN AMEIJDEN, E.J.C., VLAHOV, D., VAN DEN HOEK, J.A.R., FLYNN, C. and COUTINHO, R.A. (1996) 'A comparison of pre-AIDS morbidity among injection drug users in Amsterdam and Baltimore', paper presented at the Seventh International Conference on the Reduction of Drug Related Harm, Hobart, Australia.

WARD, J., MATTICK, R. and HALL, W. (1992) *Key Issues in Methadone Maintenance Treatment*, New South Wales: University Press.

WHALEN, C., HORSBURGH, C., HOM, D., LAHHART, C., SIMBERKOFF, M. and ELLNER, J. (1995) 'Accelerated course of HIV infection after tuberculosis', *American Journal of Respiratory and Critical Care Medicine*, **151**, pp. 129–35.

WOODFIELD, D.G., HARNESS, M., RIX-TROTT, K., TSUDA, F., OKAMOTO, H. and MAYUMI, M. (1994) 'Identification and genotyping of hepatitis C virus in injectable and oral drug users in New Zealand', *Australian and New Zealand Journal of Medicine*, **24**, pp. 47–50.

WORLD HEALTH ORGANIZATION (1992) *The ICD-10 Classification of Mental and Behavioural Disorders*, Geneva: World Health Organization.

WORLD HEALTH ORGANIZATION (1993) *Death Related to Drug Abuse*, Report on a WHO Consultation, Geneva, 22–5 November, Geneva: World Health Organization, Programme on Substance Abuse.

WORLD HEALTH ORGANIZATION INTERNATIONAL COLLABORATIVE GROUP (1994) *Multi-City Study on Drug Injecting and Risk of HIV Infection*, Geneva: World Health Organization.

ZADOR, D., SUNJIC, S. and DARKE, S. (1992) 'Heroin related deaths in New South Wales, 1992: Toxicological findings and circumstances', *Medical Journal of Australia*, **164**, pp. 204–7.

Chapter 4

Drug Injecting and HIV-1 Infection: Major Findings from the Multi-City Study

Meni Malliori, Maria Victoria Zunzunegui, Angeles Rodriguez-Arenas and David Goldberg

This chapter, based on the results of the World Health Organization Multi-City Study on Drug Injecting and Risk of HIV Infection, attempts to illuminate similarities and dissimilarities in the characteristics of injectors, in HIV-1 prevalence and in risk behaviours around the world. The findings tend to show that the commonalities manifest in the general characteristics and in the behaviour of drug injectors across the globe far outweigh the differences. Analysis of the data permits the drawing of a profile of the drug injector as likely to be male, aged in the late twenties, having initiated injection at age 19, and being of heterosexual orientation. Further similarities are apparent in frequency of injecting, drugs injected, frequency of sexual intercourse, and frequency of unsafe sexual contact. Based on these facts one would expect to see a corresponding uniform spread of HIV-1 infection. The findings, however, contradict this assumption, since a wide range of HIV-1 seroprevalence was demonstrated. The spread of low, middle and high prevalence cities prompts the examination of factors that may be playing a prominent role in the spread of HIV-1, which is explained in later chapters.

Epidemiological and behavioural data were collected from 12 cities in five continents (Appendix 1 and 2). The total sample was 6436. The centres participating in the survey were the following, the figure in parenthesis representing the sample size: Athens (400), Bangkok (601), Berlin (380), Glasgow (503), London (534), Madrid (472), New York (1478), Rio de Janeiro (479), Rome (487), Santos (220), Sydney (424) and Toronto (458). For most subjects recruited to participate in the survey (over 75 per cent), the city of recruitment was their normal place of residence. In Glasgow, New York and Rome this was the case for over 95 per cent of respondents.

The questionnaire used in the survey covered five main categories of information: demographic characteristics of injecting drug users, characteristics of drug injecting behaviour, characteristics of sexual behaviour, HIV-1 and

AIDS awareness, and HIV-1 testing prior to interview. Current HIV-1 status was assessed using salivary or blood samples.[1]

Socio-Demographic Characteristics

The main demographic characteristics of injecting drug users across the world tend to show some striking similarities despite the great diversity in the socio-cultural background of the cities participating in the study.

Injectors were found to be predominantly male, despite the relatively high proportion of females recruited in the survey (over 30 per cent in Berlin, London and Santos) (Table 4.1). Of the Bangkok sample, however, only 5 per cent were female. Based on evidence from other information available in each of the cities, these proportions are probably reasonably representative of the actual gender distributions for injecting drug users in each city.

In most centres injectors were most commonly aged between 21 and 34 years at the time of interview. However, in Glasgow, the majority of injectors were less than 25 years old, whilst in New York most were older than 34.

Regarding the participants' educational level, most injectors had received full-time education for between 10 and 14 years (Table 4.2). However, in Athens, Bangkok, Madrid, Rome and Santos, over 50 per cent of injectors had received less than 10 years of full-time education. In Santos 40 per cent had less than five years. The percentage of those injectors having pursued further education (15+ years) is small, with the exception of Rio de Janeiro where over 20 per cent received more than 15 years full-time education. The proportion of those with

Table 4.1 Gender, age at time of interview, normal place of residence (in the city sampled)

Cities	Gender %			Age %			Residence in city %	
	Male	Female	n	<20	21–34	35>	n		n
Athens	77	23	(400)	2	85	13	(392)	83	(397)
Bangkok	95	5	(601)	3	80	18	(542)	–	–
Berlin	56	44	(380)	6	83	11	(379)	82	(376)
Glasgow	71	29	(503)	15	81	3	(500)	99	(503)
London	66	34	(533)	6	79	14	(524)	86	(532)
Madrid	81	19	(466)	9	88	3	(469)	95	(463)
New York	74	26	(1477)	1	40	60	(1477)	98	(1088)
Rio	87	13	(479)	3	88	9	(479)	94	(479)
Rome	80	20	(487)	3	91	6	(484)	98	(486)
Santos	58	42	(220)	9	73	18	(220)	79	(219)
Sydney	80	20	(410)	12	76	12	(415)	77	(422)
Toronto	77	23	(444)	3	67	31	(436)	–	–
Total			(6400)				(6317)		(4965)

Figures rounded to the nearest per cent
n = sample on which percentage was calculated

Table 4.2 Years of full-time education completed, main source of income

| Cities | Years of education % | | | | Main source of income % | | | | |
	<9	10–14	15>	n	Employment	Unemployment benefit	Illegal income	Spouse/relative's income	n
Athens	51	41	9	(400)	65	1	7	27	(376)
Bangkok	65	34	2	(600)	70	0	29	1	(589)
Berlin	33	67	1	(380)	16	29	52	3	(332)
Glasgow	23	77	0.2	(500)	9	89	3	0	(496)
London	16	72	11	(526)	28	51	18	3	(516)
Madrid	71	26	2	(465)	41	9	48	1	(422)
New York	18	72	9	(1477)	22	42	30	6	(1473)
Rio	24	49	27	(477)	54	1	17	28	(459)
Rome	50	47	2	(487)	52	1	37	11	(474)
Santos	88	10	2	(217)	50	20	30	0	(218)
Sydney	26	71	4	(418)	16	78	6	0.2	(411)
Toronto	22	67	11	(441)	22	68	8	1	(427)
Total				(6388)					(6193)

Figures rounded to the nearest per cent
n = sample on which percentage was calculated

less than four years education was greatest in Bangkok, Madrid, Rio de Janeiro and Santos.

The majority of injectors were found to have been unemployed in the six months prior to interview. However, the proportions of injectors whose income came from employment varied across the centres from over 60 per cent in Athens and Bangkok to 16 per cent and less in Berlin, Glasgow and Sydney.

A high percentage of those interviewed had never been married, varying from more than 80 per cent in Glasgow and Sydney, to 50 per cent in New York and Bangkok (Table 4.3). The next highest group was of those widowed, separated, or divorced. Under 13 per cent overall were legally married at the time of interview. Only between 20 per cent and 40 per cent of injectors were living with a current sexual partner.

Between 20 per cent (Rome) and almost 70 per cent (New York) of injectors had at least one child and approximately 45 per cent and 35 per cent of respondents in New York and Santos respectively had two or more children.

In Madrid, New York, Santos, Sydney and Toronto, between 20 per cent and 35 per cent of injectors were homeless, whilst in Bangkok, Glasgow, Rio de Janeiro and Rome, over 50 per cent lived in a home which did not belong to either themselves or their partners.

In each centre more than 50 per cent of injectors had been in prison overnight at least once since they had first injected a drug, and in Glasgow, New York, and Toronto over 30 per cent had been incarcerated more than five times.

Based on the above information, the profile of a drug injecting user on a global scale would be a male, in his late twenties, unmarried, unemployed, with a permanent place of residence and a high school education. There are, however,

Table 4.3 Marital status, living circumstances, children, prison

Cities	Marital status %				Living with sexual partner %		Homeless %		Children %		Prison %		
	Widowed/ separated/ divorced	Married	Never married/ single	n	%	n	%	n	%	n	Ever	More than 5 times	n
Athens	22	14	64	(400)	39	(398)	5	(399)	29	(400)	79	25	(399)
Bangkok	35	11	54	(394)	27	(583)	5	(573)	37	(599)	70	9	(592)
Berlin	20	9	71	(379)	29	(375)	18	(372)	32	(379)	66	7	(377)
Glasgow	10	6	84	(503)	36	(501)	5	(502)	51	(502)	76	41	(470)
London	22	11	66	(532)	42	(529)	19	(529)	40	(532)	71	22	(531)
Madrid	9	10	81	(469)	23	(464)	24	(470)	26	(469)	52	10	(470)
New York	37	13	50	(1365)	30	(1476)	29	(1476)	68	(1478)	84	33	(1459)
Rio	10	13	77	(472)	19	(476)	3	(477)	41	(478)	61	9	(477)
Rome	14	10	76	(487)	18	(440)	7	(482)	23	(487)	54	11	(487)
Santos	20	6	74	(168)	29	(217)	36	(173)	54	(218)	96	22	(176)
Sydney	11	3	86	(422)	29	(417)	37	(423)	33	(423)	53	10	(423)
Toronto	29	5	65	(402)	24	(451)	29	(443)	45	(444)	76	33	(433)
Total				(5993)		(6327)		(6319)		(6409)			(6294)

Figures rounded to the nearest per cent
n = sample on which percentage was calculated

divergent figures such as the high numbers of injectors with little or no education in Bangkok, Rio de Janeiro and Santos, and the high proportion of homeless injectors in Madrid, New York, Santos, Sydney and Toronto.

Drug Injecting

Results from the survey indicate that there are marked similarities across centres in many aspects of injectors' current behaviour. The questions addressed age at first drug injection, frequency of injecting, sharing of injecting equipment, cleaning of injecting equipment, sources of injecting equipment, and travel and injecting.

Since the survey questions on current risk behaviour applied to the previous six months, it was important that injectors recruited to the study, especially those from treatment centres, had been injecting for most of this period. For most centres at least 75 per cent of respondents had injected during four to six months of the six months prior to interview.

The most common age for commencement of drug injecting was between 15 and 19 years (Table 4.4). In all cities the majority of respondents had begun injecting before the age of 25. A substantial proportion of between 10 per cent and 16 per cent of injecting drug users who started injecting at age 14 or under was found in Berlin, Glasgow, Madrid, New York, Santos, Sydney and Toronto.

Almost 60 per cent of respondents in each centre had been injecting for six years or more. New York was exceptional, where most injectors had been injecting for longer than 15 years. The minority, between 10 per cent and 20 per cent of injectors, had been injecting for less than two years, and between 15 per cent and 25 per cent of injectors for three to five years.

The comparative figures for frequency of injecting reveal a pattern that is common in most centres. With the exceptions of Rio de Janeiro (23 per cent) and Sydney (36 per cent), about 50 per cent or more of the respondents in all the centres injected daily during the previous six months. In all cities at least 70 per cent injected at least once a week. The highest frequencies of injecting were found in Berlin and Glasgow, where most injected every day.

Heroin was found to be the most commonly injected drug in the cities of Athens, Bangkok, Berlin, Glasgow, London, Madrid, New York, Rome and Sydney. Heroin injection was rare in Santos. Cocaine was the drug most commonly injected in Rio de Janeiro, Santos and Toronto (Table 4.5).

Whilst the data suggest that in a majority of the cities heroin is the main drug that is injected, and that in a minority it is cocaine that is injected, there are some interesting differences between cities. Bangkok, Santos and Rio are marked by drug users' preferences for a single drug, heroin in the case of Bangkok and cocaine in the cases of Rio and Santos. In several cities there is a preference for both heroin and cocaine, sometimes used together, but with an absence of use of other drugs, as in the case of Athens, Madrid, New York and Rome. In none of

Table 4.4 Age at first injection, number of years injecting, frequency of injection

Cities	Age at first injection %				Number of years injecting %				Frequency of injection %			
	<14	15–24	25>	n	0–5	6–15	16–45	n	Monthly (or less)	Weekly	Daily	n
Athens	3	77	20	(400)	39	52	8	(389)	11	14	75	(397)
Bangkok	2	70	28	(586)	39	51	11	(523)	7	11	82	(599)
Berlin	11	78	12	(380)	37	50	12	(379)	3	8	90	(378)
Glasgow	10	86	4	(500)	44	53	3	(498)	2	8	90	(499)
London	8	79	12	(531)	31	55	14	(518)	8	8	64	(527)
Madrid	16	77	7	(469)	35	62	3	(466)	6	16	78	(468)
New York	15	69	16	(1461)	14	28	59	(1458)	15	23	62	(1375)
Rio	5	86	9	(479)	41	48	11	(479)	30	48	23	(479)
Rome	6	88	6	(486)	30	65	5	(483)	–	–	–	–
Santos	16	69	15	(219)	42	40	18	(218)	21	35	44	(218)
Sydney	14	77	9	(420)	39	50	11	(411)	18	46	36	(421)
Toronto	14	69	17	(444)	32	34	33	(437)	19	29	52	(449)
Total				(6375)				(6259)				(5810)

Figures rounded to the nearest per cent
n = sample on which percentage was calculated
Frequency of injection reported for previous six months

Table 4.5 Any injection of heroin, cocaine, heroin and cocain, methadone, amphetamine, tranquillizers, barbiturates, during previous six months

Cities	Heroin %	Cocaine %	Heroin and cocaine %	Methadone %	Amphetamine %	Tranquillizers %	Barbiturates %	n
Athens	99	52	54	3	3	5	2	(400)
Bangkok	99.8	0.3	0	0	0.2	1	0.2	(601)
Berlin	97	56	52	4	18	19	23	(380)
Glasgow	70	10	9	5	27	57	1	(503)
London	90	34	34	16	27	25	9	(534)
Madrid	81	56	62	4	2	4	1	(472)
New York	72	66	65	1	1	1	0.3	(1478)
Rio	1	99	0	0	3	<1	0	(479)
Rome	99	49	17	0	1	3	0.2	(487)
Santos	4	94	0	4	2	2	12	(220)
Sydney	84	30	12	13	61	6	4	(424)
Toronto	54	83	24	6	4	2	12	(458)
Total								(5957)

Figures rounded to the nearest per cent (except Bangkok)
n = sample on which percentage was calculated

the aforementioned sites is the injection of methadone, amphetamine, tranquillizers or barbiturates at all common.

Other cities are characterized by polydrug use with the injection of amphetamine, tranquillizers and/or barbiturates occurring alongside (but to a lesser extent than) heroin. This is the case in Berlin, Glasgow, London, Sydney, and to some extent Toronto (where barbiturates are significant). London and Sydney are marked by the highest levels of the injection of methadone, probably reflecting diversion from legitimate prescriptions. Glasgow is marked by extremely high levels of tranquillizer injection, and (not shown in Table 4.5) the injection of buprenorphine.

Needle and Syringe Sharing

Of particular importance are the relatively low levels of needle and syringe sharing discovered through this survey compared to levels of sharing reported in many cities during the mid to late 1980s. Syringe sharing can involve injection with equipment previously *used* by others (which poses a risk of infection to the recipient) and *passing on* equipment (which poses a risk of transmission to others) (Table 4.6).

In each centre at least 45 per cent of the respondents said that they had not injected with a *used* needle and syringe in the six months before interview, and at

Table 4.6 Percentage of injectors using needles/syringes received from someone else; number of people n/s were received from; percentage of injectors who passed on n/s; number of people they passed n/s onto

Cities	Accepted used n/s %		How many people n/s were received from %			Gave n/s to others %		How many people n/s were passed onto %		
		n	2 to 5	6>	n		n	2 to 5	6>	n
Athens	49	(400)	35	11	(195)	42	(400)	39	13	(163)
Bangkok	54	(601)	48	8	(317)	53	(595)	53	5	(311)
Berlin	50	(380)	40	21	(184)	51	(378)	35	35	(187)
Glasgow	43	(502)	44	16	(209)	57	(501)	42	36	(283)
London	34	(529)	46	13	(179)	37	(526)	43	18	(197)
Madrid	45	(467)	49	24	(197)	52	(468)	48	25	(225)
New York	43	(1430)	41	12	(611)	47	(1430)	47	16	(649)
Rio	30	(473)	56	10	(140)	24	(472)	46	18	(112)
Rome	19	(458)	55	0	(85)	20	(433)	67	0	(102)
Santos	55	(218)	39	31	(114)	60	(210)	46	31	(118)
Sydney	42	(421)	38	8	(168)	32	(420)	40	19	(130)
Toronto	44	(450)	42	16	(198)	38	(450)	41	24	(171)
Total		(6329)			(2597)		(6283)			(2648)

Figures rounded to the nearest per cent
n = sample on which percentage was calculated

least 68 per cent did not inject with a used needle more often than on a monthly basis. This would indicate that the majority of injectors, most of whom inject daily, are minimizing their risk of infection, since one of the crucial factors in HIV-1 transmission is the use of a needle or syringe that has already been used by someone else.

In most centres, however, there was a minority of drug users (14 per cent in total) who were sharing used needles and syringes on a daily or weekly basis during the previous six months. Highest proportions of weekly or daily sharing were found in Santos, Berlin and Madrid. On the whole there was little difference in the frequency of sharing injecting equipment between male and female injectors.

For those who did inject with a used needle and syringe during the six months prior to interview, the majority had received the equipment from only one other person. A small core of 14 per cent obtained previously used injecting equipment from more than five other persons. The highest levels of multiple sharing were reported from Madrid, Santos and Berlin.

An almost identical profile as that seen for frequency of injecting with used needles and syringes, was observed for those injectors who *passed on* used injecting equipment to others.

Of equal importance was the evidence that injectors who used injecting equipment that had been used by someone else, reported that they nearly always cleaned their equipment before injecting themselves, even though they might employ inefficient cleaning methods (Table 4.7). Only a small minority of 5 per cent declared they never cleaned their equipment. The lowest rates of cleaning

Table 4.7 Percentage of injectors who always cleaned used needles/syringes; methods used for cleaning n/s; where clean n/s were obtained from

Cities	Always cleaned used n/s %	n	Methods of cleaning used n/s %			n	Where clean n/s were obtained from %		n
			cold water	hot water	boiling & bleach		pharmacist	needle exchange	
Athens	87	(197)	58	14	12	(187)	91	0	(381)
Bangkok	92	(324)	80	8	9	(322)	52	0	(600)
Berlin	75	(187)	33	42	23	(180)	49	8	(373)
Glasgow	88	(215)	7	41	47	(208)	49	46	(500)
London	87	(182)	14	25	56	(181)	31	22	(522)
Madrid	84	(210)	80	2	11	(199)	93	0	(470)
New York	77	(623)	17	15	32	(601)	6	3	(1395)
Rio	69	(143)	89	1	4	(111)	95	0	(479)
Rome	74	(111)	58	39	0	(109)	–	–	–
Santos	64	(118)	71	7	10	(107)	2	0	(141)
Sydney	84	(172)	30	18	48	(165)	39	51	(380)
Toronto	53	(198)	–	–	–	–	44	0.2	(449)
Total		(2680)				(2370)			(5690)

Figures rounded to the nearest per cent
n = sample on which percentage was calculated

were reported from Rio de Janeiro, Toronto and Santos. However, the cleaning methods used by injectors are often inadequate. Only in London did more than 50 per cent of injectors employ the acceptable practices of immersing injecting equipment in boiling water or bleach. In Athens, Bangkok, Madrid, Rio de Janeiro and Santos, between 60 per cent and 90 per cent of respondents used cold water only.

The above observations regarding the relatively low levels of needle and syringe sharing could be considered as encouraging, particularly in view of the widely differing levels of new needle and syringe availability (see also Appendix 2). In some centres injecting equipment can be purchased legally or obtained free of cost, while in others there are legal impediments to obtaining new injecting equipment. The results of the survey showed wide variations in the sources of needles and syringes. In Athens, Madrid and Rio de Janeiro, more than 90 per cent of drug injectors obtained needles and syringes from a pharmacist, drug store or shop. In Glasgow and Sydney, about 50 per cent reported needle/syringe exchange as the most important source. Other sources commonly indicated in the remaining centres included 'purchasing equipment on the street' (New York) and 'obtaining needles and syringes from other drug users' (Toronto).

Another aspect addressed in the questionnaire was the extent to which injectors travelled beyond their area of residence as well as their injecting behaviour outside that area. This is significant since one factor contributing to the spread of HIV-1 infection is the mobility of injectors and the mixing of different population groups. The survey findings show that about 40 per cent to 65 per cent of injectors had injected away from their city of residence in the two years prior to interview, with a proportion ranging from 10 per cent to 30 per cent having shared needles and syringes at these times (see also Chapter 7).

To summarize, with regard to drug injecting behaviour, again a more or less typical pattern emerges involving initiation of injection at an average age of 19 and similarities in frequency of injecting, drugs injected and equipment sharing and cleaning techniques. These findings have important implications for HIV-preventive strategies since they suggest that current commonalities in drug injectors' behaviour outweigh the differences established in the various centres.

Sexual behaviour

The areas investigated in this part of the survey were frequency of sexual intercourse, condom use, the sexual partner profile, female sex work, and the occurrence of men having sex with men.

There is a common belief that drug users who take opiates practice sexual intercourse less frequently than the non-user (see Chapter 2). Evidence from this study suggests that even injectors with serious drug dependence are just as sexually active, if not more so, than the general population. The issues dealt with in the questionnaire were frequency of sexual intercourse (vaginal, anal, oral) with someone of the opposite sex in the six months prior to interview, and the proportion of primary versus casual sex partners.

The frequency of sexual intercourse with someone of the opposite sex was similar for most centres, with most reporting intercourse in the last six months: only approximately 20 per cent indicated no intercourse, 30 per cent reported monthly, 35 per cent weekly and 15 per cent daily sexual intercourse (Table 4.8). The lowest rates of sexual activity were reported in Bangkok where almost 90 per cent of interviewees had sexual intercourse monthly or never. The highest rates were found in Glasgow where over 70 per cent reported having intercourse on a weekly or daily basis.

In all centres the frequency of vaginal intercourse with primary or regular partners was considerably higher than with casual partners. Indeed, between 30 per cent and 70 per cent stated they had no intercourse with any casual partners during the previous six months. On average, however, 10 per cent to 15 per cent reported intercourse with casual partners on a weekly or daily basis. Regarding anal intercourse, the great majority of injectors reported never having had anal intercourse with either primary or casual partners during the period investigated (Table 4.9). In most centres, the proportion of respondents who indicated having done so was 9 per cent or less.

The data also show that approximately 90 per cent of those who had vaginal or anal intercourse with a primary opposite sex partner in the six months prior to interview did so with no more than one partner. In contrast, the Santos data reveal about 40 per cent of injectors reporting intercourse with two or more primary partners. Across all the centres, of those who did have intercourse with

Table 4.8 Frequency of sexual intercourse (vaginal, anal, oral); frequency of vaginal intercourse with primary and with casual partners

| Cities | Frequency sexual intercourse % + | | | | | Frequency vaginal intercourse % + | | | | | |
| | | | | | | primary partners | | | casual partners | | |
	never	monthly or less	weekly	daily	n	weekly	daily	n	weekly	daily	n
Athens	25	31	33	12	(400)	39	11	(300)	7	3	(302)
Bangkok	47	43	10	1	(598)	16	1	(316)	2	1	(313)
Berlin	20	23	26	31	(379)	33	5	(301)	12	2	(301)
Glasgow	19	25	44	13	(501)	50	10	(408)	9	1	(406)
London	29	24	35	12	(528)	47	12	(375)	6	1	(377)
Madrid	32	34	27	7	(462)	47	5	(228)	9	2	(269)
New York	23	27	40	10	(1477)	44	10	(1132)	11	1	(1133)
Rio	19	34	42	5	(478)	42	5	(390)	16	0	(390)
Rome	100	0	0	0	(56)	49	10	(417)	13	1	(421)
Santos	15	15	38	33	(200)	38	20	(152)	21	11	(152)
Sydney	20	30	36	14	(423)	39	13	(334)	10	1	(325)
Toronto	17	35	35	13	(452)	33	12	(374)	16	4	(373)
Total					(5954)			(4727)			(4762)

+ *With someone of the opposite sex in the six months prior to interview*
Figures rounded to the nearest per cent
n = sample on which percentage was calculated

Table 4.9 Anal intercourse reported with primary and casual partners; anal or vaginal intercourse reported with more than two primary partners or more than two casual partners

| Cities | Anal intercourse %+ | | | | Vaginal/anal intercourse %+ | | | | |
	with primary partners	n	with casual partners	n	with 2 or more primary partners	n	with 2 or more casual partners	n
Athens	25	(297)	29	(136)	10	(225)	66	(111)
Bangkok	2	(316)	2	(309)	7	(225)	62	(82)
Berlin	11	(300)	7	(301)	12	(177)	64	(99)
Glasgow	11	(409)	3	(403)	9	(325)	67	(147)
London	18	(374)	7	(377)	13	(286)	64	(141)
Madrid	21	(214)	23	(154)	10	(158)	71	(110)
New York	15	(1131)	8	(1133)	17	(862)	73	(436)
Rio	21	(389)	28	(390)	10	(230)	89	(266)
Rome	30	(409)	13	(418)	15	(281)	68	(165)
Santos	20	(142)	21	(140)	42	(60)	90	(62)
Sydney	9	(328)	7	(166)	11	(215)	71	(79)
Toronto	11	(378)	4	(373)	14	(229)	77	(209)
Total		(4687)		(4300)		(3273)		(1907)

+ *With someone of the opposite sex in the six months prior to interview*
Figures rounded to the nearest per cent
n = sample on which percentage was calculated

casual partners of the opposite sex, between 30 per cent (Bangkok, London) and 80 per cent (Santos) had three or more partners during the six month period. Less than 40 per cent in each centre had only one casual partner.

The focus of this section of the survey was on behaviour which tends to increase or reduce the likelihood of infection through sexual transmission. It is therefore important to explore the extent to which individuals showed awareness of personal risk and knowledge of the means to reduce it, as well as the degree of risk reduction strategies actually adopted. A close correspondence was noted again in the responses from all centres to the survey questions, this time regarding condom use.

Patterns of condom use differed according to whether sexual intercourse was with a primary or casual partner (Table 4.10). The majority of injectors never used condoms with primary partners of the opposite sex. The highest rates were reported in Madrid, New York, Rome, Santos and Sydney where 15 per cent to 20 per cent said they 'always' used a condom with primary partners. The lowest rates of condom use with primary partners were found in Rio de Janeiro, Athens and Glasgow.

Condom use was found to be more commonly associated with sexual intercourse with casual partners than with primary partners. Injectors reporting 'always' using condoms with casual partners reached nearly 40 per cent in New York and Toronto, with the next highest levels of condom use with casual partners found in Bangkok, London and Rome. When comparing male with female injectors, there was little difference noted overall in the frequency of condom use with either primary or casual partners.

Table 4.10 Frequency of condom use with primary and casual partners

Cities	Condom use with primary partners %+				Condom use with casual partners %+			
	always	sometimes	never	n	always	sometimes	never	n
Athens	7	17	77	(230)	22	18	60	(113)
Bangkok	12	23	65	(226)	35	20	45	(83)
Berlin	13	17	70	(187)	21	33	46	(96)
Glasgow	8	18	75	(330)	17	32	51	(148)
London	12	18	70	(284)	31	35	34	(140)
Madrid	20	27	53	(170)	24	41	34	(116)
New York	20	26	55	(871)	37	32	31	(436)
Rio	4	12	84	(231)	10	22	68	(268)
Rome	17	31	52	(285)	31	34	35	(168)
Santos	15	14	72	(81)	23	32	45	(73)
Sydney	13	26	61	(220)	27	30	43	(83)
Toronto	–	–	–	–	36	31	33	(209)
Total				(3115)				(1933)

+ *With someone of the opposite sex in the six months prior to interview*
Figures rounded to the nearest per cent
n = sample on which percentage was calculated

The findings regarding safer sex practices show a consistency across centres despite variations in condom availability. In cities where a majority of the population subscribe to the Catholic religion like Madrid, Rio de Janeiro, Rome and Santos, cultural obstacles including attitudes of shame, sexism, prejudice and in particular the disapproval of the Catholic Church have discouraged or prevented free distribution and wide use of condoms. In other centres, such as Athens and Glasgow, it has been lack of information that has limited condom use. With such conditions preventing the large-scale adoption of condom use in certain centres, it seems that sexual transmission may become an increasingly important route of infection among injectors and from them to others.

The data obtained regarding the sexual partners of injectors support the hypothesis that risk of transmission of infection is a real possibility for the non-injecting population (see also Chapter 9). Many drug injectors reported having sexual partners who were not injectors themselves (Table 4.11). For those who had a primary opposite sex sexual partner in the six months prior to interview, the percentage with a partner who did not inject drugs ranged from just over 20 per cent in Berlin to almost 90 per cent in Bangkok. In most of the centres between 40 per cent and 50 per cent of injectors had a primary partner who was not a drug injector, with a similar pattern emerging for casual partners. The highest rates of non-injecting primary or casual partners were found in Bangkok (over 90 per cent) and Rio de Janeiro (around 80 per cent).

The data concerned with the issue of female sex work reveal that between 18 per cent (London) and 76 per cent (Berlin) of female injectors had been given money, goods or drugs by a client in return for sex in the six months before interview. Apart from Rio de Janeiro where the percentage was very low, more than 10 per cent of females who were given money, goods or drugs for sex in all

Table 4.11 Percentage of primary and casual partners who had ever injected drugs; percentage of females who had been given money, goods or drugs for sex; percentage of men who had sex with men

Cities	Primary partners (opposite sex) who had ever injected drugs %			Casual partners (opposite sex) who had ever injected drugs %			Females who were given money, goods or drugs for sex %		Men who had sex with men %+	
	0	1>	n	0	1>	n		n		n
Athens	50	50	(222)	54	46	(136)	34	(71)	8	(305)
Bangkok	87	13	(242)	92	8	(83)	29	(17)	6	(561)
Berlin	25	75	(164)	31	69	(95)	76	(156)	8	(213)
Glasgow	46	54	(322)	36	64	(143)	26	(125)	1	(355)
London	28	72	(272)	33	67	(133)	18	(143)	7	(529)
Madrid	51	49	(178)	36	64	(114)	46	(50)	6	(334)
New York	51	49	(862)	41	59	(418)	28	(305)	8	(1091)
Rio	84	16	(231)	79	21	(265)	21	(57)	26	(417)
Rome	57	43	(285)	45	55	(151)	22	(73)	4	(378)
Santos	72	28	(92)	57	43	(74)	72	(53)	38	(93)
Sydney	35	65	(201)	36	64	(83)	54	(26)	20	(118)
Toronto	45	55	(229)	38	62	(199)	–	–	14	(304)
Total			(3300)			(1894)		(1076)		(4698)

+ *Anal or oral intercourse within the last 5 years*
Figures rounded to the nearest per cent
n = sample on which percentage was calculated

centres had sexual contact with a client on a daily basis, and in Berlin the proportion was as high as 70 per cent. The number of different clients in an average month varied greatly in each centre. In Bangkok, New York, Rio de Janeiro and Sydney between 40 and 50 per cent of the women interviewed who received payment for sex had between one and five clients, whereas in Glasgow, Berlin and London between 40 per cent and 65 per cent reported seeing over 100 clients in one month. It should be taken into account, however, that some centres (for example Bangkok and Rio de Janeiro) had few women in the sample.

The final item considered in the context of sexual behaviour was the number of men having sex with men in the last five years. The average proportion mostly varied between 4 per cent (Rome) and 20 per cent (Sydney). The highest rates were found in Rio de Janeiro and Santos where 26 per cent and 38 per cent of male injectors respectively reported having practised anal or oral sexual intercourse with another man in the previous five years. In Glasgow, on the other hand, only 1 per cent indicated such activity.

When comparing the results of both sexual and injection risk behaviour, it appears that more change has occurred in injection risk behaviour than in sexual risk behaviour. The willingness of injectors to reduce injecting risk behaviour to a greater extent than sexual risk behaviour is sometimes interpreted as inconsistent. It has been suggested that such variance exists because of a lack of adequate information or awareness of risk, but this may be a simplistic conclusion. People engage in many activities involving risk, for pleasure or excitement, in full knowledge of the dangers involved. Thus it may be rational from the injector's standpoint to avoid sharing injecting equipment (since this does not reduce the pleasure experienced by injecting) but to refrain from using condoms which may decrease the pleasure associated with sexual intercourse. Therefore it may prove more difficult to initiate change in sexual risk behaviour to the same degree as injection behaviour.

HIV and AIDS Awareness

One of the questions asked in the survey with regard to HIV-1 and AIDS awareness was how often injectors talked about AIDS with others, that is with drug using friends, with their sexual partners and with their family (Table 4.12). The responses showed that injectors mostly discussed the subject with their drug using friends, less with their sexual partners and least of all with their family.

Injectors were also asked if they knew that persons with HIV-1 could look well and whether they believed that people with HIV-1 will become seriously ill. In most centres between 75 per cent and 90 per cent of injectors knew that persons with HIV-1 could look well. However, the corresponding figures in Bangkok and Rome were lower (66 per cent and 71 per cent respectively), showing that injectors in those centres were less well informed. The same applies to the question of HIV-1 and serious illness. Most injectors considered that all or most people with HIV-1 will become seriously ill. Only 10 per cent or less believed that only 'a few' persons with HIV-1 would eventually become seriously ill, except in Bangkok and Rome where about 30 per cent thought this was case.

Further, respondents were asked to report if they had made behaviour changes in response to the AIDS epidemic. In most centres, between 75 per cent and 90 per cent of injectors indicated that, since they first became aware of AIDS, they had done something to avoid catching HIV-1 themselves. The lowest reports of behaviour change were from Santos (50 per cent) and Rio de Janeiro (59 per cent).

HIV-1 Testing

Respondents were asked whether they had ever been tested for HIV-1. In most centres between 44 per cent (Bangkok) and 81 per cent (Sydney) of injectors had undergone attributable HIV-1 testing at least once prior to the interview (Table 4.13). The highest rates of previous testing were reported in Berlin (90 per cent) and Rome (94 per cent). The lowest rate was reported from Rio de Janeiro, where 27 per cent of injectors had ever been tested. There is also an observable consistency between the self-reported results of those having had a previous positive HIV-1 test and the actual HIV-1 test results, with the first being only slightly lower.

Table 4.12 Percentage who talk frequently with drug using friends, sexual partners, family members about AIDS; belief that a person can have the AIDS virus and look well; perception of numbers of people who have the AIDS virus that become seriously ill; any behaviour change to avoid catching the virus (since first hearing of AIDS)

Cities	Talk about AIDS frequently %						Belief that a person can have the AIDS virus and look well %		Perception of numbers of people who have the AIDS virus that become seriously ill %			Behaviour change to avoid getting AIDS %	
	with drug using friends	n	sexual partners	n	family	n		n	all	a few	n		n
Athens	37	(400)	37	(363)	19	(395)	76	(399)	44	3	(369)	88	(396)
Bangkok	38	(601)	22	(593)	20	(599)	66	(596)	29	31	(566)	92	(592)
Berlin	33	(380)	33	(378)	9	(380)	84	(376)	27	14	(290)	86	(379)
Glasgow	33	(502)	24	(481)	13	(498)	89	(503)	34	5	(437)	83	(498)
London	28	(526)	23	(516)	7	(523)	76	(521)	43	4	(451)	78	(524)
Madrid	24	(467)	20	(467)	19	(467)	76	(465)	41	10	(375)	72	(414)
New York	46	(1477)	42	(1415)	29	(1475)	90	(1470)	26	7	(1346)	79	(1433)
Rio	16	(479)	25	(479)	13	(479)	77	(479)	27	3	(433)	59	(465)
Rome	40	(477)	30	(472)	18	(478)	71	(418)	15	27	(357)	–	–
Santos	33	(205)	39	(205)	25	(205)	89	(205)	22	13	(194)	50	(204)
Sydney	47	(424)	41	(424)	17	(424)	91	(422)	46	6	(415)	86	(416)
Toronto	29	(448)	36	(326)	13	(410)	86	(451)	44	4	(456)	86	(458)
Total		(6386)		(6119)		(6333)		(6305)			(5689)		(5779)

Figures rounded to the nearest per cent
n = sample on which percentage was calculated

Table 4.13 Percentage who had ever been tested for HIV; percentage who self-reported as positive; percentage who tested positive

Cities	Ever had an HIV-1 test %	n	Self reported positive %	n	Tested positive %	n
Athens	55	(399)	2	(196)	1	(400)
Bangkok	44	(601)	34	(264)	34	(599)
Berlin	90	(378)	13	(325)	16	(354)
Glasgow	54	(500)	2	(249)	2	(457)
London	47	(512)	10	(216)	13	(491)
Madrid	77	(432)	51	(293)	60	(146)
New York	51	(1467)	29	(405)	48	(847)
Rio	27	(475)	22	(120)	34	(131)
Rome	94	(484)	29	(453)	20	(186)
Santos	68	(218)	59	(122)	63	(214)
Sydney	81	(411)	5	(310)	2	(424)
Toronto	74	(443)	5	(292)	5	(446)
Total		(6320)		(3245)		(4695)

Figures rounded to the nearest per cent
n = sample on which percentage was calculated

HIV-1 Antibody Test Results

On assessing the actual prevalence of HIV-1 infection as identified through study testing at each centre, a surprisingly wide variation was observed. HIV-1 prevalence rates of 5 per cent or less were found in Athens, Glasgow, Sydney and Toronto. Medium rates of between 10 per cent and approximately 20 per cent were identified in Berlin, London and Rome. High rates of approximately 60 per cent were seen in Madrid and Santos. HIV-1 test results were available on over 90 per cent of the sample in each centre apart from Madrid (31 per cent), New York (57 per cent), Rio de Janeiro (72 per cent) and Rome (38 per cent). In these four centres, especially Madrid, Rome and Rio de Janeiro, the lack of HIV-1 test data available on such large proportions of the samples, is cause for considerable caution when interpreting their HIV-1 prevalence rates.

Conclusion

On examining the comparative data as presented in this chapter, it has been possible to highlight some marked similarities in the general characteristics and in the current behaviour of drug injectors from the 12 cities participating in the survey. A convergence of data is evident in terms of age, sex, injecting habits and frequencies, as well as in sexual behaviour, despite the heterogeneous socio-cultural background of each population. One would consequently expect to find corresponding levels of HIV-1 seroprevalence in the centres. Yet the data on current HIV-1 status strongly contradict this assumption and lead to the conclusion that there are additional factors influencing HIV-1 transmission which should be further explored. The polarization between low, middle and high prevalence cities, whether industrial or developing, may suggest a complex of factors contributing to the level of HIV-1 infection. These areas of investigation remain to be analyzed more expansively so as to permit implementation of more effective interventions. Factors influencing HIV-1 prevalence are examined in further chapters.

Note

1 The complete questionnaire and fuller dataset (including raw numbers) will be found in World Health Organization International Collaborative Group (1994) *Multi-City Study on Drug Injecting and Risk of HIV Infection* (WHO/PSA/94.4), Geneva: World Health Organization.

Chapter 5

New Injectors and HIV-1 Risk

Samuel R. Friedman, Patricia Friedmann, Paulo Telles, Francisco Bastos, Regina Bueno, Fabio Mesquita and Don C. Des Jarlais

Most persons who inject drugs for the first time are likely to be uninfected with HIV-1 unless they are men who have sex with men or residents of a country characterized by very high rates of heterosexual transmission. Indeed, there is a considerable literature showing that new drug injectors are less likely to be infected with HIV-1 than longer-term injectors (De Rossi *et al.*, 1988; Friedman *et al.*, 1989; Lima *et al.*, 1994; van den Hoek *et al.*, 1988; Vlahov *et al.*, 1990; Zunzunegui-Pastor *et al.*, 1993). It has been suggested that the seroconversion rates of new injectors may vary in a complicated relationship with the overall seroprevalence and seroconversion rates of an area (Friedman *et al.*, 1994a), with new injectors having higher seroconversion rates than longer-term injectors in cities with high but stable seroprevalence (Ciaffi *et al.*, 1992), lower seroconversion rates in cities of medium-to-high but increasing seroprevalence, and equally low seroconversion rates in cities with low seroprevalence. New male injectors seem to become infected later in their injection careers than do women in New York, as well as in some (but not all) other American cities (Des Jarlais *et al.*, 1994; Friedman *et al.*, 1993, 1994a; Neaigus *et al.*, 1995).

Existing data indicate that new injectors may be less aware of AIDS risks than longer-term injectors, and that they may also engage in higher levels of risk behaviour (Friedman *et al.*, 1989; Kleinman *et al.*, 1990).

It seems, then, that people who begin to inject drugs should be prime targets for prevention activities, since they are mostly still uninfected but are at high risk.

This chapter analyzes the data concerning new injectors in the World Health Organization Multi-City Study on Drug Injecting and Risk of HIV Infection. It examines each participating city's relative proportions of new injectors (by gender), their HIV-1 seroprevalence for new and for longer-term injectors, and how this varies by gender; and presents data on risk behaviours and their correspondence with years of injection.

Methods

Participants in the WHO study included both out-of-treatment and in-treatment drug injectors (Appendix 1). Years of injection are defined by subtracting age at first injection from current age. Unless otherwise specified, 'new' injectors are defined as those who have been injecting for six years or less, while 'old' injectors are defined as those who have been injecting for more than six years.

Cities were classified by seroprevalence as low (Athens, Glasgow, Sydney and Toronto, where seroprevalence was 5 per cent or less), medium (Berlin, London and Rome, where seroprevalence was 13 per cent to 20 per cent), and high (Bangkok, Madrid, New York, Rio de Janeiro and Santos, where seroprevalence was 34 per cent to 63 per cent).

One of the important analyses in this chapter is the estimated proportion of new injectors in the various cities. This needs to be interpreted cautiously, since several factors can affect the measured proportion of new injectors. These factors include:

1 *The initiation rate of new injectors* as a proportion of the total city population — which is a measure of the extent to which the population is generating potential new recruits for parenteral exposure to HIV-1 and other blood-borne viruses.

2 *The prior 'stock' of old injectors.* For example, New York City has a much higher proportion of injectors who began injecting in the 1960s and 1970s than other cities in this study, because New York experienced a big influx into injection at that time (WHO Collaborative Study Group, 1993).

3 *Recruitment procedures* may have differed in different cities. For example, if a city recruited the street sample using old heroin users as fieldworkers, but most new injectors were cocaine users, this would tend to decrease its measured proportion of new injectors. Similar results might be produced if the treatment sample were recruited at a methadone programme where most of the local new injectors have eschewed opioids.

4 *Geographical factors.* If the project has mainly recruited subjects from areas with long-term injecting drug users, but there are other neighbourhoods with larger proportions of new injectors, this will tend to underestimate the true proportion new injecting drug users.

5 Differing proportions of *truly hidden new users.* In a New York study that attempted to recruit large numbers of new injectors, it was found that an unknown, but possibly large, number of persons may begin to inject, but then will avoid having much, if any, presence in visible drug-dealing scenes for several years thereafter. Should they continue to inject, there is a very high chance that they will eventually be drawn to the main centres of drug injecting life, but an *unknown* proportion remain hidden, either because they stop injecting drugs or, perhaps, because they maintain controlled levels of use over many years and thus avoid the main centres of drug dealing. Differences in police enforcement, differing degrees of stigmatization of drug

use, and different occupational or industrial distributions may also cause different proportions of injecting drug users to remain hidden, which may affect the measured proportion of new injectors.

Results

Prevalence of New Injectors

Table 5.1 gives data on the distribution of respondents by years of injection. In the 12 cities altogether, 38 per cent of subjects had been injecting for six years or less. In 10 of the cities, the proportion of new injectors ranged from 37 per cent to 50 per cent; while Glasgow had 56 per cent, and New York had only 16 per cent.

A higher proportion of women than men were new injectors (see Table 5.2, 43 per cent versus 36 per cent). In Glasgow, 69 per cent of the women were new injectors (as compared to 51 per cent of the men), and in New York these proportions were 25 per cent and 12 per cent respectively.

HIV-1 Seroprevalence and Years of Injection

As Table 5.3 shows, new injectors were less likely to be infected with HIV-1 than old injectors (15 per cent versus 28 per cent). Given that new injectors have had less potential exposure time, and that they often inject with other new injectors (Friedman *et al.*, 1994b), this is hardly surprising. The study data indicate that new injectors were significantly less likely to be infected than old injectors in seven of the cities surveyed (Bangkok, Berlin, Glasgow, Madrid, New York, Rio

Table 5.1 New and old injectors, by site and total sample (New injectors have been injecting drugs for 6 years or less; old injectors for more than 6 years.)

Cities	New injectors		Old injectors	
	n	%	n	%
Athens	180	46	208	54
Bangkok	227	43	296	57
Berlin	175	46	204	54
Glasgow	280	56	217	44
London	217	42	299	58
Madrid	194	42	269	58
New York	229	16	1228	84
Rio de Janeiro	223	47	256	53
Rome	176	37	306	63
Santos	107	50	108	50
Sydney	190	47	218	53
Toronto	160	37	277	63
Total	2358	38	3886	62

Figures rounded to the nearest per cent

Table 5.2 Percentage of new injectors, by gender, by site and by total sample (New injectors have been injecting drugs for 6 years or less; old injectors for more than 6 years. Probabilities are by x^2 unless otherwise indicated.)

Cities	New injectors %		
	Men	Women	p
Athens	49	39	.113
Bangkok	43	43	.994
Berlin	43	50	.222
Glasgow	51	69	.000
London	39	49	.032
Madrid	43	39	.509
New York	12	25	.000
Rio de Janeiro	46	53	.259
Rome	35	41	.264
Santos	50	49	.935
Sydney	45	57	.049
Toronto	36	38	.810
Total	36	43	.000

Figures rounded to the nearest per cent

Table 5.3 Percentage HIV seropositive of new injectors and old injectors, by site and by total sample (New injectors have been injecting drugs for 6 years or less; old injectors for more than 6 years. Probabilities are by x^2 unless otherwise indicated.)

Cities	New injectors		Old injectors		
	%	n	%	n	p
Athens	1	(180)	0	(208)	.127
Bangkok	29	(225)	37	(296)	.040
Berlin	11	(161)	20	(192)	.017
Glasgow	0	(253)	4	(198)	.024*
London	13	(205)	13	(271)	.721
Madrid	45	(73)	75	(71)	.000
New York	25	(130)	52	(702)	.000
Rio de Janeiro	21	(43)	41	(88)	.024
Rome	7	(61)	28	(123)	.001
Santos	66	(106)	59	(103)	.309
Sydney	2	(190)	2	(218)	.604
Toronto	6	(156)	4	(273)	.272
Total	15	(1783)	28	(2743)	.000

Figures rounded to the nearest per cent
n = sample on which percentage was calculated
* Probability by Fisher's exact test

de Janeiro and Rome); and in three of the others (Athens, Sydney and Toronto) seroprevalence is too low for differences to appear. In London and Santos, however, prevalence does not seem to differ by years of injection. Indeed, even when comparisons were made between 'very new injectors' (defined as those who had been injecting for three years or less) and those who had injected for more than three years, the seroprevalences were equal (in London, very new injectors were 16 per cent seropositive versus 12 per cent for other injectors; in Santos the proportions were 63 per cent vs. 62 per cent). Thus, drug injectors in these two cities seemed to be equally as likely to be infected very early in their injection careers as more experienced injectors. The equal prevalence of new and older injectors in Santos, a city with high prevalence and perhaps high seroconversion rates, implies that the relationship between overall seroprevalence, overall seroconversion rates, and the relative seroprevalence rates of new and older injectors may be more complex than was previously suggested by Friedman *et al.* (1994a).

In order to determine why years of injection were not related to seroprevalence in London and Santos, comparisons were made between the characteristics of new (and very new) injectors in each of these cities, with those in other cities that displayed similar proportions of HIV-seropositive injectors, new injectors, and women. Thus, Santos was compared with Rio de Janeiro and Madrid, and London with Berlin and Rome. In these comparisons, there were a number of variables showing differences among the cities. Notably, new or very new injectors in Santos were more likely than those in Rio de Janeiro and Madrid to inject with used syringes, engage in same-sex sexual intercourse, to be women, to be homeless, and not to have engaged in deliberate risk reduction to avoid AIDS. In London, new or very new injectors were more likely than those in Berlin or Rome: (a) to talk about AIDS with family members; (b) to talk about AIDS with drug-injecting friends; (c) to have previously been tested for HIV-1 infection; and (d) to receive unemployment benefits.

Further analyses were conducted to determine whether, among drug injectors in London and in Santos, there might be an association between HIV-1 serostatus and years of injection within categories of some of these variables. These analyses did not help clarify why new (and very new) injectors in London were as likely to be infected as their more experienced colleagues. They were more helpful in Santos. In Santos, among those who had made behaviour changes in order to protect themselves from AIDS, significant differences were observed between very new and longer-term injectors. Very new injectors who had made behaviour changes were 68 per cent seropositive, but only 44 per cent of longer-term injectors who had modified their behaviour were seropositive (p<0.04). Among those who had *not* tried to protect themselves, 64 per cent of very new injectors and 80 per cent of longer-term injectors were seropositive (p=.1205). This suggests that longer-term injectors who had tried to protect themselves (with 'only' 44 per cent infected) were more likely to benefit from such efforts than very new injectors (since 68 per cent of these very new injectors were infected, as compared with 64 per cent of those who had not tried to protect themselves). These data suggest that, while behaviour change generally is protective, many of the very new injectors in Santos may have tried to protect themselves too late or, due to inexperience, ineffectively. Specifically, we would suggest that they might have become involved in high-prevalence networks early in their injection careers, and began to take steps to protect themselves only thereafter. It is not clear, however, why similar processes might not have been operative in Madrid or Rio de Janeiro. Furthermore, other factors, such as the much smaller size of Santos (450 000 persons in approximately 40 square kilometres) as compared with Madrid or Rio de Janeiro, might lead to differences in social networks that might affect the relationships between new and older injectors. More research is needed to investigate these issues in greater depth.

HIV-1 Seroprevalence and Gender Among New Injectors

Table 5.4 presents data on seroprevalence by gender among new injectors. Men and women seemed to have similar infection rates among the total sample of new injectors. Women, however, were more likely to be infected among new injectors in Berlin, New York, and Athens (where the small number of seropositives among new injectors, too, indicates a need for caution). Further research on why women are more likely to be infected early in their injection careers in some cities — and why this is not true in others — may help us understand why, in some cities, men seem to be relatively protected and women seem to be at higher risk. In the meantime, it is clear that any obstacles to women making use of harm-reduction programmes, drug treatment services, and other prevention resources should be eliminated.

Table 5.4 Percentage HIV seropositive by gender among new injectors, by site and by total sample (New injectors have been injecting drugs for 6 years or less; old injectors for more than 6 years. Probabilities are by x^2 unless otherwise indicated.)

Cities	Men		Women		
	%	n	%	n	p
Athens	0	(147)	6	(33)	.033*
Bangkok	29	(215)	20	(10)	.728*
Berlin	5	(84)	17	(77)	.012*
Glasgow	1	(158)	0	(95)	1.00*
London	14	(123)	13	(82)	.934
Madrid	47	(64)	33	(9)	.445*
New York	18	(74)	34	(56)	.032
Rio de Janeiro	23	(31)	17	(12)	.669
Rome	4	(52)	22	(9)	.100*
Santos	65	(62)	68	(44)	.695
Sydney	2	(141)	0	(45)	1.00*
Toronto	8	(118)	0	(38)	.120*
Total	15	(1269)	16	(510)	.429

Figures rounded to the nearest per cent
n = sample on which percentage was calculated
* Probabilities by Fisher's exact test

Risk and Other Behaviours

Table 5.5 presents data on a number of behaviours for the total sample and for subsets of low, medium and high seroprevalence cities. This allows investigation of whether the differences in behaviours between new and old injectors might be related to the prevalence of HIV-1 infection in each drug-injecting population.

Approximately 43 per cent of drug injectors interviewed had injected with syringes that others had used in the prior six months, and an approximately equal proportion had passed used syringes on to others during this same period. There was considerable overlap between the two groups (r=0.497). Syringe sharing did not vary with years of injection, with one possible exception: in medium seroprevalence cities, old injectors may be slightly more likely to report having injected with a used syringe than new injectors (p=0.057).

Patterns of consistent condom use were more diverse, although rates of condom use were not high in any of the subsets examined. It seems at first glance that old injectors were more likely to report consistent condom use with both casual and primary partners than new injectors. These relationships, however, are most evident in high seroprevalence cities rather than indicative of the sample as a whole. Thus, consistent condom use did not vary significantly by length of injection in either low or medium seroprevalence cities. In high seroprevalence cities, on the other hand, consistent condom use with both primary and casual partners was more common among old injectors than among new injectors.

Old injectors were slightly more likely to have a primary sex partner who injects drugs than new injectors. This difference between old and new injectors was primarily concentrated in the high seroprevalence cities.

Among men, new injectors were more likely to report having had sex with another man (in the five years before the interview) than longer-term injectors.

For drug injectors, talking about AIDS is an important part of the process of learning about the disease, and of then taking steps to reduce or avoid risk (Des Jarlais et al., 1995; Neaigus et al., 1994). Injectors were asked to what extent they talked about AIDS with: (a) drug-using friends, (b) sex partners, and (c) family. For the total sample, about 5 per cent more of old injectors than of new injectors reported that they talked about AIDS with each of these groups of people. The difference between old and new injectors in talking with these groups was greatest in high seroprevalence cities.

Old injectors were also more likely than new injectors to know that a person who looks healthy can be infected with HIV-1 (at least in medium and high seroprevalence cities, where such knowledge is most likely to be based on experience).

Even though longer-term injectors have had more time to change their behaviour in order to reduce the risk of becoming infected with HIV-1 than new injectors, there were no significant differences by years of injection in risk reduction behaviour, with approximately 80 per cent of all subjects reporting that they had tried to reduce their risk of becoming infected.

Table 5.5 Percentage who engaged in risk behaviours in prior six months for new injectors and old injectors, by city seroprevalence (New injectors have been injecting drugs for 6 years or less; old injectors for more than 6 years. Probabilities are by x^2 unless otherwise indicated.)

	All cities Injectors			Low* Injectors			Medium* Injectors			High* Injectors		
	new	old	p	new	old	p	new	old	p	new	old	p
Injected with used syringe	41 (2338)	43 (3824)	.176	43 (809)	45 (917)	.380	31 (561)	36 (786)	.057	45 (968)	44 (2121)	.700
Passed used syringe on to others	44 (2318)	43 (3799)	.319	45 (807)	42 (917)	.225	38 (549)	34 (769)	.180	47 (962)	46 (2113)	.751
Always used condoms with primary partners	11 (1167)	16 (1884)	.000	9 (398)	8 (366)	.415	13 (301)	15 (442)	.373	11 (468)	19 (1076)	.000
Always used condoms with casual partners	24 (721)	29 (1192)	.009	28 (250)	25 (292)	.423	28 (159)	30 (247)	.786	18 (312)	31 (653)	.000
Has primary partner who is an IDU	25 (2306)	27 (3799)	.045	32 (791)	33 (891)	.609	31 (555)	36 (785)	.086	15 (960)	21 (2123)	.000
Men: Any male/male sex in prior 5 years	13 (1518)	8 (2764)	.000	10 (520)	6 (634)	.006	5 (264)	5 (417)	.825	17 (734)	9 (1713)	.000
Talks about AIDS with drug-using friends	77 (2334)	81 (3868)	.000	75 (809)	78 (917)	.227	79 (559)	84 (801)	.047	77 (966)	82 (2150)	.000
Talks about AIDS with sexual partners	63 (2254)	68 (3688)	.000	66 (746)	68 (805)	.322	70 (552)	73 (791)	.260	57 (956)	66 (2092)	.000
Talks about AIDS with family	45 (2322)	50 (3831)	.000	38 (796)	41 (886)	.290	40 (561)	36 (798)	.226	54 (965)	59 (2147)	.007
Knows that an HIV-infected person can look healthy	79 (2300)	84 (3822)	.000	86 (808)	86 (919)	.914	73 (528)	80 (764)	.001	77 (964)	84 (2139)	.000
Has changed behaviour to protect self from AIDS	79 (2117)	80 (3483)	.730	87 (802)	85 (911)	.292	79 (389)	84 (497)	.070	73 (926)	77 (2075)	.052
Has previously been tested for HIV	54 (2312)	64 (3827)	.000	56 (794)	74 (911)	.000	69 (561)	81 (791)	.000	44 (957)	54 (2125)	.000
Has previously tested positive for HIV	12 (1096)	26 (2068)	.000	4 (397)	3 (624)	.727	7 (370)	27 (616)	.000	28 (329)	42 (828)	.000

Figures rounded to the nearest per cent
Figure in parenthesis is the sample on which percentage was calculated
* Low seroprevalence cities are Athens, Glasgow, Sydney and Toronto; medium are Berlin, London and Rome; high are Bangkok, Madrid, Rio de Janeiro and Santos

It appears that old injectors have had more opportunity to decide to be tested than new injectors. Ten per cent fewer new injectors than old injectors had been tested. This difference was significant within low, medium, and high seroprevalence cities. Similarly, old injectors were more likely to report having previously tested seropositive for HIV-1 than new injectors in the total sample, and in the medium and high seroprevalence cities.

Conclusions and Discussion

Preventing Initiation

The measured variation among cities in the proportion of new injectors needs to be interpreted cautiously, as was discussed in the section on Methods. Nevertheless, it is clear that large numbers of persons have begun to inject drugs in many of the cities studied since the beginning of the AIDS era. Furthermore, although in cities with mature HIV-1 epidemics several years may elapse between the time of initiation into injection and the time when the initiates' probability of infection reaches that of the longer-term injectors, new injectors are at high risk of HIV-1 infection and other blood-borne infections. Thus, it is clearly urgent that effective methods be developed to reduce the extent of initiation into injecting drug use. Such methods might take any of several forms. First, they might involve personal interventions with individuals likely to become drug injectors. One experimental project used intensive group work with heroin sniffers and significantly reduced the proportion who went on to injection during the follow-up period (Casriel *et al.*, 1990; Des Jarlais *et al.*, 1992a). More effective programmes need to be developed and evaluated to work with school-age youth — both in school and out — to help them resist becoming 'hard-drug' users and/ or injectors. One question that needs to be addressed is the extent to which such programmes should also provide 'harm reduction' education, so that those youths who go on to use drugs in spite of the intervention will at least be more able to protect themselves against HIV-1 and other risks. It is likely that such education would be most effective and accepted by the general public if it were targeted at those youths at greatest risk.

Programmes should also be developed and tested that focus on drug injectors who are likely to be initiators of others into drug injecting. Such interventions should attempt to enlist current users' aid in refusing to initiate others. (Anecdotal evidence from drug injectors has shown that many already try to protect others by refusing to initiate them even when asked.) Another aim of such programmes should be to encourage potential initiators to teach anyone who approaches them (or whom they approach) about initiation into the practical application of harm-reduction techniques. Finally, such programmes should try to discourage participants from *ever* sharing syringes with anyone they might initiate. Further studies of the social-network environments of drug injectors at the time of initiation may help in finding ways to recruit potential subjects for such programmes, and in devising appropriate programme materials.

Another approach to preventing the onset of drug injection is drug treatment. Specifically, it must be made easy and appealing to enter drug-treatment programmes for persons at high risk of initiating injection because of their non-injecting use of injectable substances, or because of their use of other (late-)precursor drugs. The failure of many nations to have provided a massive increase in drug treatment availability may have allowed potentially preventable initiations into drug injection as well as preventable HIV-1 infections among those who have already begun to inject.

Further, we need to consider macrosocial and macroeconomic causes of initiation into drug use and drug injection, and policies and programmes that might target this level. Research is clearly needed to help ascertain such causes. If drug enforcement policies, racial or gender inequality, economic disadvantage and/or hopelessness, or widespread sexual abuse contribute to initiation, or if other large-scale forces contribute to initiation, then we need to consider how these can be eliminated or at least reduced.

Preventing HIV-1 Infection among New Injectors

In spite of efforts to prevent initiation of additional persons into drug injecting, large numbers of persons in both developed and developing countries are likely to start injecting (see also Chapter 1). The data presented in this chapter clearly indicate that new injectors are at considerable behavioural risk for HIV-1. Two-fifths reported that in the six months prior to interview they had injected with syringes or needles that others had used. Condom use was low, and approximately one-third of new injectors had primary partners who injected drugs, while about one in seven of male new injectors had engaged in sex with other men. More encouragingly, about three-quarters of new injectors reported they talked about AIDS with their drug-using friends, almost two-thirds did so with sex partners, and almost half did so with their family. This widespread 'AIDS talk' may help explain the high proportion of new injectors who knew that a healthy-looking person can be infected with HIV-1, as well as the high proportion who reported having made behavioural changes to protect themselves against HIV-1. Nonetheless, since such discussion seems to be an important part of the process of risk reduction (Des Jarlais *et al.*, 1995; Neaigus *et al.*, 1994), further programmes to increase the extent to which new drug injectors discuss AIDS within their social networks seem likely to be useful.

One issue is the extent to which special HIV prevention programmes for new injectors are needed. Available evidence suggests that although new injectors have higher rates of HIV-1 seroconversion in cities with stable high seroprevalence, this is not true in low seroprevalence cities or in cities where seroprevalence is rapidly increasing (Friedman *et al.*, 1994a). It is probable that the value of special programming for new injectors will vary among cities as a function of patterns of social association among injectors of different ages and, perhaps, of the perceived need for secrecy on the part of new initiates. Research on this issue is needed.

Although almost two-thirds of the new injectors had previously been tested for HIV-1, it should be useful to increase the availability of these services to new injectors. It may be that there was recruitment bias operating, such that those new injectors who were most likely to be recruited for the study may also have been those most likely to seek or to be recruited for HIV-1 counselling and testing.

Some new injectors are particularly hard to recruit for prevention activities such as HIV-1 testing, syringe exchange, or other harm reduction efforts. This is often a result of their fear of becoming known as engaging in stigmatized and, in some nations, punishable drug using behaviours. Efforts should be made to develop new ways of seeking any 'hidden' new injectors in a locality and, where they exist, to find ways to make preventive services available to them in spite of their perceived need (and ability) to remain undetected as drug injectors.

A Growing Tragedy

There are an estimated five million drug injectors in the world (Chapter 1). The data presented in this chapter from the WHO Study suggest that one-third or more of the planet's drug injectors began to inject after the risk of AIDS had become known. Indeed, this proportion of new injectors is almost certainly an underestimate by now — in spite of all the uncertainty in attempting such an estimate, as discussed above. This would be true for two reasons:

First, the gathering of data for the WHO study was completed in 1992. This means that a further five years have since elapsed, during which additional scores of thousands of persons have begun to inject drugs — in spite of the fact that injection-related HIV-1 infection has become a publicly known, worldwide catastrophe.

Second, drug injection has continued to disperse geographically, to areas that were not well-represented at the time of this study (Chapter 1). Drug injection has now spread to many parts of South-east and southern Asia, to East Europe, to new regions of South America, and to Africa. This extensive spread of injection means that scores — perhaps hundreds — of thousands of additional people have begun injecting in the recent past. In some of these areas, furthermore, such as Myanmar, Vietnam, and north-east India, HIV-1 has spread exceedingly rapidly, such that 50 per cent to 90 per cent of drug injectors in some communities are now infected (Stimson, 1994). To some extent, this rapid spread of HIV-1 may be due to the lack of local traditions of injecting drug use.

There are a number of mechanisms that may help explain the international spread of injecting drug use. The use of therapeutic injections in countries such as Pakistan, India and Thailand has enabled drug users to learn about drug injecting from health workers. Through the mixing of cultures, such as foreign soldiers and refugees associated with the Vietnam war, whole populations have been exposed to new patterns of drug use. Also, changes in the availability of traditionally used drugs in countries such as Myanmar, China and Columbia have contributed to a transition to the use of injectable drugs. In such developing countries, not only are new injectors confronted with problems similar to those experienced by new injectors in developed countries (where drug injector networks already exist), but they are also likely to be confronted by a drug using subculture that does not have a tradition of drug injection, with no drug injection rituals and a lack of 'wisdom' based on networks of older drug injectors. Such a lack of a drug injection culture may hamper prevention activities which rely on peer education and norms. Furthermore, prevention and treatment agencies in such countries have limited experience in responding to the problem of drug injection. Not only are all injecting drug users new injectors in these settings, but policy makers, researchers and interventionists are also new to the situation.

There is no way to be sure how representative the sample of cities in this study is in terms of the percentage of new injectors who have become infected. It includes large centres of drug injection such as New York City and Bangkok, but excludes rural injectors and those in southern Asia and South-east Asia to whom HIV-1 spread after it reached Bangkok. If we assume (a) that the 15 per cent HIV-1 infection rate among new injectors in the WHO study is a 'best guesstimate' of the proportion of 'AIDS-era-initiate' new injectors who have become infected with HIV-1; and (b) that one-third of the estimated drug injectors in the world have begun to inject since HIV-1 became known, then approximately *a quarter of a million* people have become infected with this fatal disease during a period when harm reduction policies with adequate funding could probably have reduced new infections significantly. Furthermore, many other new injectors have undoubtedly become infected with other potentially fatal blood-borne pathogens such as hepatitis B and hepatitis C. Indeed, in localities where either HBV or HCV are widespread among older injectors, they can spread among new injectors even more rapidly than HIV-1; thus, in Baltimore, approximately 15 per cent of new injectors were infected with HIV-1 — but 50 per cent were infected with hepatitis B and 75 per cent with hepatitis C — within the first eight months of their injection careers (Vlahov, 1994).

This growing public health problem is composed of several components. To some extent there has been a failure of research and science. Those who have conducted research in these areas have not succeeded in finding sufficiently adequate ways to keep drug injection from spreading to new countries, to keep young people from becoming drug injectors, or to keep them from becoming infected if they do inject. Where there has been progress in developing programmes (such as syringe exchanges and methadone treatment), there has been a failure of many countries' political systems to implement them.

This lack of knowledge may have been a component in a more general failure of policy that has allowed (or inadvertently contributed to) the spread of drug injection to new countries (Des Jarlais *et al.*, 1992b), and that may have failed to prevent new initiations into drug injection either in countries where this practice was well-established before the HIV-1 epidemic or in countries to which injecting has since spread. Most countries have also failed to expand drug treatment services and to implement widespread harm reduction programmes.

These failures of science and of policy themselves raise additional issues for research and action. First, can science be made more effective? Second, are there economic and political restraints in current national and economic systems that contribute either to the seeming intractability of the problem of drug injection or the policy inadequacies discussed above? In conclusion, while research and action on these deeper questions is extremely difficult, and likely to prove somewhat controversial, the large number of persons who have begun to inject drugs, the large number who have become infected, and, indeed, the data presented in this book as a whole suggest that this research is long overdue.

Acknowledgments

We would like to acknowledge support from the World Health Organization; from United States National Institute on Drug Abuse grant R01 DA03574; from FAPERJ (Foundation for the Development of Science, Rio de Janeiro), Oswaldo Cruz Foundation; and from Projeto Brasil, sponsored by the STD/AIDS Division of the Brazilian Ministry of Health.

References

CASRIEL, C., DES JARLAIS, D.C., RODRIGUEZ, R., FRIEDMAN, S.R., STEPHERSON, B. and KHURI, E. (1990) 'Working with heroin sniffers', *Journal of Substance Abuse Treatment*, **7**, pp. 1–10.

CIAFFI, L., NICOLOSI, A., CORREA-LEITE, M.L., *et al.* (1992) 'Incidence of HIV infection in intravenous drug users from Milan and Northern Italy, 1987–91', Abstract No. ThC 1552, paper presented at the Eighth International Conference on AIDS, Amsterdam, the Netherlands.

DE ROSSI, A., BORTOLOTTI, F., CADROBBI, P. and CHIECO-BIANCHI, L. (1988) 'Trends of HTLV-1 and HIV infection in drug addicts', *European Journal of Cancer and Clinical Oncology*, **24**, pp. 279–80.

DES JARLAIS, D.C. (1996) 'HIV epidemiology and interventions among injecting drug users', *International Journal of STD & AIDS*, **7**, suppl. 2, pp. 57–61.

DES JARLAIS, D.C., CASRIEL, C., FRIEDMAN, S.R. and ROSENBLUM, A. (1992a) 'AIDS and the transition to illicit drug injection — results of a randomized trial prevention program', *British Journal of Addiction*, **87**, pp. 493–8.

DES JARLAIS, D.C. FRIEDMAN, S.R., CHOOPANYA, K., VANICHSENI, S. and WARD, T.P. (1992b) 'International epidemiology of HIV and AIDS among injecting drug users', *AIDS*, **6**, pp. 1053–68.

DES JARLAIS, D.C., FRIEDMAN, S.R., SOTHERAN, J.L., WENSTON, J., MARMOR, M., YANCOVITZ, S.R., FRANK, B., BEATRICE, S. and MILDVAN, D. (1994) 'Continuity and change within an HIV epidemic: Injecting drug users in New York City, 1984 through 1992', *Journal of the American Medical Association*, **271**, pp. 121–7.

DES JARLAIS, D.C., FRIEDMAN, S.R., FRIEDMANN, P., WENSTON, J., SOTHERAN, J.L., CHOOPANYA, K., VANICHSENI, S., RAKTHAM, S., GOLDBERG, D., FRISCHER, M., GREEN, S., LIMA, E.S., BASTOS, F.I. and TELLES, P.R. (1995) 'HIV/AIDS-related behavior change among injecting drug users in different national settings', *AIDS*, **9**, pp. 611–17.

FRIEDMAN, S.R., DES JARLAIS, D.C., NEAIGUS, A., ABDUL-QUADER, A., SOTHERAN, J.L., SUFIAN, M., TROSS, S. and GOLDSMITH, D. (1989) 'AIDS and the new drug injector', *Nature*, **339**, pp. 333–4.

FRIEDMAN, S.R., JOSE, B., NEAIGUS, A., GOLDSTEIN, M., CURTIS, R. and DES JARLAIS, D.C. (1993) 'Female injecting drug users get infected with HIV sooner than males', Session 3137, 121st Annual Meeting of the American Public Health Association, San Francisco, CA.

FRIEDMAN, S.R., DES JARLAIS, D.C., JOSE, B., NEAIGUS, B. and GOLDSTEIN, M. (1994a) 'Seroprevalence, seroconversion, and the history of the HIV epidemic among drug injectors', in NICOLOSI, A. (Ed) *HIV Epidemiology: Models and Methods*, pp. 137–50, New York: Raven Press.

FRIEDMAN, S.R., DOHERTY, M.C., PAONE, D. and JOSE, B. (1994b) *Notes on Research on the Etiology of Drug Injection*. Consultant report to the United States National Academy of Sciences.

KLEINMAN, P.H., GOLDSMITH, D.S., FRIEDMAN, S.R., HOPKINS, W. and DES JARLAIS, D.C. (1990) 'Knowledge about and behaviors affecting the spread of AIDS: A street survey of intravenous drug users and their associates in New York City', *International Journal of the Addictions*, **25**, pp. 345–61.

LIMA, E.S., FRIEDMAN, S.R., BASTOS, F.I., TELLES, P.R., FRIEDMANN, P., WARD, T.P. and DES JARLAIS, D.C. (1994) 'Risk factors for HIV-1 seroprevalence among drug injectors in the cocaine-using environment of Rio de Janeiro', *Addiction*, **89**, pp. 689–98.

NEAIGUS, A., FRIEDMAN, S.R., CURTIS, R., DES JARLAIS, D.C., FURST, R.T., JOSE, B., MOTA, P., STEPHERSON, B., SUFIAN, M., WARD, T.P. and WRIGHT, J.W. (1994) 'The relevance of drug injectors' social networks and risk networks for understanding and preventing HIV infection', *Social Science & Medicine*, **38**, pp. 67–78.

NEAIGUS, A., FRIEDMAN, S.R., GOLDSTEIN, M., ILDEFONSO, G., CURTIS, R. and JOSE, B. (1995) 'Using dyadic data for a network analysis of HIV infection and risk behaviors among injecting drug users', in NEEDLE, R.H., COYLE, S.L., GENSER, S.G. and TROTTER, R.T. (Eds), *Social Networks, Drug Abuse and HIV Transmission* [NIDA Research Monograph 151] pp. 20–37, Rockville, MD: National Institute on Drug Abuse.

STIMSON, G.V. (1994) 'Reconstruction of sub-regional diffusion of HIV infection among injecting drug users in southeast Asia: Implications for early intervention', *AIDS*, **8**, pp. 1630–2.

STIMSON, G.V., ADELEKAN, M.L. and RHODES, T. (1996) 'The diffusion of drug injecting in developing countries', *International Journal of Drug Policy*, **7** (4), pp. 244–55.

VAN DEN HOEK, J.A.R., COUTINHO, A., VAN HAASTRECHT, H.J.A. *et al.* (1988) 'Prevalence and risk factors of HIV infections among drug users and drug-using prostitutes in Amsterdam', *AIDS*, **2**, pp. 55–60.

VLAHOV, D. (1994) Untitled presentation at the Panel on Injection Drug Users and the

HIV Epidemic, 2 November, Session 3115, 122nd Annual Meeting of the American Public Health Assn., Washington, DC.

VLAHOV, D., MUNOZ, A., ANTHONY, J.C. *et al.* (1990) 'Association of drug injection patterns with antibody to human immunodeficiency virus type 1 among intravenous drug users in Baltimore, Maryland', *American Journal of Epidemiology*, **132**, pp. 847–56.

WHO COLLABORATIVE STUDY GROUP (1993) 'An international comparative study of HIV seroprevalence and risk behaviour among drug injectors in 13 cities', *Bulletin on Narcotics*, **45**, pp. 19–46.

ZUNZUNEGUI-PASTOR, M.V., RODRÍGUEZ-ARENAS, M.A. and SARASQUETA EIZAGUIRRE, C. (1993) 'Drogadicción intravenosa y riesgo de infección por VIH en Madrid, 1990', *Gaceta Sanitaria*, **7**, pp. 2–11.

Chapter 6

The Structure of Stable Seroprevalence HIV-1 Epidemics among Injecting Drug Users

Don C. Des Jarlais, Kachit Choopanya, Peggy Millson, Patricia Friedmann and Samuel R. Friedman

In many areas, the introduction of HIV-1 into the local population of injecting drug users (IDUs) was followed by extremely rapid dissemination within this group. Rapid HIV-1 spread has occurred both in industrialized and developing countries, and in very large cities such as New York (Des Jarlais *et al.*, 1989), moderate-sized cities such as Edinburgh (Robertson *et al.*, 1986) and in semi-rural areas such as the state of Manipur, India (Naik *et al.*, 1991) (also see: Des Jarlais *et al.*, 1992; Friedman and Des Jarlais, 1991).

Fortunately, there have also been examples of localities in which HIV-1 was introduced into a local population of IDUs, but where HIV-1 seroprevalence has subsequently remained low and stable, such as Glasgow (Scotland), Lund (Sweden), Tacoma (Washington, USA), Toronto (Canada) and Sydney (Australia) (Des Jarlais *et al.*, 1995a). Understanding the factors which account for the differences between localities where HIV-1 spreads very rapidly among IDUs and localities in which HIV-1 has basically remained under control among IDUs, is one of the most important questions in the field of HIV-1 epidemiology. The World Health Organization Multi-City Study on Drug Injecting and Risk of HIV Infection has provided a unique opportunity to address this question (Appendix 1). This chapter examines what is currently known about the structure of high- and low-HIV seroprevalence epidemics among IDUs, using the WHO dataset as a whole, with special emphasis on two high-seroprevalence cities — New York and Bangkok — and three low-seroprevalence cities — Glasgow, Toronto and Sydney.

Introduction of HIV-1 into the Local IDU Population

HIV-1 can be introduced into local IDU populations in several ways. In some cities, such as New York (Des Jarlais *et al.*, 1989), Sydney (Ross *et al.*, 1992) and

Rio de Janeiro (Lima *et al.*, 1994), HIV-1 was probably introduced into a local area by men who have sex with men (MSM), and then spread to IDUs who also were MSM, and then to other IDUs. In this sense, MSM IDUs can be considered a 'bridge population' between non-injecting MSM and the IDU population as a whole. HIV-1 infection among women IDUs who have sex with women is also an important topic for additional research, as the role of such persons within the larger spread of HIV-1 has not been determined (Jose *et al.*, 1993; Reardon *et al.*, 1992).

Moreover, contrary to the popular stereotype, a substantial proportion of IDUs do travel. Indeed, substantial numbers of subjects in each of the 13 cities in the WHO Study reported having injected outside of their home city within the previous two years (see Chapter 7). Some of this travel can be considered 'drug tourism' — that is drug users going to a different locality where drugs are less expensive (Simons, 1994) — while some of the travel may simply be a part of the drug distribution business, with the drug users carrying drugs from one city to another. When drug injectors do travel from one city to another, they are unlikely to carry injection equipment with them because of the possibility of difficulties with customs officials. Drug users who travel may have considerable difficulties in obtaining their own sterile injection equipment while in unfamiliar cities. Travelling drug injectors may thus be particularly likely to inject with equipment which has been previously used — and will be subsequently used — by other injectors.

In the case of Bangkok, although it has not been determined how HIV-1 was first introduced here, it is likely that it was brought in by travelling HIV-infected IDUs. Because Bangkok is located on a heroin distribution route from the nearby Golden Triangle, the street prices of heroin in Bangkok are generally quite low, and therefore may attract IDUs from outside the area.

Potential Rapid Spread of HIV-1 among IDUs

Among the WHO Study cities, well documented very rapid transmission of HIV-1 occurred among IDUs in New York City and in Bangkok. In New York, HIV-1 seroprevalence among IDUs increased from under 10 per cent in 1978 to approximately 50 per cent by 1983 (Des Jarlais *et al.*, 1989), with an estimated rate of 13 new HIV-1 infections per 100 person-years at risk. In Bangkok, HIV-1 seroprevalence among IDUs increased from approximately 2 per cent in the first quarter of 1988 to over 40 per cent in the third quarter of 1988, with an estimated rate of four new HIV-1 infections per 100 person-months at risk (Vanichseni and Sakuntanaga, 1990).

In both New York and Bangkok, the rapid spread of HIV-1 was associated with multi-person use of injection equipment ('sharing') and occurred through rapid and efficient mixing of the IDUs who were sharing needles and syringes. Another factor contributing to the period of rapid spread in New York was the use of 'shooting galleries', where a drug injector could rent a needle and syringe, inject with it, and then return it to the operator of the shooting gallery. There was usually no (or at most, minimal) cleaning of the injection equipment between uses by different IDUs. Such cleaning as did occur was merely to prevent the needle and syringe from becoming so clogged that they could no longer be used.

In Bangkok, rapid dissemination of HIV-1 was associated with sharing among large numbers of IDUs; use of needles and syringes kept by drug dealers (who would lend the needle and syringe to different customers); and being incarcerated (Choopanya *et al.*, 1991). Whether the incarceration risk factor was a result of actually sharing equipment while injecting in prison (Wright *et al.*, 1994) or whether incarceration led IDUs to form new soical networks with other IDUs (with whom they only subsequently shared injection equipment after being released from prison) has not yet been determined.

Very rapid dissemination of HIV-1 among IDUs should not be seen simply as a consequence of any multi-person use of injection equipment, but rather as resulting from occasions when IDUs share with large numbers of other IDUs within short time periods and outside of naturally occurring friendship networks.

Behaviour Change/Risk Reduction among IDUs

Contrary to the popular sterotype that IDUs are not at all concerned about their health and therefore will not change their injection behaviour to avoid HIV/ AIDS, evidence, mainly from developed countries, indicates that the great majority have shown that they actually will and do change their behaviour in response to concerns about AIDS. Again, the WHO Study has provided an excellent opportunity to study cross-national aspects of AIDS risk reduction among IDUs, including the validity of the self-reports of behaviour change/risk reduction. The WHO data actually contain some of the strongest evidence to date for the validity of self-reported HIV/AIDS behaviour change/risk reduction among IDUs (Des Jarlais *et al.*, 1994a). Moreover, there is now strong biological evidence for the validity of the self-report data from Bangkok in particular (Chitwood, 1994; Des Jarlais *et al.*, 1994b).

Table 6.1 presents the percentage of subjects who, when asked: 'Since you first heard of AIDS, have you done anything to avoid getting AIDS?', reported that they had changed their behaviour. The cities are grouped by current HIV-1 seroprevalence, and there is no direct linkage between seroprevalence and the percentage of IDUs who have changed their behaviour. Large majorities of IDUs have changed their behaviour in almost all of the cities. While a majority of subjects reported that they had changed their behaviour in response to concerns about AIDS, there is also substantial variation across the different cities, with a low of 50 per cent in Santos and a high of 92 per cent in Bangkok. Determinants of the differences in the percentages of IDUs who have changed their behaviour because of concerns about AIDS have yet to be established, but are likely to be related to the types and intensity of the HIV-1 prevention efforts for IDUs in the different cities, and the amount of time that had elapsed in each city between

Table 6.1 Number and percentage of persons reporting behaviour change when asked 'Since you first heard of AIDS, have you done anything to avoid catching the virus yourself?'

		Reported behaviour change
Low seroprevalence cities:	Athens	347 (88%)
	Glasgow	412 (83%)
	Sydney	357 (86%)
	Toronto	395 (86%)
Medium seroprevalence cities:	Berlin	326 (86%)
	London	411 (78%)
	Rome	Not available
High seroprevalence cities:	Bangkok	542 (92%)
	Madrid	300 (72%)
	New York	1133 (79%)
	Rio de Janeiro	276 (59%)
	Santos	103 (50%)

Seroprevalence: low, under 5%; medium, 5–20%; high, over 20%

initiation of local prevention efforts and the moment when the WHO Study data were collected (see also Chapter 12).

More detailed analyses of the specific types of behaviour change have been conducted for Bangkok, Glasgow, New York and Rio de Janeiro (Des Jarlais *et al.*, 1995b). In all four of these cities, changes in drug-injection behaviour occurred in a significantly larger percentage of subjects than did changes in sexual behaviour. The most frequent change in injection behaviour was to 'stop or reduce sharing' of injection equipment, while the most frequent sexual behaviour changes were increased use of condoms, fewer sexual partners and greater selectivity in choosing sexual partners.

Stabilization of HIV-1 Seroprevalence

Although the amount of data available varies across the different cities, it is likely that stabilization of HIV-1 seroprevalence has by now occurred in all of the WHO Study cities. The data on stabilization of HIV-1 seroprevalence is particularly strong for Bangkok, Glasgow, New York, Sydney and Toronto.

In Bangkok, seroprevalence surveys have been conducted at least annually among IDUs at the Bangkok Metropolitan Administration drug abuse treatment programmes. In the autumn of 1988, seroprevalence was approximately 40 per cent, and this had not changed by the end of 1993 (Choopanya, unpublished data).

In Glasgow, seven serial cross-sectional studies conducted among 2300 of Glasgow's estimated 8500 IDUs found HIV-1 seroprevalence rates ranging from

1 per cent to at most 5 per cent, but with no increasing trend over time from 1986 to 1992 (Frischer *et al.*, 1992).

In New York, studies of IDUs entering drug treatment and IDUs recruited from street sources show stabilization of HIV-1 seroprevalence at approximately 50 per cent from 1984 to 1994 (Des Jarlais *et al.*, 1989, 1994c).

In Sydney, seven serial cross-sectional studies conducted among 2700 of an estimated 7800 IDUs found HIV-1 seroprevalence rates ranging from 0.5 per cent to at most 5 per cent. Significantly higher rates were evident among MSM IDUs (from 13 per ent to 44 per cent), but there was no discernible trend towards an increase in overall seroprevalence rates from 1984 to 1991 (Kaldor *et al.*, 1993).

In Toronto, seven serial cross-sectional studies conducted among 1300 of an estimated 8000 IDUs found HIV-1 seroprevalence rates ranging from 0.8 per cent to 3.3 per cent, but again, with no increasing trend from 1988 to the end of 1992 (Millson *et al.*, 1993).

It is important to note that stabilization of HIV-1 seroprevalence among a population of IDUs does *not* imply an absence of new HIV-1 infections (Des Jarlais *et al.*, 1994c). Populations of IDUs are dynamic groups, with some IDUs leaving the population (due to death or ceasing to inject) and with an influx of new persons beginning to inject drugs. Since HIV-infected IDUs are particularly likely to die from HIV-related illnesses, and since almost all persons will probably not be HIV-infected as of the time they start to inject drugs, an absence of new HIV-1 infections would lead to a declining HIV-1 seroprevalence in the IDU population over time.

Continuing Risk Behaviour

While behaviour change/risk reduction has probably been a very important factor in the stabilization of HIV-1 seroprevalence among IDUs in the WHO Study cities, this stabilization has not occurred through an elimination of all risk behaviour. Table 6.2 shows the percentage of IDUs in each city who reported any injecting with equipment that had been previously used by someone else (that is any receptive sharing) in the six months prior to the interview. While the determinants of the variation across cities in Table 6.2 have yet to be identified, it is clear that nothing close to complete risk elimination has occurred among IDUs in the WHO Study cities and that there is no direct relationship between any risky injections and current seroprevalence.

Estimated Seroconversions

What happens after HIV-1 seroprevalence reaches certain levels in an IDU population is another critical question for which the WHO Multi-City Study has provided important leads. Although the WHO Study was conducted as a cross-

Table 6.2 Number and percentage of injecting drug users who reported injecting with equipment previously used by someone else ('sharing') during the six months prior to interview

		Reported any sharing
Low seroprevalence cities:	Athens	197 (49%)
	Glasgow	215 (43%)
	Sydney	175 (42%)
	Toronto	198 (44%)
Medium seroprevalence cities:	Berlin	189 (50%)
	London	181 (34%)
	Rome	89 (19%)
High seroprevalence cities:	Bangkok	325 (54%)
	Madrid	208 (45%)
	New York	622 (44%)
	Rio de Janeiro	144 (30%)
	Santos	119 (55%)

Seroprevalence: low, under 5%; medium, 5–20%; high, over 20%

sectional behaviour and serostatus survey, it is possible to develop an estimate of HIV-1 seroconversion among the IDUs who participated in the study in the different cities. One of the questions in the survey asked whether the subject had previously been tested for HIV-1, and a follow-up question asked about the results of the most recent HIV-1 test.

Since blood or saliva samples were collected and tested as part of the WHO Multi-City Study, subjects who had previously been tested HIV-negative, and who were HIV-positive on the blood/saliva sample collected as part of the study itself, can be considered as possible HIV-1 seroconverters. In Bangkok, the records of the drug abuse treatment programmes were checked, and documentation was found of a previous seronegative test for all of the 17 persons who had both reported a previous negative test and who also had tested positive at the time of the WHO Multi-City Study (Des Jarlais *et al.*, 1994a). For New York City, the estimated seroconversion rates were compared by using the outcomes of this 'report of previous negative test' as measured against other estimates of HIV-1 seroconversion derived from two large cohort studies of IDUs in New York City. It was found that this method produces somewhat high, but still reasonably compatible estimates for HIV-1 seroconversion (Des Jarlais, unpublished data).

However, using this 'report of a previous negative test' method when comparing estimated seroconversions across different cities, clearly requires great caution, particularly in regard to the characteristics of previously tested IDUs, which may vary across cities. Also, the duration of time since the most recent negative test may differ, and the accuracy in the reports of previous tests may vary. Table 6.3 presents the number and percentage of previously tested subjects, the number and percentage of subjects with reported previous negative

Table 6.3 Seroconversion analysis based on previous self-reported negative HIV-1 test and positive HIV-1 test when surveyed

		Previously tested	Previously tested neg*	% Apparent seroconversion
Low seroprevalence cities:	Athens	220 (55%)	193 (98%)	0 (0.0%)
	Glasgow	270 (54%)	243 (98%)	0 (0.0%)
	Sydney	331 (81%)	296 (95%)	1 (0.3%)
	Toronto	327 (74%)	278 (95%)	5 (1.8%)
Medium seroprevalence cities:	Berlin	340 (90%)	284 (87%)	12 (4.4%)
	London	242 (47%)	194 (90%)	11 (6.0%)
	Rome	453 (94%)	323 (71%)	6 (4.8%)
High seroprevalence cities:	Bangkok	265 (44%)	174 (66%)	17 (9.8%)
	Madrid	331 (77%)	145 (49%)	16 (39.0%)
	New York	752 (51%)	288 (71%)	50 (29.8%)
	Rio de Janeiro	128 (27%)	94 (78%)	5 (9.4%)
	Santos	148 (68%)	50 (41%)	22 (45.8%)

Seroprevalence: low, under 5%; medium, 5–20%; high, over 20%
* Denominator for percentages is the number of people who were previously tested and who knew their HIV-1 test result.

tests, as well as the number and percentage of possible seroconverters (as a percentage of all persons with a reported previous negative test) in the various cities.

Despite the uncertainties in using this method of identifying possible HIV-1 seroconverters, there is a striking pattern in the findings. The cities for which data are available clearly fall into three clusters associated with the current HIV-1 seroprevalence in the cities. Low, medium and high seroprevalence cities have correspondingly low, medium and high seroconversion rates.

A strong relationship between background HIV-1 seroprevalence among IDUs and current HIV-1 seroconversion was also observed in a study of 15 US cities from 1988 to 1992. In that study, seroconversion rates in cities with seroprevalence below 10 per cent ranged from zero to 3.8 per 100 person-years at risk, while seroconversion rates in cities with seroprevalence above 20 per cent ranged from 3.7 to 8.1 per 100 person-years at risk (Friedman *et al.*, 1995).

Conclusions

The WHO Multi-City Study offers the first opportunity to systematically compare HIV-1 epidemics among IDUs in different areas, including comparison of epidemics in industrialized and developing countries. The WHO data show that a large percentage of IDUs in all study cities will change their behaviour in response to concerns about HIV and AIDS. This large-scale behaviour change has been followed by stabilization of HIV-1 seroprevalence in all cities for which data are available. The behaviour change is not, however, elimination of all risk behaviour. There appears to be a substantial residual level of risky injections among IDUs in all cities. New HIV-1 infections are a product not only of the frequency of risk behaviour of individual IDUs, but also of the likelihood that the risk behaviour will occur among IDUs with different HIV-1 status. Thus, in low HIV-1 seroprevalence cities, the residual risk behaviour appears to lead to very low numbers of new HIV-1 infections, while in moderate to high HIV-1 seroprevalence cities, the residual risk behaviour appears to lead to moderate to high numbers of new HIV-1 infections. The critical factor in control of HIV-1 epidemics among injecting drug users therefore, would seem to be initiating large-scale behaviour change/risk reduction while HIV-1 seroprevalence is still at very low levels.

References

CHITWOOD, D.D. (1994) 'Annotation: HIV risk and injection drug users — evidence for behavioural change', *American Journal of Public Health*, **84**, pp. 350.

CHOOPANYA, K., VANICHSENI, S., PLANGSRINGARM, K., SONCHAI, W., CARBALLO, M., FRIEDMANN, P., FRIEDMAN, S.R. and DES JARLAIS, D.C. (1991) 'Risk factors and HIV seropositivity among injecting drug users in Bangkok', *AIDS*, **5**, pp. 1509–13.

DES JARLAIS, D.C., FRIEDMAN, S.R., NOVICK, D., SOTHERAN, J.L., THOMAS, P., YANCO-VITZ, S., MILDVAN, D., WEBER, J., KREEK, M.J., MASLANSKY, R., BARTELME, S., SPIRA, T. and MARMOR, M. (1989) 'HIV-1 infection among intravenous drug users in Manhattan', *Journal of the American Medical Association*, **261**, pp. 1008–12.

DES JARLAIS, D.C., FRIEDMAN, S.R., CHOOPANYA, K., VANICHSENI, S. and WARD, T.P. (1992) 'International epidemiology of HIV and AIDS among injecting drug users', *AIDS*, **6**, pp. 1053–68.

DES JARLAIS, D.C., FRIEDMAN, S.R., SOTHERAN, J.L., WENSTON, J., CARBALLO, M., CHOOPANYA, K. and VANICHSENI, K. (1994a) 'Reliability and validity in cross-national research on AIDS risk behaviour among injecting drug users', in NICOLOSI, A. (Ed.) *HIV ELpidemiology: Models and Methods*, pp. 65–75, New York: Raven Press.

DES JARLAIS, D.C., CHOOPANYA, K., VANICHSENI, S., PLANGSRINGARM, K., SONCHAI, W., CARBALLO, M., FRIEDMAN, P. and FRIEDMAN, S.R. (1994b) 'AIDS risk reduction and reduced HIV seroconversion among injecting drug users in Bangkok', *American Journal of Public Health*, **84**, pp. 452–5.

DES JARLAIS, D.C., FRIEDMAN, S.R., SOTHERAN, J.L., WENSTON, J., MARMOR, M., YANCOVITZ, S.R., FRANK, B., BEATRICE, S. and MILDVAN, D. (1994c) 'Continuity and change within an HIV epidemic: Injecting drug users in New York City, 1984 through 1992', *Journal of the American Medical Association*, **271**, pp. 121–7.

DES JARLAIS, D.C., HAGAN, H., FRIEDMAN, S.R., FRIEDMANN, P., GOLDBERG, D., FRISCHER, M., GREEN, S., TUNVING, K., LJUNGBERG, B., WODAK, A., ROSS, M., PURCHASE, D., MILLSON, M.E. and MYERS, T. (1995a) 'Maintaining low HIV seroprevalence in populations of injecting drug users', *Journal of the American Medical Association*, **274**, pp. 1226–31.

DES JARLAIS, D.C., FRIEDMAN, S.R., FRIEDMANN, P., WENSTON, J., SOTHERAN, J.L.,

CHOOPANYA, K., VANICHSENI, S., RAKTHAM, S., GOLDBERG, D., FRISCHER, M., GREEN, S., LIMA, E.S., BASTOS, F.I. and TELLES, P.R. (1995b) 'HIV/AIDS-related behaviour change among injecting drug users in different national settings', *AIDS*, **9**, pp. 611–17.

FRIEDMAN, S.R. and DES JARLAIS, D.C. (1991) 'HIV among drug injectors: The epidemic and the response', *AIDS Care*, **3**, pp. 239–50.

FRIEDMAN, S.R., JOSE, B., DEREN, S., DES JARLAIS, D.C., NEAIGUS, A. and NATIONAL AIDS RESEARCH CONSORTIUM (1995) 'Risk factors for HIV seroconversion among out-of-treatment drug injectors in high- and low-seroprevalence cities', *American Journal of Epidemiology*, **142**, pp. 864–74.

FRISCHER, M., GREEN, S., GOLDBERG, D., HAW, S., BLOOR, M., McKEGANEY, N., TAYLOR, A., COVELL, R., GRUER, L., FOLLETT, E., KENNEDY, D. and EMSLIE, J. (1992) 'Estimates of HIV infection among injecting drug users in Glasgow from 1985–1990', *AIDS*, **6** (11), pp. 1371–5.

JOSE, B., FRIEDMAN, S.R., CURTIS, R. GRUND, J-P.C., GOLDSTEIN, M.F., WARD, T.P. and DES JARLAIS, D.C. (1993) 'Syringe-mediated drug-sharing (backloading): A new risk factor for HIV among injecting drug users', *AIDS*, **7**, pp. 1653–60.

KALDOR, J., ELFORD, J., WODAK, A., CROFTS, J.N. and KIDD, S. (1993) 'HIV prevalence among IDUs in Australia: A methodological review', *Drug and Alcohol Review*, **12**, pp. 175–84.

LIMA, E.S., FRIEDMAN, S.R., BASTOS, F.I., TELLES, P.R., FRIEDMANN, P., WARD, T.P. and DES JARLAIS, D.C. (1994) 'Risk factors for HIV-1 seroprevalence among drug injectors in the cocaine-using envrionment of Rio de Janeiro', *Addiction*, **89**, pp. 689–98.

MILLSON, P., MYERS, T., RANKIN, J., MAJOR, C., FEARON, M. and RIGBY, J. (1993) 'Trends in HIV seroprevalence and risk behaviour in IDUs in Toronto, Canada', Abstract PO–C15–2936, presented at the Ninth International Conference on AIDS, Berlin, Germany.

NAIK, T.N., SARKAR, S., SINGH, H.L., BHUNIA, S.C., SINGH, Y.I., SINGH, P.K. and PAL, S.C. (1991) 'Intravenous drug users — A new high-risk group for HIV infection in India', *AIDS*, **5**, pp. 117–18.

REARDON, J., WILSON, M.J., LEMP, G.F., GAUDINO, J.A., SNYDER, D., ELCOCK, M. and NGUYEN, S. (1992) 'HIV-1 infection among female injection drug users (IDU) in the San Francisco Bay Area, California 1989–1991', Abstract No. ThC 1553, presented at the Eighth International Conference on AIDS, Amsterdam, the Netherlands.

ROBERTSON, J.R., BUCKNALL, A.B.V., WELSBY, P.D., ROBERTS, J.J.K., INGLIS, J.M., PEUTHERER, J.F. and BRETTLE, R.P. (1986) 'Epidemic of AIDS-related virus (HTLV-III/LAV) infection among intravenous drug users', *British Medical Journal*, **292**, pp. 527–9.

ROSS, M.W., WODAK, A., GOLD, J. and MILLER, M.E. (1992) 'Differences across sexual orientation on HIV risk behaviours in injecting drug users', *AIDS Care*, **4**, pp. 139–48.

SIMONS, M. (1994) 'Drug floodgates open, inundating the Dutch', *New York Times*, 20 April, A4.

VANICHSENI, S. and SAKUNTANAGA, P. (1990) 'Results of three seroprevalence surveys for HIV in IVDU in Bangkok', Abstract No. F.C.105, presented at the Sixth International Conference on AIDS, San Francisco, CA.

WHO COLLABORATIVE STUDY GROUP (1993) 'An international comparative study of HIV prevalence and risk behaviour among drug injectors in 13 cities', *Bulletin on Narcotics*, **45**, pp. 19–46.

WRIGHT, N.H., VANICHSENI, S., AKARASEWI, P., WASI, C. and CHOOPANYA, K. (1994) 'Was the 1988 HIV epidemic among Bangkok's injecting drug users a common source outbreak?', *AIDS*, **8**, pp. 529–32.

Chapter 7

Mobility and the Diffusion of Drug Injecting and HIV Infection

Martin Frischer

The use of substances to achieve purely psychic effects is widespread in human societies. Throughout documented history there is evidence of drug cultivation, production and consumption around the world. The discovery of ever more efficient methods for producing drugs has enabled more widespread consumption.

The increase in contact between societies beginning with the European voyages of discovery from the fifteenth century onwards introduced new substances to different cultures, such as tobacco, which rapidly became widespread in Europe. Coca was produced in Peru and Bolivia many centuries before the Inca empire. During the Spanish conquest of the region, farming activity in the region increased and the coca trade rapidly expanded. Opium and hashish are thought to have originated in Asia and reached the American continent either through Europe or directly across the Pacific. During the twentieth century the flow of drugs from producer areas in the developing world to countries in the developed world has greatly increased and patterns of drug trafficking are continually expanding and diversifying (International Narcotics Control Board, 1995). However, there is also a considerable flow of psychoactive drugs in the other direction involving the commercial sale of alcohol products, tobacco, hypnosedatives, solvents and amphetamines.

This global diffusion of psychic substances is sometimes portrayed as an 'internationalization of drug addiction' (Berlinguer, 1992) on the grounds that effects are more harmful when drugs alien to local traditions are widely used. There are well-documented instances of this in the twentieth century, such as the introduction of alcohol to native Americans and Eskimos (Westmayer, 1992). However, the widespread introduction and use of opium in early nineteenth century Britain was not considered to be problematic, and excessive use was taken as evidence of an individual's bad habits (Stimson and Oppenheimer, 1982).

Prior to the twentieth century, the diffusion of drugs was primarily through importation and exportation. However, the massive increase in international travel, particularly since 1950, means that increasing numbers of people are being exposed to new diseases, as well as social practices and products, in comparison to previous eras. The supposition that an increase in international travel created the conditions for the global spread of disease has been well documented for HIV-1 (Hawkes *et al.*, 1994). While there has been considerable debate on the merits of considering drug use a 'disease', it can be argued that, at least to some extent, the diffusion of drug use can be modelled using concepts borrowed from epidemiology.

Individual and Geographical Diffusion of Drug Use

Hunt and Chambers (1976) consider that peer pressure is the common factor for explaining new and sustained patterns of drug use. For drug use to become established within a group, the theoretical simulations and empirical data presented in their book, *The heroin epidemics*, indicate that it is necessary to have a number of initiators coming into a social group. Single initiators are unlikely to facilitate substantial drug epidemics since each initiator has a fairly low probability of introducing new users, who in turn will initiate a still smaller number of individuals. Nevertheless, rapid growth of incidence (microdiffusion) is dependent on 'the new user and not the confirmed addict'.

De Alarcon (1969) reported that heroin injecting was introduced to Crawley, England, in the 1960s (Figure 7.1) by local youths who had acquired the habit while visiting or living in other towns. The link between the initiators and the initiated was either long-standing, such as schools and neighbourhoods, or more recent, for example drinking venues (pubs) and dance halls. Outsiders from neighbouring towns probably played a role either by bringing in supplies or accompanying Crawley youths to London and other locations. Thus the spread of new forms of drug use involves geographical mobility of a relatively small number of initiators and depends on the size and cohesion of their home community.

However, Hunt and Chambers (1976) note that while there is relative isolation among groups (for example young people in different cities), there nevertheless appears to have been, at least in the United States during the 1970s, a process of diffusion across the country. This phenomenon, which they call *macrodiffusion*, is a hierarchical process characterized by a tendency for peak incidence to occur in large cities and subsequently in progressively smaller cities and towns.

Hunt and Chambers argue that, although there is no obvious mechanism for macrodiffusion, this process is seen in many innovations, for example the spread of television stations in the United States between 1940 and 1965. It is difficult to evaluate this hypothesis with regard to drug use, because of the lack of reliable incidence and prevalence data.

Hunt and Chambers use data on peak use (from drug treatment pro- grammes) to map the diffusion of epidemics of heroin use in the late 1960s and early 1970s. This indicates that the first stage of the epidemic of US heroin use occurred on the north-east coast along the megalopolitan chain of cities from

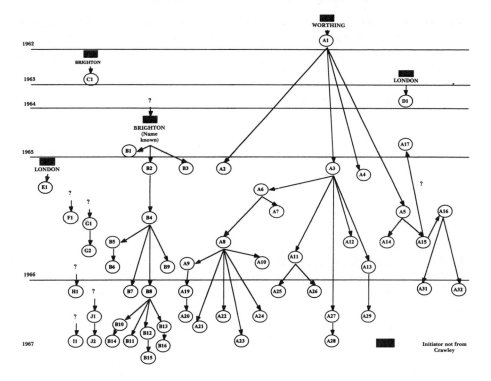

Figure 7.1 The spread of heroin use among 58 people living in Crawley, England, during 1967
Source: De Alarcon, 1969

Boston to Washington, and in southern California. Large inland and Gulf coast cities were also early centres of epidemic use. From these continental margins, heroin use seems to have moved to the interior, spreading sequentially from cities in regions of high population density to those of lower density. Other data suggest that the same principle holds true within states.

The concepts of micro- and macrodiffusion of drug use have not been developed or subjected to further empirical testing since the pioneering work of Hunt and Chambers. It is clear, however, that since the 1980s there has been a further type of diffusion, of an international character, which includes elements of micro- and macrodiffusion but which also has unique characteristics. One such characteristic is law enforcement activity which causes changes to trafficking routes. As the authorities in Iran, Pakistan and Turkey have tightened controls on their borders, traffickers have found it easier to transport illicit consignments of heroin and cannabis through the states of central Asia where border controls have been weakened since the disintegration of the Soviet Union. Local drug markets may be created along new routes, one reason being that with increased surveillance of money laundering in many parts of the developed world, traffickers have to establish local markets to realize their profits. The emergence of the former Soviet Central Asian republics as independent states with uncertain economic prospects could herald a massive expansion of drug cultivation in this region over the next few years.

The social and economic changes which have occurred since the mid-1980s are already reported to have been accompanied by rapid growth in illicit drug use and trafficking, especially in the European part of the former union (Lee, 1992). This phenomenon can be seen in terms of macrodiffusion, although there are insufficient data to map temporal and geographical trends within this region. While current demand is being met with supplies from within the former USSR, rapid expansion of trade, travel and economic ties could result in the former USSR participating, both as a consumer and supplier, in the international drugs market.

During 1994 many African states recorded increased seizures of illicit drugs and the arrest and prosecution of large numbers of persons for drug-related offences. Increasing use of heroin in Africa has been attributed to spillover of transit traffic from producer countries in south-east and south-west Asia (United Nations Economic and Social Council, 1995).

The important point is that the available data on micro- and macrodiffusion indicate that heroin epidemics are not indigenous, but dependent on a variety of economic, social and political factors. Diffusion also depends on individuals' predispositions to experiment with psychoactive substances. In Western Europe increasing levels of post-war drug use have been attributed to greater individualism and consumerism. Psychological factors also may play an important role due to the weakening of family relationships and lengthening periods of adolescence (Rutter and Smith, 1995).

Migration and Tourism

High levels of growth in international travel and, in some areas of the world, greater freedom of movement, have enabled drug users to migrate to, or visit, new areas. One of the best documented examples is that of Italian drug injectors moving to London in the late 1980s and early 1990s (Lipsedge, Dianin and Duckworth, 1993). The movement of over 1000 injectors in this period occurred as the Italian response to problems of harmful drug use and HIV was largely based on law enforcement and compulsory drug-free residential treatment. In contrast, during the same period, the UK emphasis was on harm reduction. However, interviews with Italian injectors in London (Table 7.1) revealed a variety of reasons for moving rather than a single major factor.

The majority of those questioned did not know how long they would remain in the UK and many respondents had come to London as part of a tour of several European countries. The overall socio-economic status of Italian injectors interviewed declined following migration to London as indexed by a 50 per cent increase in unemployment and substantial reductions in financial support from family of origin. Although Italian injectors may notionally move to London to avail themselves of harm reduction facilities, the outcome is often contrary to

Table 7.1 Factors influencing migration of Italian drug injectors to London (194 injectors interviewed in 1990, 1991)

Push Factors	Pull Factors
Unemployment	Hope of overcoming drug problems by change of environment
Family–housing–legal problems	Finding work and accommodation
Lack of treatment services and medical care	Opportunities for enjoyment
	To learn English

stated intentions. High levels of drug use, HIV risk behaviour and criminal activity were reported by the Italian migrants. Self-reported HIV-1 prevalence was 30 per cent compared to about 6 per cent among British injectors living in London.

Another, and very different, example of large-scale migration of drug users is the movement of recovering urban drug users from the New York City–Philadelphia corridor to the small town of Williamsport, Pennsylvania (Milofsky *et al.*, 1993). Extensive fieldwork indicated that by 1990 there were about 2000 mostly African-American recovering drug users and their relatives living among the 70 000 population. Between about 1982 and 1990 a variety of public and private service providers created a therapeutic environment with great appeal to urban drug users seeking to change their behaviour. The major factor in relocating to Williamsport seems to have been the 'good news' about the town passed on through 'interpersonal networks facilitated by membership in Alcoholics and Narcotics Anonymous'.

Local attitudes to these incomers have been predictably varied. While some officials have argued that the character of Williamsport will ultimately be destroyed by the town's hospitality, others have pointed to the integration of the incomers and the fact that there is little evidence to suggest that serious crime is increasing or that the quality of medical care is declining.

As with the Italian migrants to London, the vast majority of recovering drug users in Williamsport are not permanent incomers. Many 'recovery immigrants' stay only for a few months. A smaller number who flourish in the town stay on, often with their families. One of the main factors which facilitated the expansion of treatment provision in Williamsport was under-utilized low-cost housing. It seems likely that treatment provision will stabilize or decline as the availability of this type of housing is rapidly diminishing while other immigrants move to Williamsport from relatively close large conurbations.

Nowhere has the phenomenon of inward-migrant drug users been more prominent or received more attention than Amsterdam, capital city of the Netherlands. After World War Two, drugs were used in Amsterdam by such diverse groups as American sailors and jazz musicians from the Caribbean. However, the phenomenon became more widespread with the advent of youth tourism during the 1960s. The changing face of drug tourism in Amsterdam since then has been documented by Korf (1994). By the 1980s the assumption made by many authorities was that foreign drug users came to Amsterdam because of the city's liberal climate, low drug prices and methadone programmes.

However, in a study of 382 drug tourists conducted in 1985/6, the pull factors did not fully explain trends in heroin tourism. Most of the reasons given were not drug specific and as with the Italian injectors in London, many respondents had visited a number of European cities. The vast majority had a long history of drug use and on arriving in Amsterdam they tended to live among people of their own nationality or language. Overall, one-third were short-term visitors, almost two-thirds were long-term visitors and a small percentage visited Amsterdam six or more times per year.

From the mid-1980s, official policy has been to reduce the number of foreign heroin users in Amsterdam. Examples of this policy include the funding of an ecumenical agency which helped German drug users living in Amsterdam to return to their native cities and discouraged foreigners from participating in methadone programmes. However, because drug-pull factors are not the only, or even major, determinant of drug user tourism and migration, foreign heroin users continue to travel to cities such as Amsterdam and London.

Travel to Purchase Drugs

The 'coffee houses' of Amsterdam provide a rare example of a location where an illicit drug (cannabis) can be purchased without fear of prosecution. On the other hand, purchasing opiates and stimulants has become more difficult in Amsterdam, and German drug users are now more likely to visit towns close to the Dutch–German border to buy these drugs. Dutch heroin users in rural areas often buy small quantities of heroin in their home town and will travel greater distances for larger quantities, although they rarely go to Amsterdam unless there are good public transport connections (Korf *et al.*, 1990).

In Glasgow, Scotland, 210 young drug users were asked where they would go to buy different types of drugs in the city (Forsyth *et al.*, 1992). As with other consumer products, respondents indicated that they would travel further to buy more expensive drugs. Most drugs were reported to be available in areas characterized by social deprivation and there was a trend for drug consumers to travel from less deprived areas to purchase drugs. However, it has also been reported that being distant from an area where a desired drug is obtainable (for example heroin) could increase the likelihood of drug users switching to a substance more readily available locally (for example buprenorphine). MDMA, which was identified as the most expensive drug (per unit cost), did not fit this pattern as a high percentage of subjects purchased the drug in city centre nightclubs.

Transportation of drugs can also have an impact on transit countries where some drugs leak out to the local market (Hartnoll, 1989). For some drug users or drug couriers who are not themselves users, attempting to import drugs by internally concealing the drugs in packages within the body (body-packing), can have tragic consequences. Several countries have reported deaths among people attempting to import drugs in this way (Frischer, Green and Goldberg, 1994). Ramrahka and Barton (1993) draw attention to the particular dangers of using this method for smuggling cocaine.

The Role of Drug Injector Mobility in HIV/AIDS

Another aspect of drug users' mobility is the risk of importing and exporting infection, either through sharing of injecting equipment or sexual contact. A survey of 250 injectors recruited at a methadone clinic in Tel Aviv, Israel, during 1988/9, revealed that 2.6 per cent were HIV-1 positive (Dan *et al.*, 1992). There were no significant differences in mean age or duration of injecting between HIV positive and negative injectors, but the former were more likely to have injected abroad, particularly in North America and Western Europe. HIV-1 among injectors in Tel Aviv has remained low and stable since 1986 (2 per cent) and risk behaviours within Israel occur at fairly low rates. The authors conclude that 'most seropositive Israeli injectors continue to acquire their infection abroad'.

In Ohio, the HIV-1 prevalence rate among 855 injectors recruited in non-treatment settings during 1989/90 was 1.5 per cent (Seigal *et al.*, 1991). Research among this group indicated that variables typically associated with HIV infection in high seroprevalence areas, such as needle sharing and frequency of injection, had little predictive power. However, seropositive subjects were more likely to have travelled to north-eastern areas of the United States where HIV-1 is 'hyperendemic' among injectors. Similar findings have been reported among injectors from Michigan who visit high prevalence areas (Chandrasekar, Molinari and Kruse, 1990). An analysis of over 32 000 injectors in 60 US cities (Erickson, Stevens and Estrada, 1992) found that over 40 per cent reported injecting drugs and having sex in other cities (which were often AIDS epicentres).

In north-east Malaysia, 62 (30 per cent) out of 210 injectors recruited in detoxification wards in 1991/2 were HIV-1 positive (Singh and Crofts, 1993). One hundred and fifty-nine injectors had travelled to Thailand in the preceding five years, 32 per cent of whom were positive. Although 26 per cent of those who had not left Malaysia were also positive, the injector population is very mobile within the country. Those injectors who were residents of border towns had higher HIV-1 rates and the clear implication of this study is that HIV-1 infection is being imported from higher prevalence regions in Thailand.

In China, the introduction of heroin injection to local Chinese culture by visitors from Myanmar in the 1980s is thought to be the source of HIV-1 among injectors in south-west China (Zheng *et al.*, 1994).

In south-east Asia, diffusion across international borders has been associated with the microdiffusion of injecting as a new route of drug administration. The rapid increase of injecting with limited understanding of blood-borne transmission of infection has resulted in a number of HIV epidemics among drug injectors in this area (Poshyachinda, 1993). Geographical proximity and known migration patterns appear to have been responsible for epidemic spread in this region (Stimson, 1994). The first cases of HIV-1 among drug injectors in Bangkok were identified in 1987 and by early 1988, HIV-1 prevalence was around 30 per cent. In less than a year similar epidemic spread was repeated in southern Thailand and in northern Malaysia. By 1990, cases of HIV-1 among drug injectors were being reported in Singapore.

In a study undertaken in 1990/1, 1311 Puerto Rican injectors were interviewed in four north-eastern states in the USA and 1692 injectors in San Juan, the capital city of Puerto Rico. All groups reported substantial rates of HIV risk behaviour while visiting or staying in out-of-state locations (Colon *et al.*, 1993). The island group reported US coastal states as the most likely destinations. In each of the five sites, more than 50 per cent of those who travelled did so to one or more of the other four states. Geographical clustering into a small number of cities and frequent travel between these cities suggest intensive within-group interactions among this mobile population.

In these studies, it would appear that HIV-1 is being imported from high prevalence to low prevalence areas, although respondents were not asked about their risk behaviour outside their area of residence. This hypothesis strongly resembles the macrodiffusion hypothesis discussed above, although, while a drug epidemic requires a considerable influx of new users, a very small number of injectors importing HIV-1 may be sufficient to generate an HIV epidemic.

This hypothesis is supported by data from Edinburgh, Scotland. Of 379 injectors who received treatment in Edinburgh between 1985 and 1987, 101 (26 per cent) had shared needles and syringes in 140 locations outside the city (Jones *et al.*, 1988). One injector who had shared in Edinburgh and southern Europe was retrospectively found to have seroconverted in January 1983 soon after returning to Scotland. Furthermore, this person shared with other Edinburgh injectors who seroconverted later that year. The authors concluded that while 'it is unlikely that only one individual introduced the virus to Edinburgh . . . this information provides a mechanism to explain the unexpected pockets of HIV infection in northern Europe'.

This case study highlights the importance of obtaining travel histories from infected and uninfected injectors in order to understand HIV spread across geographical boundaries. Another source (cited in Gossop, 1992) reports that during 1982 a small family group of drug users from Edinburgh lived in Oxford where they shared injecting equipment with undergraduates and American air force personnel. The family returned to Edinburgh where they played an active part in the local drug scene. Two of the family were later found to be HIV-1 positive.

Of 113 heterosexual HIV-1 positive cases seen at St Thomas's Hospital in London to May 1991, 52 were injectors and 13 were contacts of injectors (Mitchell *et al.*, 1991). Forty to 65 of the cases were not born in the UK, although only four cases could be described as non-UK residents (that is intending to return home in three months). The authors conclude that foreign drug injectors make a substantial contribution to the UK figures for heterosexual transmission of HIV-1. However, in these cases it has not been suggested that foreign injectors are transmitting HIV-1 to indigenous injectors within the UK.

Other locations where mobility has been identified as an HIV risk factor among drug injectors are Portugal (Nossa *et al.*, 1993) and Italy (Rezza and Greco, 1987). In Brazil, the spread of drug use to indigenous peoples has been linked to the social and cultural degradation which has been caused by drug trafficking (Eluf, 1992). Unfortunately the role of drug injecting in transmitting HIV had not been clearly recognized in South America, and Libonatti *et al.* (1993) report that HIV prevalence among injectors increased rapidly in Brazil and Argentina during the late 1980s and early 1990s.

HIV Risk Behaviour: Comparative Data from 12 Cities

The topic of drug user mobility and HIV risk behaviour was addressed in the World Health Organization Multi-City Study on Drug Injecting and Risk of HIV Infection. In total, 6436 drug injectors were interviewed in 12 cities, of whom over 90 per cent were normally resident in the study locations (see Appendix 1 for study details). Respondents were asked 'Have you injected outside [the study area] in the last two years?' If the answer was affirmative, they were then asked 'Could you tell me all the different places where you have injected drugs?' Up to five locations were recorded. This procedure was then repeated for 'sharing needles and syringes'. (The study interview manual states that respondents should be informed that sharing in this context refers to sharing with people they met in these locations and *not* to fellow travellers.) Respondents were not questioned further about sharing events, for example with regard to frequency or cleaning of injecting equipment.

Table 7.2 shows that in nine of the 12 cities over 40 per cent of respondents reported out-of-city injecting and in Berlin and Sydney the proportion was over 60 per cent. Conversely, New York and Bangkok were the only cities where out-of-city injecting was reported by less than 30 per cent of respondents. In six of the 12 centres, over 10 per cent of respondents also reported out-of-city sharing. Both in absolute terms and as a proportion of out-of-city injecting, Santos, Brazil had the highest level of out-of-city sharing followed by Berlin, London, Rio de Janeiro, Sydney and Toronto. Low proportionate sharing rates were observed in Athens, Bangkok, Glasgow, Rome and New York.

Unfortunately the merged data set does not contain information on locations where injecting and sharing took place. However, analysis of locations visited by the injectors interviewed in Glasgow, Scotland (Goldberg *et al.*, 1994), reveals that a considerable number of respondents engaged in HIV risk behaviour in the UK cities of Edinburgh and London where HIV-1 prevalence is much higher than in Glasgow.

Table 7.3 shows the relationship between injecting and sharing outside the

Table 7.2 Proportion of respondents in the WHO Study reporting injecting, and sharing needles and syringes, outside study city in previous two years

Cities	Total n	Injecting %	Sharing %
Athens	(400)	59.3	6.7
Bangkok	(601)	22.9	4.8
Berlin	(380)	62.7	20.1
Glasgow	(503)	45.7	6.5
London	(534)	51.5	16.2
Madrid	(472)	50.6	7.8
New York	(1478)	12.7	3.1
Rio	(479)	37.8	9.6
Rome	(487)	44.7	5.6
Santos	(220)	48.2	25
Sydney	(424)	61.2	15.5
Toronto	(458)	47.7	14.6

Table 7.3 Injecting, and sharing needles and syringes, outside study city, by risk behaviour and selected attributes

	Behaviour out of the study city			
	Injected %	Not injected %	Shared %	Not shared %
Daily injector*	68.8	60.8	65.2	70.1
Sharing equipment*	46.9	38.8	77.4	37.4
Passing on equipment*	49	39.1	69.5	42.7
Sex with casual partners*	48.2	40.8	55	45.9
Previous HIV test	69.3	54.4	70.8	69.4
HIV positive	18.2	26.2	25.1	15.3
City usual residence	84.2	96.1	75.6	86.6

* = *during previous six months*

study area in the previous two years and current behaviour and attributes. Respondents who reported injecting outside the study area were significantly more likely (p<0.05) to be daily injectors, to inject with and pass on previously used equipment, and to have sex with casual partners, than those who did not inject outside the study area. They were more likely to have had a previous HIV-1 test but *less* likely to be HIV-1 positive. Out-of-city injectors were also less likely to be normally resident in the study area.

The findings with regard to sharing outside the study area were similar with two exceptions: there was no significant difference in terms of daily injecting or previous HIV test, and those who shared outside the study area were significantly *more* likely to be HIV positive compared to non-sharers.

The finding that injecting and sharing outside the study area are associated

Table 7.4 Proportion HIV-1 positive by injecting and equipment sharing outside of study area in the previous two years

Cities	n	HIV positive %			
		Injected outside the study area		Shared outside the study area	
		no	yes	no	yes
Athens	(400)	0	0.8	1.0	0
Bangkok	(601)	33.5	36.5	*29.3*	*58.6*
Berlin	(380)	*20.5*	*12.8*	*17.8*	*6.9*
Glasgow	(503)	1.2	2.4	2.2	3.6
London	(534)	11.7	14.1	*10.9*	*20.3*
Madrid	(472)	55.9	63.6	62.1	66.7
New York	(1478)	48.5	41.3	42.3	36.7
Rio	(479)	*24.0*	*48.2*	43.2	57.9
Rome	(487)	17.0	23.6	*18.8*	*43.8*
Santos	(220)	*54.6*	*71.7*	*58.8*	*78.2*
Sydney	(424)	1.2	2.3	2.8	1.5
Toronto	(458)	3.4	6.2	6.2	6.6
Total	(6436)				

Bold italicized figures indicate a significant difference in HIV-1 prevalence between injecting yes/no or sharing yes/no (p<.05)

with HIV-1 prevalence in different directions is explored in more detail in Table 7.4. The overall *negative* association between injecting and HIV-1 prevalence is primarily due to the large sample size in New York. In the two Brazilian cities, being HIV-1 positive was associated with out-of-city injecting. In these two cities, as well as in Bangkok and London, out-of-city sharing was associated with being HIV-1 positive, although in Berlin it was associated with being HIV-1 *negative*.

The potential for HIV-1 transmission is illustrated by further comparisons of some of the cities highlighted in Table 7.4. In Rio de Janeiro, HIV-1 prevalence among those injecting outside the city was 48 per cent compared to 24 per cent among those injecting only within the city. Significantly higher percentages of the former group also use (44 vs. 21 per cent) and pass on (41 vs. 14 per cent) previously used injecting equipment. In Bangkok, HIV-1 prevalence among those who shared equipment outside the city was 58 per cent compared to 28 per cent among those injecting only within the city. A significantly higher percentage of the former group reported current casual sex (47 vs. 18 per cent). In London, injectors who had shared outside the city had an HIV-1 prevalence rate of 20.3 per cent compared to 10.9 per cent of those only sharing within London. Only 67 per cent of the former group were London residents compared to 80 per cent of the latter group.

From the point of view of HIV prevention, these findings are discouraging since they indicate the existence of a large number of mobile drug injectors moving between areas with varying HIV-1 prevalence levels, and engaging in higher levels of 'at-home' risk behaviour than their less mobile peers who inject only within their home area.

Summary and Conclusions

The ever-increasing pace of social and cultural change provides opportunities for people to engage in diverse activities in new settings. In many areas of the world traditional patterns of drug use are being supplemented or replaced by new practices. The mechanisms of diffusion are diverse: introduction of new practices by a small number of new users, tourism and migration, cross-border contact, drug transportation, and increasing opportunities for economic and international contact.

Prior to the HIV/AIDS era, information on diffusion of drug use practices was scarce and the theoretical model developed by Hunt and Chambers has lain in abeyance since the 1970s. It would appear that the main problem is the lack of epidemiological data with which to test and refine the theory. With the coming of the HIV/AIDS epidemic, the situation has changed somewhat and there are an increasing number of drug prevalence studies carried out throughout the world. Several social and behavioural studies of drug users in the HIV/AIDS area have noted patterns of travel which could account for the importation of HIV from high prevalence to low prevalence areas. However, there has been almost no data comparing the risk behaviour of static and mobile injectors to enable assessment of their combined roles in the transmission of HIV-1.

The findings from the World Health Organization Multi-City Study on Drug Injecting and Risk of HIV Infection show that mobility is not equally distributed among those interviewed, but is relatively concentrated among higher risk injectors. Although there are now many reports of risk reduction by drug users around the world (Des Jarlais *et al.*, 1992), the activity of considerable numbers of injectors could be sufficient to ignite new epidemics in areas of low prevalence and maintain HIV-1 prevalence rates in areas where the majority of injectors are taking effective risk reduction measures.

The analogy between the spread of drug use and the spread of infection is now widely accepted, mainly because of HIV/AIDS and, as the WHO study shows, the two phenomena are often highly interrelated. While the study also highlighted the patterning of injectors' mobility, further work is needed to investigate the reasons for travel and the out-of-city contexts in which drug use takes place.

Acknowledgments

Thanks to Liz Moore for help in obtaining source material.

References

BERLINGUER, G. (1992) 'The interchange of disease and health between the old and new worlds', *American Journal of Public Health*, **82**, 10, pp. 1407–13.

CHANDRASEKAR, P.H., MOLINARI, J.A. and KRUSE, J.A. (1990) 'Risk factors for human immunodeficiency virus among parenteral drug abusers in a low prevalence area', *Southern Medical Journal*, **83**, 9, pp. 996–1001.

COLON, H., ROBLES, R., MATOS, T. and SAHAI H. (1993) 'HIV transmission and travel patterns of Puerto Rican drug injectors', *International Aids Conference*, **9**, 2, PO–C15–2958.

DAN, M., CHANA, A., FINTSI, Y. and BAR-SHANY, S. (1992) 'Human immunodeficiency virus infection among intravenous drug addicts in Israel; stable low prevalence over 34 months', *International Journal of Epidemiology*, **21**, 3, pp. 561–3.

DE ALARCON, R. (1969) 'The spread of heroin abuse in a community', *Bulletin of Narcotics*, **21**, pp. 17–22.

DES JARLAIS, D.C., FRIEDMAN, S.R., CHOOPANYA, K., VANICHSENI, S. and WARD, T.P. (1992) 'International epidemiology of HIV and AIDS among injecting drug users', *AIDS*, **6**, pp. 1053–68.

ELUF, L.N. (1992) 'Environment and narcotics trafficking in Brazil', *Bulletin of Narcotics*, **44**, 2, pp. 21–5.

ERICKSON, J.R., STEVENS, S. and ESTRADA, A. (1992) 'Risk for HIV among homeless male and female intravenous drug users in the United States', *International AIDS Conference*, PoC 4317.

FORSYTH, A.J.M., HAMMERSLEY, R.H., LAVELL, T.L. and MURRAY, K.J. (1992) 'Geographical aspects of scoring illegal drugs', *British Journal of Criminology*, **32**, 4, pp. 292–309.

FRISCHER, M., GREEN, S. and GOLDBERG, D. (1994) *Substance abuse related mortality: a worldwide review*, Vienna: United Nations International Drug Control Program.

GOLDBERG, D., FRISCHER, M., TAYLOR, A., GREEN, S., MCKEGANEY, N., BLOOR, M., REID, D. and COSSAR, J. (1994) 'Mobility of Scottish injecting drug users and risk of HIV infection', *European Journal of Epidemiology*, **10**, pp. 387–92.

GOSSOP, M. (1992) *Living with drugs*, England: Ashgate Press.

HARTNOLL, R. (1989) 'The international context', in MACGREGOR, S. (Ed.) *Drugs and British Solciety*, pp. 36–51, London: Routledge.

HAWKES, S., HART, G.J., JOHNSON, A.M., SHERGOLD, C., ROSS, E., HERBERT, K.M., MORTIMER, P., PARRY, J.V. and MABEY, D. (1994) 'Risk behaviour and HIV prevalence in international travellers', *AIDS*, **8**, pp. 247–52.

HUNT, L.G. and CHAMBERS, C.D. (1976) *The heroin epidemics*, New York: Spectrum Publications.

INTERNATIONAL NARCOTICS CONTROL BOARD (1995). *Report of the International Narcotics Control Board for 1994*, Vienna: United Nations.

JONES, G., DAVIDSON, J., BISSET, C. and BRETTLE, R. (1988) 'Mobility of injecting drug users as a means of spread for the human immunodeficiency virus', *ANSWER (AIDS News Supplement, CDS Weekly Report)*, A76, pp. 1–4.

KORF, D.J. (1994) 'Drug tourists and drug refugees', in OEUW, E. and MARSHALL, I.H. (Eds) *Between prohibition and legalization: the Dutch experiment in drug policy*, Amsterdam: Kugler Publications.

KORF, D.J., VAN AALDEREN, H., HOOGENHOUT, H.P. and SANDWIJK, J.P. (1990) *Gooise Geneugten*, Amsterdam: SPCP.

LEE, R.W. (1992) 'Dynamics of the Soviet illicit drug market', *Crime, Law and Social Change*, **17**, 3, pp. 177–233.

LIBONATTI, O., LIMA, E., PERUGA, A., GONZALEZ, R. and ZACARIAS, F. (1993) 'Role of drug injection in the spread of HIV in Argentina and Brazil', *International Journal of STD and AIDS*, **4**, 3, pp. 135–41.

LIPSEDGE, M., DIANIN, G. and DUCKWORTH, E. (1993) 'A preliminary survey of Italian intravenous heroin users in London', *Addiction*, **88**, 11, pp. 1565–72.

MILOFSKY, C., BUTTO, A., GROSS, M. and BAUMOHL, J. (1993) 'Small town in mass society: Substance abuse treatment and urban-rural migration', *Contemporary Drug Problems*, **20**, 3, pp. 433–70.

MITCHELL, S., BAND, B., BRADBEER, C. and BARLOW, D. (1991) 'Imported heterosexual HIV infection in London', *British Medical Journal*, **337**, pp. 1614–15.

NOSSA, P., CRUZ, M., POMBO, V., CRAVIDAO, R.C. and SILVESTRE, A. (1993) 'Social behaviour and mobility of HIV patients', *International AIDS Conference*, P0–C31–3305.

POSHYACHINDA, V. (1993) 'Drugs and AIDS in south-east Asia', *Forensic Science International*, **62**, (1–2), pp. 15–28.

RAMRAKHA, P.S. and BARTON, I. (1993) 'Drug smugglers' delirium: suspect cocaine intoxication in travellers with fever and bizarre mental states', *British Medical Journal*, **306**, pp. 470–1.

REZZA, G. and GRECO, D. (1987) 'Drug addicts, homosexual males and international travel', *AIDS*, **1**, 3, p. 191.

RUTTER, M. and SMITH, D. (1995) *Psychosocial disorders in young people*, London: Academia Europaea.

SIEGAL, H.A., CARLSON, R.G., FALCK, R., LI, L., FORNEY, M.A., RAPP, R.C., BAUMGARTEN, K., MYERS, W. and NELSON, M. (1991) 'HIV infection and risk behaviours among intravenous drug users in low seroprevalence areas in the midwest', *American Journal of Public Health*, **81**, 12, pp. 1642–4.

SINGH, S. and CROFTS, N. (1993) 'HIV infection among injecting drug users in north-east Malaysia', *AIDS Care: Psychological and socio-medical aspects of AIDS/HIV*, **5**, 3, pp. 273–81.

STIMSON, G.V. (1994) 'Reconstruction of subregional diffusion of HIV infection among drug injectors on southeast Asia: implications for early intervention', *AIDS*, **8**, 11, pp. 1630–2.

STIMSON, G.V. and OPPENHEIMER, E. (1982) *Heroin addiction: treatment and control in Britain*, London: Tavistock Publications.

UNITED NATIONS ECONOMIC AND SOCIAL COUNCIL (1995) *Illicit drug traffic and supply, including reports from subsidiary bodies and evaluation of their activities*, Vienna: United Nations.

WESTMAYER, J. (1992) 'Cultural perspectives: native Americans, Asians and new immigrants', in LOWINSON, J.H., RUIZ, P., MILLMAN, R.B. and LANGROD, J.G. (Eds) *Substance abuse: a comprehensive textbook*, Baltimore: Williams & Wilkins.

ZHENG, X., TIAN, C., CHOI, K.H., ZHANG, J., CHENG, H., YANG, X., LI, D., LIN, J., QU, S., SUN, X., HALL, T., MANDEL, J. and HEARST, N. (1994) 'Injecting drug use and HIV infection in southwest China', *AIDS*, **8**, 2, pp. 1141–7.

Chapter 8

Modelling the HIV-1 and AIDS Epidemic among Drug Injectors

Carlo A. Perucci, Damiano Abeni, Massimo Arcà, Marina Davoli and Andrea Pugliese

The use of mathematical models in the analysis of the spread of infectious diseases goes back to pioneering works by Ross (1911) and by Kermack and McKendrick (1927), and has developed into a very rich body of theories and applications, as shown for instance in the monographs by Bailey (1975) and Anderson and May (1991). The goals of mathematical modelling may be very diverse: Hethcote and Van Ark (1992) list fifteen purposes, and three limitations, of epidemiological modelling. At one extreme, one may study simple and general models in order to identify the main mechanisms that underlie the epidemic dynamics, and to define concepts and quantities, such as the 'basic reproductive ratio' (Diekmann, Heesterbeek and Metz, 1990), that crucially determine the final outcome of an epidemic. At the other extreme, one may build a very detailed model for the spread of a specific disease in a specific population in order to predict accurately the future trends.

The literature on models for the transmission dynamics of HIV-1 is very rich, certainly more than for any other infectious disease. Various transmission routes have been considered in these models, either in isolation or within integrated frameworks: these include sexual transmission among homosexual men, heterosexual transmission, parenteral transmission among drug injectors through needle sharing, and mother-to-newborn transmission. We refer readers to Castillo-Chavez (1989) and Gupta, Anderson and May (1993) for a survey of models and to Hethcote and Van Ark (1992) for a study of HIV-1 transmission in the United States, in which transmission among different risk groups and spatial scales are integrated. We have to note, however, that, with a few exceptions, discussed below, modellers have neglected HIV-1 transmission among drug injectors.

In this chapter, we stress two aims of mathematical modelling. The first is to identify and to quantify the importance of the main routes through which the spread of HIV-1 infections are likely to have occurred and to occur in the near future; the second aim is to perform 'thought experiments' on possible or conceivable control programmes. Our choice of the models used to study the

HIV-1 epidemic among drug injectors, and from them to other groups, has been guided by these aims.

How can a model be built to answer these questions? First of all, one has to decide whether one needs to consider HIV-1 transmission among the total population, or whether one can restrict consideration to drug injectors; the answer can only be pragmatic. In our case, we have chosen to disregard sexual transmission among homosexual men, due to the limited number of AIDS cases among homosexual men in Italy, but to consider heterosexual transmission of HIV-1 infection.

Then, there are several choices for the mathematical representation of the population. We will stay within the framework of 'compartmental models' in which the total population is divided into a number (usually small) of discrete categories, which relate to the social and behavioural status of the individuals as well as to the disease status (for example susceptible, infectious, infected but not infectious, immune). There is a trade-off in the number of compartments in such a model: too few compartments may disregard important heterogeneities of the populations; too many compartments will cause an explosion in the number of parameters to be estimated. Moreover, there will be so few individuals in any compartment that any trend will be overwhelmed by statistical fluctuations.

Finally, there are choices in the representation of the epidemic dynamics. For instance, to discuss HIV-1 transmission among drug injectors, Kaplan (1989) emphasizes the role of needles as disease vectors; Capasso et al. (in press) consider needle sharing groups. Our choice, as in Blower et al. (1991) and Iannelli et al. (1992), has been to neglect the peculiarities of parenteral transmission, and to model HIV-1 transmission through needle-sharing using the 'mass-action law' usual in epidemic disease modelling.

Once the model, as a tool, has been devised, one must assign parameter values, and initial values of the state variables. These can be obtained either from independent observations, or from fitting the model to observed data. Clearly, the 'validation' of a model against observational evidence is more satisfactory if one has obtained independent parameter estimates than if the parameter values have been estimated from the same observations. On the other hand, a model can be used just to obtain estimates of parameters that could otherwise be very difficult to obtain; for instance, the number of sexual partners of an 'average' individual might be more accurately estimated from data on disease spread than from interview reports, where several biases may occur.

As stated above, most choices in modelling will be pragmatic, guided by available observational evidence. The results of a model must then be checked against appropriate observations. Of course, one must keep in mind that what we call 'observations' are also based on models and assumptions; for instance, 'data' on AIDS cases include corrections for reporting delays, under-reporting, and so on; 'data' on HIV-1 infection depend on many more assumptions.

Despite all the more or less arbitrary choices involved in model building, and the inherent limitations, we believe that HIV-1 transmission models can give public health decision-makers important clues for setting intervention priorities and allocating resources.

Models of HIV-1 Transmission among Drug Injectors

As reported elsewhere in this book, significant prevalence levels of HIV-1 infection among drug injectors have been reported in many countries in which this behaviour has been identified. This characterizes drug injectors as a 'core group' in the AIDS epidemic. The observed values of HIV-1 prevalence range widely, with significant differences often arising, even at the regional level. Although these differences can be ascribed, in most cases, to different behavioural patterns and/or different drug policies, in some instances they remain unexplained.

Transmission of HIV-1 among drug injectors can occur either through the sharing of the injecting equipment, which we will refer to as 'needle sharing', or through sexual activity. Drug injectors can share needles in shooting galleries (that is with strangers), in groups (of three or more), with a friend (who may or may not be also a sexual partner). Sexual activity can be homosexual or heterosexual and it includes regular partnerships, casual contacts, and prostitution (sex for money, drugs, or other goods). The interweaving of these behaviours, which usually occur concurrently, creates a rather complex transmission dynamic, where different modelling options are possible.

Kaplan (1989) developed and analyzed a mathematical model of HIV-1 transmission among drug injectors through the use of shared needles in shooting galleries. He used this model to investigate the impact on the epidemic dynamics of the sharers-to-needle ratio, heterogeneous sharing rates, and frequency of using bleach to decontaminate syringes. In Kaplan's words, 'the model demonstrated that policies such as the distribution of cleansing solutions and/or injection equipment among drug addicts could slow or stop intravenous transmission of HIV-1 in shooting galleries'. More recently, using the same model framework and data from the New Haven, Connecticut, legal Needle Exchange Program, Kaplan was able to estimate the infectivity of a single contaminated syringe (Kaplan and Heimer, 1992) and to credit the programme implementation with a significant decrease in HIV-1 prevalence among New Haven drug addicts (Kaplan and Heimer, 1994).

Capasso *et al.* (in press) adapted the Kaplan 'needles that kill' model to the Italian situation where, although needle sharing among drug injectors played (and still plays) a crucial role in the transmission dynamics of HIV-1, shooting galleries do not exist. In his representation, Capasso substituted shooting galleries with sharing groups, and assumed grouping to occur according to a Poisson process, with a Poisson-distributed group size. Published work includes qualitative analysis of the model equations, while parameter estimation and model validation, mainly based on data collected in the Northern Italian Seronegative Drug Addicts study (Rezza *et al.*, 1994), are still in progress.

A different approach to modelling the transmission of HIV-1 among drug injectors has been adopted by Iannelli *et al.* (1992). On one hand, they chose to summarize the whole needle sharing process in a single parameter, the contact rate, to be interpreted as the mean number of drug injectors a susceptible drug injector borrows needles from, in a time unit. On the other hand, their model takes into account explicitly the time elasped since the moment of infection, and allows the individual's infectiousness to depend on it. Checking the model solutions against the data on AIDS incidence among drug users in Lazio (Italy), Iannelli *et al.* (1992) evaluated the effect of including in the representation the heterogeneity in contact rates, reduction in contact rates through time, delayed progression to AIDS and reduced infectiousness as effects of systematic therapy, and heterosexual transmission of HIV-1 among drug injectors.

Multi-population Models of the Transmission Dynamics of HIV-1 that include Drug Injectors as a Subgroup

The sexual interaction between drug injectors and those who do not inject drugs is substantial. This is mainly due to three factors. First, the large majority of drug users are at a sexually active age; second, the male-to-female ratio among drug users is usually much greater than one (in Italy it is estimated to be between four and five) so it follows that male drug injectors are bound to find most of their sexual partners among non-drug-using females; third, prostitution (sex for money, drugs, or other goods) is fairly common among female drug injectors. Consequently, although needle sharing and sexual contact between drug users account for nearly all the HIV-1 infections among drug injectors, in most countries outside Africa the majority of new infections in heterosexuals (of both sexes) can be ascribed to sexual contact with infected drug injectors.

Mathematical modelling can help in studying the characteristics of this interaction and its effects on the transmission dynamics of HIV. Published work includes analyses based on different approaches (Williams and Anderson, 1994; Blower *et al.*, 1991; Van Druten *et al.*, 1990; Arcà, Spadea and Perucci, 1992; Stigum *et al.*, 1991). The authors of these studies conclude that every prediction made on the basis of the available information on behaviours and mixing patterns remains largely imprecise, and they recommend better data collection.

A Model of the Transmission Dynamics of HIV-1 in Lazio, Italy

In Italy, as in most industrialized countries, data from AIDS surveillance systems (Centro Operativo AIDS, 1995) document a steady increase in the number of newly diagnosed people with AIDS who report heterosexual contact as the transmission route. Although in many cases information on the risk category of the infected partner is missing, sexual contact with a partner who injects, or used to inject, drugs is overall the most frequently reported exposure (59 per cent among females and 24 per cent among males), exceeded, among males, by sexual contact with sex workers (43 per cent of male heterosexual cases). Females reporting sex with bisexual partners, as well as reports of contact with partners from endemic areas, such as Sub-Saharan Africa, are much less frequent (2 per cent and 1 per cent, respectively).

Individual data on newly diagnosed HIV-1 infections have been collected in Lazio, the region of central Italy which surrounds and includes Rome, for a decade (Brancato *et al.*, 1997). Despite their limited validity with respect to assessment of exposure, these data confirm the growing trend for new cases of HIV-1 attributable to heterosexual transmission. It is not immediately clear, however, how closely this 'heterosexual epidemic' relates to the transmission dynamics of HIV-1 among drug injectors. Thus, it is of interest to estimate the proportion of heterosexually transmitted infections due to 'direct contact' with a drug injector, and to assess the plausibility of a large viral spread among non-drug-injecting heterosexuals. Such estimates may help to quantify the potential effect of behavioural changes among drug injectors and to compare this effect with the effect of a generalized change in sexual behaviours. In a recent paper, Arcà, Spadea and Perucci (1992) have given qualitative insights into some of these questions, based on the analysis of a mathematical model of the transmission dynamics of HIV-1 in Italy. They conclude that 'the occurrence of a purely heterosexual epidemic seems unlikely' and that 'the role of IDUs as an infection reservoir will continue to be substantial'.

In order to move towards more quantitative results, we made some changes in the structure of Arcà's mathematical model, which thereafter we will refer to as *StMe8*. Below, we summarize the main features of this modified model:

1 The model considers the population aged 15 to 44 years, stratified in four groups with respect to sex (male/female) and injecting drug use (yes/no). In this model, HIV-1 can be transmitted either through needle sharing among drug injectors or through heterosexual contact; given the epidemiological situation in Italy, and for the sake of simplicity, the model does not consider homosexual transmission.

2 We do not represent the early stage of the epidemic, and set the starting point for all the numerical simulations at 1 January 1991. This choice exempts us from taking into account the behavioural changes that occurred before this date, in response to the emergence of the AIDS epidemic, or independently from it. The 1991 starting point provides an 'initial scenario', which includes the estimated prevalence of HIV-1 in each of the interacting groups, and thus becomes an important determinant of the model solutions.

3 In drawing the initial scenario, we make large use of the results of the survey of 487 drug injectors, carried out in Rome in 1990 within the framework of the WHO Multi-City Study of Drug Injecting and HIV Infection. As

detailed below, drug users are stratified with respect to their behaviours (needle sharing and prostitution), and many parameters describing these behaviours are estimated.

4 We use the available evidence from observational studies to estimate the parameters describing the distribution of sexual behaviours among non-drug-injecting heterosexuals (D'Arcangelo, Marasca and Vitiello, 1990), the probability of transmitting HIV-1 associated with various behaviours (Jewell and Shiboski, 1990; Kaplan and Heimer, 1992), and the distribution of the incubation period (defined as the period between infection with HIV-1 and the onset of severe symptoms leading to AIDS diagnosis) (Longini *et al.*, 1989; Mariotto *et al.*, 1992).

5 The number of prevalent cases of HIV-1 in Lazio as of 1 January 1991, overall and with respect to the main groups considered in the model, is estimated from data from the regional surveillance system, carried out by the Osservatorio Epidemiologico since 1985 (Brancato *et al.*, 1997).

Survey Data and Model Parameters

The first task, in building the initial scenario, is to estimate the total number of drug injectors and, among them, the male-to-female ratio. The application of different estimation techniques, such as the mark-recapture method and the multiplier formula, to the incomplete data at hand (deaths due to overdose, drug users who refer to treatment centres, police reports) suggests a significant increase in the prevalence of drug use in Lazio in the years around 1990, especially among males (Perucci *et al.*, 1994). On the basis of these results, we have increased the estimate of just under 15 000 regular injectors, used in *StMe8* for the early 1980s (at the beginning of the virus spread) to a more realistic value of 25 000 as of 1 January 1991. Moreover, we have increased the male-to-female ratio from 3.5 to 4.8. The resulting HIV-1 prevalence rates among injectors are 20 per cent among males and 33 per cent among females.

The survey of drug injectors is not based on a probabilistic sample of its target population. By comparing the data on the interviewed injecting drug users (IDUs) with the information they provided on other IDUs they knew, we concluded that those IDUs not in touch with treatment centres were under-represented in the survey. In fact, 19 per cent of those interviewed, irrespective of sex, reported not having had treatment in the year before the interview, while 26 per cent of nominated males and 34 per cent of nominated females were reported as not receiving treatment in the same period. Since drug injectors who had been treated in the year before the interview reported behaviours associated with HIV-1 transmission more frequently than others, we used the percentages above to compute weighted estimates of the behavioural parameters. For example, in estimating the proportion of female drug injectors who had shared needles in the six months before the interview, we combined the values of 0.52 among treated and 0.33 among non-treated IDUs, to obtain:

$$P_{sha-f} = 0.52 * 0.66 + 0.33 * 0.34 = 0.46$$

The weighted estimate is slightly lower than the proportion of females who shared needles (0.48) observed in the sample as a whole. Using the same technique, we estimated other parameters of IDUs' behaviours, relevant to the transmission dynamics of HIV. These are summarized in Table 8.1:

On the basis of the above data, we stratified male IDUs into two subgroups, according to needle sharing status, and female IDUs into four groups, according to needle sharing and prostitution status.

From self-reported data on HIV-1 status, validated by immune-enzymatic tests of saliva specimens in a sub-sample of 124 IDUs, we derived the relative rates of HIV-1 prevalence associated with needle sharing (RR=2 among males, RR=2.5 among females) and prostitution (RR=2.4), and used these ratios to estimate the initial HIV-1 prevalence in the six IDU subgroups.

In Rome, the survey of IDUs' behaviours was repeated in 1992 (and again in 1995, data under process), using the same methods as in 1990. Data collected suggest a significant reduction in needle sharing, particularly by IDUs who knew they were infected, and a possible decrease in the number of females IDUs who are given money, goods or drugs for sex. No evidence of change was found with respect to sexual activity (rate of partner change, proportion of non-drug-using partners, condom use) (Davoli *et al.*, 1995). We introduced these elements in the model by allowing the relevant parameters to decrease in the first two

Table 8.1 Behavioural parameters of IDUs in Rome estimated from the WHO Multi-City Study results

	male	female
Needle sharing		
Proportion of needle sharers (lenders and/or borrowers)	.33	.46
Rate of sharing partner change (average number of		
different people sharers borrow needles from, per year)	2.64	3.47
Average number of borrowings per sharing partnership	18	23
Proportion of borrowed needles which are cleaned	.3	.3
Sexual behaviour		
Rate of sexual partner change (per year, including		
primary and casual, excluding prostitution)	2.68	2.06
Proportion of sexual partners who do not inject drugs	.8	.5
Frequency of condom use by HIV-negative	.2	.2
Frequency of condom use by HIV-positive	.46	.46
Prostitution (females)		
Proportion of female IDUs who are given money, goods		
or drugs for sex		.31
Average number of clients they have sex with, per year		750
Frequency of condom use with clients		.99

years as an effect of both 'old' IDUs improving their behaviours and 'new' IDUs being less prone to sharing.

As for non-drug-injecting heterosexuals (NDIH), prevalence rates of HIV-1 as of 1 January 1991, estimated from surveillance data, are 0.8 per thousand among males and 1.3 per thousand among females. In the model, both sexes are stratified with respect to the rate of sexual partner change, based on data collected in a probabilistic sample of the Italian population aged 18 to 30 years (D'Arcangelo, Marasca and Vitiello, 1990), and the relative rate of HIV-1 prevalence associated with high sexual activity is assumed to equal, in each sex, the relative rate of partner change.

We derived data on entries in the study population (people reaching the age of 15 and immigration) and exits from it (people reaching the age of 45, deaths and emigrations) from the official vital statistics. We assumed a tenfold increase in mortality among male IDUs and a twenty-fold increase among female IDUs, in agreement with the results of a cohort study of Rome IDUs (Perucci *et al.*, 1991). We did not allow for further increases in the total number of IDUs after 1991 and assumed a 2 per cent turnover between IDUs and NDIHs every year.

As for mixing patterns (Arcà, Spadea and Perucci, 1992), we assume proportionality with respect to needle exchange and a 'preference' of low-sex-activity heterosexuals for establishing partnerships with their like. The Jewell and Shiboski (1990) estimates of the probability of transmitting HIV-1 through sexual contacts, and the Kaplan and Heimer (1992) estimate of the infectivity from a used needle were used. In the model, the distribution of the incubation period from HIV to AIDS diagnosis is a generalized Gamma (median = 10 years and mean = 12 years), obtained by partitioning the 'infected' compartment in three sub-compartments and assuming constant rates of transition out of each of them.

Results of Basic Simulations

By submitting the described set of parameters to the transmission model, and assuming them to drive the epidemic dynamics up to the year 2000, we obtained the projected incidence and prevalence trends displayed in Figures 8.1 and 8.2. We found that the number of incident cases of HIV-1 among IDUs will continue to decline, as a result of both the saturation of the high risk subgroups and the persistence of the changes introduced in the behavioural parameters.

The predicted number of incident cases of HIV-1 among NDIHs was higher, from the beginning and especially among females, than was expected on the basis of surveillance data, suggesting the presence of many undetected infections. In fact, although the model predicted this variable to reach a plateau in 1993 and then to decline slowly, the number of newly diagnosed HIV-1 cases actually kept rising in both sexes during 1994 and 1995.

The decrease in prevalence of HIV-1 infection among IDUs (Figure 8.2) predicted from 1993 is more than balanced by the increase predicted among non-

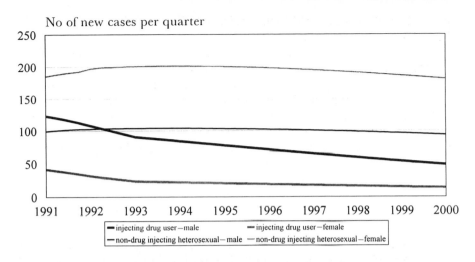

Figure 8.1   Incident cases of HIV-1 infection, by group

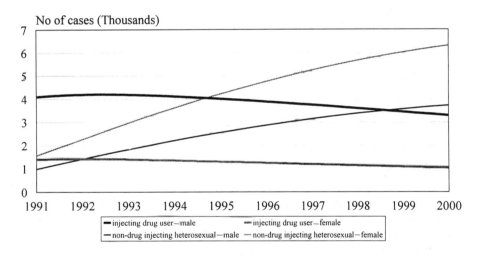

Figure 8.2   Prevalent cases of HIV-1 infection, by group

drug-injecting heterosexuals where, by the year 2000, prevalence rates reach the values of 3.3 per thousand in males and 5.5 per thousand in females. Also by the year 2000, the total number of prevalent cases of HIV-1 grows to 14 352, and only 30 per cent of these are IDUs.

In Table 8.2 the model results are arranged in a different way. The predicted total number of HIV-1 infections transmitted in the first two years (1991 and 1992) are classified with respect to affected group and transmission

Table 8.2 Predicted new HIV-1 infections in 1991 and 1992 by group and transmission route

| Transmission route | Drug injectors | | | | Non-drug-injecting heterosexuals | | | |
| | male | | female | | male | | female | |
	n	%	n	%	n	%	n	%
Needle sharing	(781)	89	(164)	62	–	–	–	–
Sex with an IDU	(79)	9	(90)	34	(74)	9	(1270)	82
Sex with a NDIH	(9)	1	(3)	1	(212)	26	(279)	18
Sex for money	(9)	1	(8)	3	(531)	65	–	–
Total	(878)		(265)		(817)		(1549)	

IDU = Injecting drug user
NDIH = Non-drug-injecting heterosexual

route. This can be needle sharing (for IDUs only), sex with an IDU, sex with an NDIH, and sex for money (for female IDUs and both IDU and NDIH males).

In the simulated transmission dynamics, 89 per cent of the infections acquired by male IDUs and 62 per cent of those acquired by female IDUs are attributable to needle sharing. Among female IDUs, one incident case out of three is due to sexual contact with an IDU partner. Sex with IDU partners accounts for more than 80 per cent of the HIV-1 incidence among non-drug-injecting females and sex for money with female IDUs accounts for two-thirds of the infections acquired by non-drug-injecting males. Overall, 27 per cent of new infections are acquired through needle sharing, and 73 per cent sexually. Of these, four out of five are transmitted by people who currently inject drugs.

Comparing the Likely Effects of Different Prevention Strategies

The results of the basic simulations support the hypothesis that in countries like Italy, where HIV-1 infection is highly prevalent among IDUs, heterosexual contact is currently the commonest route of transmission. Needle sharing, although significantly reduced, is still likely to cause several hundreds of new infections every year. Among non-drug-injecting heterosexuals, females are at higher risk than males, because of both the high male-to-female ratio among IDUs, and the different probabilities of transmission. At the same time, prostitution among female IDUs is a strong determinant of new infections among non-drug-injecting males.

In such a setting, what kind of prevention strategy is likely to give the best cost/effectiveness ratio? We tried to answer this question by using mathematical modelling as a tool for conducting 'thought experiments'. First, we modified the model parameters to simulate the effects of a 'harm reduction' strategy, focused on IDUs' behaviours. We assumed that, starting from 1 January 1993:

(a) 20 per cent of those who inject drugs stopped injecting;

(b) 20 per cent of female IDUs who have sex for money, goods or drugs stopped doing so;

(c) both needle sharing partner rates and mean number of sharing per partnership decreased by 30 per cent;

(d) in the remaining needle sharings, bleach use increased from 30 to 60 per cent; and

(e) condoms were used in 60 per cent of the intercourses which involved one (or two) IDUs.

Behavioural changes (a) and (b) could be achieved as an effect of controlled administration of substances such as methadone; needle exchange programmes and free availability of cleansing kits could result in changes described in (c) and (d). Programmes based on outreach strategies, effective counselling, and free of charge condom distribution, are required to achieve objective (e).

Figures 8.3 and 8.4 illustrate the predicted effect of this harm reduction programme on HIV-1 prevalence in the four groups considered. Two comments are worthy: first, no prevention is possible for those who are already infected; even assuming no incident HIV-1 cases after 1 January 1993, we should expect more than 5000 prevalent cases as of the end of 1999; the proposed programme would prevent 31 per cent of the 14 000 preventable cases. Second, even though no behavioural changes are explicitly assumed among non-drug-injecting heterosexuals, the programme effects are larger in this group than among drug injectors.

The quantitative impact of the simulated programme on IDUs' behaviours is summarized below:

(a) 1098 drug injectors should stop injecting;

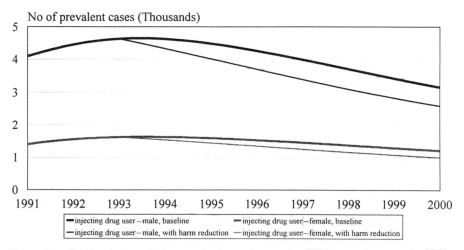

No of prevalent cases (Thousands)

- injecting drug user—male, baseline
- injecting drug user—female, baseline
- injecting drug user—male, with harm reduction
- injecting drug user—female, with harm reduction

Figure 8.3 Predicted effect of a harm reduction programme on HIV-1 prevalence among IDUs

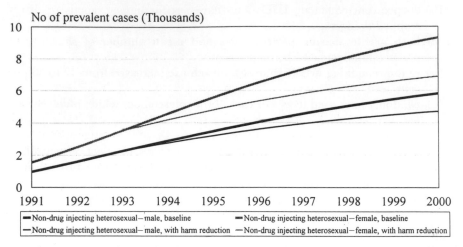

Figure 8.4 Predicted effect of a harm reduction programme on HIV-1 prevalence among NDIHs

(b) 186 drug injecting women should cease to have sex for money, goods or drugs; with (a) and (b), the new parameter values should be maintained by the new drug users;

(c) every year, in 126 000 drug injections a sterile syringe should be used instead of a used one;

(d) the overall consumption of bleach should not change (twice the cleansing on half the sharing); and

(e) every year, an extra 246 000 condoms should be used by IDUs.

We compared these data with the simulated impact of two alternative prevention strategies, both aimed at modifying the sexual behaviours in the 'general population':

(a) generalized increase in condom use; and
(b) generalized reduction in partner change rates.

To obtain, as of the end of the century, the same reduction in overall HIV-1 prevalence as that achieved through the harm reduction strategy, massive changes should occur, namely:

(a) an extra 13 400 000 condoms should be used every year; or
(b) 501 400 fewer partnerships should be established every year.

Thus, the application of our mathematical model to the Italian scenario strongly suggests that pragmatic programmes targeted at IDUs are more likely to be cost-effective than generalized information campaigns.

126

Conclusion

In this chapter, we have moved from 'pure' observational data to the development of a conceptual tool, aimed to improve our understanding of the transmission dynamics of HIV-1 in populations where drug injectors represent a significant reservoir of infection. Using this tool, and an estimate of the Lazio prevalence scenario at the beginning of 1991, we have estimated the amount of infections acquired in the first years of this decade by IDUs and NDIHs, with respect to sex and transmission route. We then predicted the epidemic trends up to the year 2000, and performed a 'thought experiment', in a field where a real experiment would have been simply impossible, obtaining results which strongly suggest priorities for prevention programmes.

However, since every model, as a crude simplification of the real world, results from choices (for example which interactions to represent, how to represent them, which values to assign to the key parameters), we must keep in mind that these results can be affected by limits and uncertainties. We investigated the relative influence that the parameters used in the model have on the predicted outcomes, through a sensitivity analysis based on the Latin hypercube sampling scheme and the partial rank correlation coefficients (Arcà, 1994). The results point to the parameters describing the probability of transmitting HIV-1 (per sex act, per partnership, male-to-female vs. female-to-male, per infected needle re-used) and to those describing the behaviours of IDUs potentially associated with HIV-1 transmission. Transmission parameters are relatively stable in time, but extremely difficult to estimate and possibly biased because of the selection of the observable populations.

As for IDUs' behaviours, the experience of the WHO Multi-City Study demonstrates that valuable data can be gathered, if an appropriate study design is adopted (for example including recruitment outside of treatment centres), standardized questionnaires prepared, and interviewers properly trained. Known limits are: the impossibility of selecting a probabilistic sample; the consequent difficulty in interpreting difference through time as behavioural change; and the need to repeat the survey every few years to take into account the mobility of the IDU population, as well as their changing behaviours (as an effect of the epidemic spread, or independently from it).

References

ANDERSON, R.M. and MAY, R.M. (1991) *Infectious diseases of humans*, Oxford: Oxford University Press.

ARCÀ, M. (1994) 'Modelli matematici eprevisioni dell'epidemia di infezione da HIV: Partire dall'evidenza, misurare l'incertezza', *Statistica Applicata*, **6**, pp. 67–78.

ARCÀ, M., SPADEA, T. and PERUCCI, C.A. (1992) 'The epidemic dynamics of HIV-1 in Italy: Modelling the interaction between intravenous drug users and heterosexual population', *Statistics in Medicine*, **11**, pp. 1657–84.

BAILEY, N.T.J. (1975) *The mathematical theory of infectious diseases*, London: Griffin.

BLOWER, S.M., HARTEL, D., DOWLATABADI, H. *et al.* (1991) 'Drug, sex and HIV: A mathematical model for New York City', *Philosophical Transactions of the Royal Society, London, Series B*, **321**, pp. 171–81.

BRANCATO, G., PERUCCI, C.A., ABENI, D.D.C. *et al.* (1997) 'The changing epidemiology of HIV infection. Ten years of HIV surveillance in Lazio, Italy, 1985–1994', *American Journal of Public Health*, **87**, 1, in press.

CAPASSO, V., VILLA, M. *et al.* (in press) 'Multistage models of HIV transmission among injecting drug users via shared drug injection equipment', *Proceedings of the 4th International Conference on Mathematical Population Dynamics*.

CASTILLO-CHAVEZ, C. (Ed) (1989) 'Mathematical and statistical approaches to AIDS epidemiology', *Lecture Notes in Biomathematics*, **83**, Berlin: Springer-Verlag.

CENTRO OPERATIVO AIDS (COA) (1995) 'Aggiornamento dei casi di AIDS notificati in Italia al 31 marzo 1995', *Notiziario dell'Istituto Superiore di Sanità*, **8**, 6, suppl.

D'ARCANGELO, E., MARASCA, G. and VITIELLO, C. (1990) 'I comportamenti sessuali della popolazione giovanile italiana in riferimento alla problematica AIDS. Primi risultati di un'indagine nazionale', *Dipartimento di Statistica, Probabilitá e Statistica Applicata. Universitá di Roma 'La Sapienza' Serie A-Ricerche*, **22**.

DAVOLI, M., PERUCCI, C.A., ABENI, D.D.C. *et al.* (1995) 'HIV risk-related behaviors among injection drug users in Rome: differences between 1990 and 1992', *American Journal of Public Health*, **85**, pp. 829–32.

DIEKMANN, O., HEESTERBEEK, J.A.P. and METZ, J.A.J. (1990) 'On the definition and the computation of the basic reproduction ratio Ro in models for infectious diseases in heterogeneous populations', *Journal of Mathematical Biology*, **28**, pp. 365–82.

GUPTA, S., ANDERSON, R.M. and MAY, R.M. (1993) 'Mathematical models and the design of public health policy: HIV and antiviral therapy', *SIAM Review*, **35**, pp. 1–16.

HETHCOTE, H.W. and VAN ARK, J.W. (1992) 'Modeling HIV transmission and AIDS in the United States', *Lecture Notes in Biomathematics*, **95**, Berlin: Springer-Verlag.

IANNELLI, M., LORO, R., MILNER, F. *et al.* (1992) 'An AIDS model with distributed incubation and variable infectiousness: application to IV drug users in Latium', *European Journal of Epidemiology*, pp. 585–93.

JEWELL, N.P. and SHIBOSKI, S.C. (1990) 'Statistical analysis of HIV infectivity based on partner studies', *Biometrics*, **46**, pp. 1133–50.

KAPLAN, E.H. (1989) 'Needles that kill: Modelling human immunodeficiency virus transmission via shared drug injection equipment in shooting galleries', *Review of Infectious Diseases*, **11**, p. 672.

KAPLAN, E.H. and HEIMER, R. (1992) 'A model-based estimate of HIV infectivity via needle sharing', *Journal of Acquired Immune Deficiency Syndromes*, **5**, pp. 1116–18.

KAPLAN, E.H. and HEIMER, R. (1994) 'A circulation theory of needle exchange', *AIDS*, **8**, pp. 567–74.

KERMACK, W.O. and McKENDRICK, A.G. (1927) 'Contributions to the mathematical theory of epidemics', *Proceedings of the Royal Society, London, Series A*, **115**, pp. 700–21.

LONGINI, I.M., CLARK, W.S., BYERS, R.H., LEMP, G.F., WARD, J.W., DARROW, W.W. and HETHCOTE, H.W. (1989) 'Statistical analysis of the stages of HIV infection using a Markov model', *Statistics in Medicine*, **8**, pp. 831–43.

MARIOTTO, A., MARIOTTI, S., PEZZOTTI, P. *et al.* (1992) 'Estimation of the AIDS incubation period in intravenous drug users: A comparison with male homosexuals', *American Journal of Epidemiology*, **135**, 4, pp. 428–37.

PERUCCI, C.A., DAVOLI, M., RAPITI, E., ABENI, D. and FORASTIERE, F. (1991) 'Mortality of intravenous drug users in Rome: A cohort study', *American Journal of Public Health*, **81**, pp. 1307–10.

PERUCCI, C.A., DAVOLI, M., PAPINI, P. *et al.* (1994), 'Evidence of increasing numbers of intravenous drug users (IVDUs) in Lazio, Italy, 1988–1992', *Proceedings of the 5th International Conference on reduction of drug-related harm*, Toronto, Ontario, Canada.

REZZA, G., NICOLOSI, A., ZACCARELLI, M. *et al.* (1994) 'Understanding the dynamics of the HIV epidemic among Italian intravenous drug users: a cross-sectional versus a longitudinal approach', *Journal of Acquired Immune Deficiency Syndromes*, **7**, pp. 500–3.

ROSS, R. (1911) *The prevention of malaria*, London: Murray.

STIGUM, H., GRONNESBY, J.K., MAGNUS, P. *et al.* (1991) 'The potential for spread of HIV in the heterosexual population in Norway: a model study', *Statistics in Medicine*, **7**, pp. 1003–25.

VAN DRUTEN, J.A., REINTJES, A.G.M., JAGER, J.C. *et al.* (1990) 'HIV infection dynamics and intervention experiments in linked risk groups', *Statistics in Medicine*, **9**, pp. 721–36.

WILLIAMS, J.R. and ANDERSON, R.M. (1994) 'Mathematical models of the transmission dynamics of human immunodeficiency virus in England and Wales: mixing between different risk groups', *Journal of the Royal Statistical Society*, **157**, pp. 69–87.

Chapter 9

Drug Injecting and Sexual Safety: Cross-national Comparisons among Cocaine and Opioid Injectors

Tim Rhodes, Ted Myers, Regina Bueno, Peggy Millson and Gillian Hunter

As drug users in many countries continue to reduce their individual harms directly associated with injecting drug use, sexual transmission is becoming increasingly important in determining the future dynamics of how HIV-1 infection is spread. In many developed and developing countries, the next stage of HIV-1 epidemic spread among drug injectors is likely to be significantly associated with whether or not, and with whom, sex is safe.

Drawing on survey findings from the World Health Organization (WHO) Multi-City Study on Drug Injecting and the Risk of HIV Infection, this chapter describes the sexual behaviour of opioid and cocaine injectors in London (United Kingdom), Toronto (Canada) and Santos (Brazil). Each of these cities give slightly different pictures of drug injecting. In London, the primary drug of choice among injectors is heroin, although polydrug use is common. In Toronto, the primary drug of choice is as likely to be cocaine as heroin, and polydrug use is also common. In Santos, the primary drug of choice is cocaine, and there is little use or injection of opioids.

Not only are there behavioural differences in patterns of drug injecting between injecting drug users (IDUs) in these cities, but there are also social, cultural and economic differences. Most importantly, Santos is a city within a 'developing' country where public health resources and infrastructures are constrained in ways which are uncommon to either London or Toronto. These differences at the city level allow for a comparative description of the sexual risk behaviour of drug injectors in different behavioural and cultural contexts. First, comparisons can be made between the sexual risk behaviour of opioid and cocaine injectors in the light of differing norms and expectations which may exist about condom use and sexual safety. Second, the implications of these findings for sexually transmitted HIV-1 infection can be discussed in the context of how best to generate HIV prevention interventions in both developed and developing countries.

Drug and Sex-related Harms

Among injecting drug users, harm reduction research and intervention have focused overwhelmingly on the harms associated with the sharing of needles, syringes and other injecting paraphernalia. This is understandable, given the public health imperative to prevent the potential rapid spread of HIV-1 infection associated with needle and syringe sharing, and the known efficacy of blood-to-blood transmission of HIV-1.

One objective of harm reduction interventions continues to be to maximize the availability and accessibility of sterile needles and syringes to drug injectors. This is particularly the case in cities or countries where availability is poor and where HIV-1 prevalence remains high among drug injectors. As has been pointed out, where availability of sterile equipment is good, levels of sharing and HIV-1 prevalence tend to be lower than where syringe availability is poor (Watters, 1996).

While there clearly remain problems of injection equipment availability in developed countries (syringe exchange is outlawed, for example, in San Francisco, Chicago and New York; see Watters, 1996), the political and resource obstacles to the establishment of effective needle and syringe distribution and exchange in many developing countries are particularly acute. In countries where organizational infrastructures and/or political impediments to responding to the public health problems associated with drug injecting are weak, it is imperative that syringe exchange be a fundamental part of intervention strategy and policy.

In cities where there exist infrastructures for HIV prevention initiatives — such as syringe exchange and community outreach — the extent to which injecting drug users have reduced their syringe sharing is encouraging. In the major cities of many developed countries, syringe sharing is no longer the norm among opioid injectors. Qualitative research among London heroin users, for example, has shown that sharing is no longer viewed as 'acceptable' behaviour, except in certain closed social networks or among sexual partners (Rhodes and Quirk, 1996). Where needle and syringe availability is adequate, the act of sharing takes on a different meaning for injectors in the age of AIDS. To some extent these social changes can be seen to have encouraged a shift from injecting cultures of ritualistic sharing symbolizing reciprocity between sharing partners towards a culture of mutual and collective responsibility about the risk and harms associated with drug injection.

In marked contrast, there is only scant evidence of sexual behaviour change among drug injectors. Surveys, most of which have been conducted in developed countries, repeatedly show that drug injectors have changed, or are changing, their injecting behaviour but have made few changes in their sexual behaviour (Des Jarlais *et al.*, 1992; van den Hoek, van Haastrecht and Coutinho, 1992; Myers *et al.*, 1995a). The only exceptions to this appear to be in sex work situations (van Ameijden *et al.*, 1994) and in primary relationships where drug injectors know themselves to be HIV-1 antibody positive (Sidthorpe, 1992;

Rhodes *et al.*, 1993; Friedman *et al.*, 1994). In these contexts, evidence suggests that sexual behaviour change can be both achieved and sustained among drug injectors and their sexual partners.

Qualitative studies have not only supported the contention that few drug injectors have changed their sexual behaviour, but have also lent additional insights into why sexual behaviour change has been less likely to occur than changes in injecting drug use. Ethnographic work recently undertaken in London shows that there are marked differences in how opioid injectors perceive the risks related to injection in comparison with the risks related to unprotected sex (Rhodes and Quirk, 1996). Not only were injection risks given higher priority because equipment sharing was often perceived to be a more efficient HIV-1 transmission route, but they were also viewed as more immediate, more likely and thus more important.

Whereas in London, as in many developed city contexts, sharing injecting equipment is generally viewed by opioid injectors to be unacceptable and unnecessary, unprotected sex may be viewed as an 'acceptable risk' (Rhodes and Quirk, 1996). Many opioid users view unprotected sex as *normal* in heterosexual sexual encounters, particularly if these encounters take place in the context of long-term relationships. In London, and in many other cities where harm reduction initiatives exist, perceived norms among heroin users tend to encourage *safer* injecting practices yet *unsafe* sexual practices (Rhodes and Quirk, 1995). To a large extent the social norms, rules and routines of heterosexual behaviour sustain a culture which legitimizes unprotected sex as an important and meaningful part of relationships. This is likely to be the case among injecting as well as non-injecting and non-drug using populations.

International Epidemiology and Sexual Transmission

There are some countries where injecting drug use is the major mode of HIV-1 transmission (for example, Malaysia). There are others, such as Thailand, Myanmar and Brazil, where injecting drug use and the shared use of injecting equipment have clearly played a critical role in determining the current and future spread of HIV-1 infection (Stimson, 1993; Lima *et al.*, 1994). There are others still, such as Colombia, Nigeria and some Eastern European countries, where the diffusion of injecting drug use and associated HIV-1 infection are either undocumented or appear comparatively recent.

Injecting drug use has been, and will remain, a pivotal determinant of the extent and distribution of HIV-1 epidemic spread, particularly in developing countries. But it is equally important to recognize the significance of sexual transmission. Sexual transmission is the primary route of HIV-1 transmission worldwide and is becoming increasingly significant in shaping the future course of HIV-1 infection among people who inject drugs and their sexual partners.

It is imperative that HIV prevention interventions targeting drug injectors do not underestimate the role of sexual transmission. In cities or countries where drug injectors do not have adequate access to sterile needles and syringes, the spread of HIV-1 infection may be particularly rapid, given that opportunities remain for the creation of new HIV-1 transmission networks through a combination of injection equipment sharing and unprotected sex. In places where sharing is no longer 'normal' or acceptable behaviour, HIV-1 will increasingly be sexually transmitted through the assortative and disassortative mixing patterns of injectors and their sexual partners.

The sexual networks of HIV-1 transmission created among injectors and their (often non-injecting) sexual partners give rise to what some have termed the 'real heterosexual epidemic' (Moss, 1987). There are good epidemiological foundations for this view. In the United States, it is estimated that drug injectors are the source of HIV-1 infection in as many as 70 to 80 per cent of heterosexually transmitted cases of AIDS (Lewis and Watters, 1991; Des Jarlais *et al.*, 1992). One recent estimate in New York City suggests that 89 per cent of heterosexually transmitted AIDS cases among non-injectors involved an IDU source (Friedman *et al.*, 1994). Estimates in Brazil also indicate that a high proportion of heterosexually transmitted cases of AIDS may be associated with unprotected sex with IDUs. In the State of Sao Paulo, for example, 40 per cent of all female heterosexual transmission cases of AIDS are reported to be sexual partners of male IDUs (Santos *et al.*, 1994).

In cities where HIV-1 prevalence is lower among injectors than that in New York or Santos (estimated at 48 per cent in 1990 in New York and 63 per cent in 1990 in Santos; Chapter 4), disassortative sexual HIV-1 transmission between injectors and their non-injecting sexual partners may be less likely. Nonetheless, in the United Kingdom — where HIV-1 prevalence has stabilized at about 8 per cent among injectors (Stimson, 1995) — a drug injecting partner is reported for over 60 per cent of first generation cases of heterosexual HIV-1 transmission (Evans *et al.*, 1992).

In addition, there remains epidemiological uncertainty about the extent of sexual transmission relative to transmission via injection equipment sharing among drug injectors. Most studies in developed countries, particularly those conducted throughout the late 1980s and early 1990s, suggest that injecting risk behaviour is the primary means of HIV-1 transmission, at least among current injectors (Battjes *et al.*, 1990). More recently, however, studies have suggested that unprotected sex is independently associated with HIV-1 transmission among people who inject drugs (Soloman *et al.*, 1993; Battjes *et al.*, 1994). In some cities, HIV-1 transmission among drug injectors is increasingly as likely to be associated with sexual transmission as with syringe sharing (Moss *et al.*, 1990; Lewis and Watters, 1991). The 'second decade' of AIDS among drug injecting and non-injecting populations is likely to continually remind us of the public health importance of sexually transmitted HIV-1 disease. As noted by Des Jarlais (1992): 'In most areas where HIV-1 has spread among injecting drug users, the drug users have become the source for both heterosexual and perinatal transmission of HIV-1.'

Add to this the higher than usual prevalence of sexually transmitted diseases transmission among drug injectors (Ross *et al.*, 1991) — and particularly among female drug injectors who exchange sex for money, drugs or other goods (van Ameijden *et al.*, 1994) — the relatively high prevalence of unplanned pregnancy (Robertson and Bucknall, 1986) and the sexual relationship problems commonly associated with opioid and injecting drug use (Mirin *et al.*, 1980), and it becomes abundantly clear that future interventions should not continue to neglect the sexual risk and health behaviour of people who inject drugs. A brief review of epidemiological research on the sexual risk behaviour of IDUs serves to reiterate this point. Key findings from this literature are summarized in Figure 9.1, together with findings from the WHO Multi-City Study of Drug Injecting and the Risk of HIV Infection.

Most IDUs have sex
Most studies find over 75 per cent of IDUs to be sexually active. In the WHO study, over 70 per cent of IDUs reported having had sex with an opposite sex partner in a six-month period in all 12 cities except Bangkok, Madrid and Rome. The frequency of vaginal sex was highest in Santos where over 70 per cent reported sex at least once a week. Over 90 per cent of those having sex with primary partners reported only one primary partner in the six months, except in Santos, where approximately 40 per cent reported two primary partners. Of those having sex with casual partners, over 60 per cent in each of 12 cities reported at least two casual partners, with the highest number reported among Santos IDUs where approximately 80 per cent reported three or more partners.

Most IDUs never use condoms with primary partners
Approximately two-thirds of drug injectors report never using condoms with their primary sexual partners. In the WHO study, the proportions reporting 'never' condom use with opposite primary partners ranged from 50 per cent (Rome) to 82 per cent (Rio de Janeiro), was least likely in Rio, Athens and Glasgow and most likely in Rome, Madrid and New York.

Many IDUs never use condoms with casual partners
Approximately one-third of drug injectors report never using condoms with their casual partners. In the WHO study, the proportions reporting 'never' condom use with opposite casual partners ranged from 30 per cent (New York) to 66 per cent (Rio de Janeiro), was least likely in Rio, Athens and Glasgow and most likely in New York and Toronto.

Dissasortative sexual mixing is high
Many IDUs (usually in the region of 50 per cent) report having non-injecting or non-using sexual partners. In the WHO study, it was most common for IDUs to have non-injecting primary partners in Bangkok, Rio and Santos (over 70 per cent) and least common in Berlin, London and Sydney (under 40 per cent). Similar trends were reported with non-injecting casual partners.

Many female IDUs work as sex workers
Most studies show that between 15 and 25 per cent of female IDUs report an involvement in sex work, although street samples have suggested higher estimates. Similar proportions of female sex workers report an involvement in injecting drug use. In the WHO study, the proportions of female IDUs exchanging sex for money or drugs ranged from between 20 to 25 per cent (London, Rio, Rome) to over 70 per cent (Berlin, Santos).

There is little or no sexual behaviour change
There are few follow-up studies of sexual behaviour change among IDUs. These studies generally show little or no marked change over time either in the number of reported sexual partners or in condom use with casual or primary partners.

Figure 9.1 Key findings on IDUs' sexual risk behaviour (For research reviews see Rhodes, Stimson and Quirk (1996) and Des Jarlais *et al.* (1992). WHO findings were collected in 1990.)

Social Epidemiology and Social Context

Like all social interaction, sexual encounters are context dependent. This means that sexual interactions are linked to the specific social and cultural environments in which they occur. The key findings from epidemiological research summarized in Figure 9.1 give an indication of the extent of reported sexual risk behaviour among drug injectors. They do not tell us how or why these behaviours occur. Taken in isolation, they cannot explain why there has been so little sexual behaviour change among IDUs despite there having been considerable changes in injecting risk behaviour. It is not the purpose of this chapter to explore the social dynamics of sexual risk behaviour among IDUs (see Rhodes, Stimson and Quirk, 1996). But it is nonetheless important to highlight the general observation that individual actions to avoid sexual risks are influenced by a variety of factors exogenous to individuals themselves. These can be seen to operate at associated interpersonal, social, cultural and political levels.

First, individual actions to avoid sexual risk are influenced by the actions of *other* individuals. The sexual transmission of a virus normally requires the participation of at least two people. This points to the important fact that protected and unprotected sex are the outcome of 'negotiated actions'. Individuals' capacity to exercise 'choice' in sexual encounters much depends on who has the control or power over the direction sexual encounters take.

Second, individual actions to avoid sexual risk are influenced by what is considered appropriate or acceptable sexual behaviour. Interpersonal negotiations towards safer sex are made considerably easier where condom use is the norm. If using condoms is a usual and expected feature of sexual encounters then such actions need not require explicit 'negotiation'. Conversely, where there exists a norm of non-condom use, it is more likely that explicit negotiation is required. It is more difficult to break norms than to conform to them. Sexual norms have an important bearing on how individuals negotiate safe and unsafe sex interpersonally.

Third, social norms about sexual behaviour are themselves context dependent. Different norms exist in different contexts. This is as likely across distinct social networks and subcultures as it is across different cultures or countries. The capacity that individuals, groups of individuals, and people in general, have in exercising choice over condom use is situationally, socially, and culturally dependent. It is difficult to encourage individuals to use condoms, for example, if there is no cultural norm of condom use.

Similarly, it is difficult to encourage risk reduction behaviour in cultures or situations where there exist punitive legal policies, unsupportive health policies or a lack of economic resources and infrastructures to encourage health behaviour change. In the city of Santos, for example, the price of condoms (at approximately US$ 0.50) is very high in the context of minimum monthly salaries (of approximately US$ 100). This may act as a disincentive to condom use, particularly in the context of female sex work, where clients may negotiate above average payments for penetrative sex without condoms (average payment is approximately US$ 10).

Last, perceptions of sexual risk are context dependent. Risk is a relative concept. When there are more important and more immediate risks in everyday life than the dangers of sexually transmitted disease or the dangers of HIV-1 infection, sexual behaviour change may not be seen as a priority (Rhodes and Quirk, 1996). The dangers associated with injecting, for example, might be seen to outweigh the dangers associated with sexual behaviour, just as the immediate dangers associated with living and surviving day to day on the streets might be seen to outweigh the dangers of HIV-1 infection.

These points serve as reminders that epidemiological findings cannot be divorced from the social contexts in which they are produced (Myers *et al.*, 1994). What is needed in future research is not just an epidemiology but a '*social epidemiology*' of drug injecting and risk behaviour. A cross-city comparison of the type discussed here cannot fully capture the social dynamics of drug use and sexual activity, but it is nonetheless important to highlight how particular social contexts of drug use may influence sexual risk behaviour as much as individuals' health beliefs and their use or injection of particular drugs.

The Drug Injecting, City and Sample Context

The remainder of this chapter draws on survey data among 1204 drug injectors in London, Toronto and Santos. These data were collected as part of the ongoing WHO Multi-City Study on Drug Injecting and the Risk of HIV Infection in the period 1991 to 1992 among 505 IDUs in London (May to December 1992), 479 IDUs in Toronto (May 1991 to April 1992) and 220 IDUs in Santos (April 1991 to December 1992). The data reported in this chapter are thus more recent (1991–2 compared with 1990) than comparative data reported elsewhere in this book and in previous WHO reports (WHO, 1994).

As was common to all cities participating in the WHO study, all respondents were current injectors and had injected in the two months prior to survey interviews. Respondents were recruited from a combination of treatment and non-treatment community-based settings in each of the three cities. Unless otherwise stated, all findings reported below relate to behaviours occurring in the six-month period prior to interview. A full methodological description of the study is provided elsewhere (WHO, 1994; see also Appendix 1).

Drug Injecting and City Context

Distinct differences in patterns of drug injecting exist in each of the three cities. In London, there were an estimated 20 000 to 30 000 opioid users in 1984 and while polydrug use is probably the norm, the most commonly injected drug is heroin. In Toronto there were an estimated 8000 to 10 000 drug injectors. There, too, polydrug use is common, although cocaine is a more commonly injected drug than in London. Surveys of Toronto drug injectors show that similar proportions of drug injectors view cocaine as much their primary drug of choice as heroin (Millson *et al.*, 1995). In Santos there were an estimated 8000 drug injectors. Almost all of them use cocaine. There is little heroin available and polydrug use is relatively uncommon.

A comparison between London, Toronto and Santos is thus methodologically desirable. This is particularly the case as far as sexual behaviour is concerned, given the increasing, yet contradictory, research evidence which tends to suggest that the regular and recreational use of cocaine is associated with a higher likelihood of sexual activity, sexual partner change and unsafe sex than the use of heroin and other opioids (Chitwood and Comerford, 1990; Chirwin *et al.*, 1991; Chaisson *et al.*, 1991).

The sample

Of the 1204 respondents, the majority in each city were male (68 per cent in London, 78 per cent in Toronto, and 60 per cent in Santos). The mean age of respondents at interview was 30.8 years in London (SD=6.2), 31.2 years in Toronto (SD=7.5) and 28.3 years in Santos (SD=7.4). Respondents had a slightly higher mean age at first injection in London (20.1, SD=4.3) than in Toronto (19.8, SD=6.2) or Santos (19.0, SD=5.1), although respondents' mean length of injecting career was slightly shorter in Santos (9.4 years, SD=7.5) than in London (10.8 years, SD=6.7) or Toronto (11.4 years, SD=8.0).

The majority of respondents were recruited outside of treatment settings (76 per cent [384] in London, 71 per cent [342] in Toronto, and 86 per cent [189] in Santos). Despite this, the majority in London (82 per cent, 414) and Toronto (70 per cent, 312) reported having had a history of drug treatment. Drug injectors in Santos, a minority of whom had a history of drug treatment (22 per cent, 50), were more likely than injectors in London and Toronto to report never having had treatment for their drug use (77 per cent in Santos compared with 18 per cent in London and 30 per cent in Toronto).

The most commonly used and injected drug in Santos was cocaine, whereas in London it was heroin, and in Toronto both cocaine and heroin. As shown in Figure 9.2, whereas 99 per cent (219) of Santos injectors reported using and 95 per cent (207) reported injecting cocaine in the six-month study period, only 5 per cent (11) reported heroin use and 4 per cent (8) heroin injection. In contrast, while 56 per cent (281) of London injectors reported using cocaine, only 34 per cent (171) reported injecting, whereas 89 per cent (446) reported heroin use and 87 per cent (436) reported heroin injection. In Toronto, 90 per cent (414) reported cocaine use, 77 per cent (356) cocaine injection, 57 per cent (271) heroin use and 55 per cent (265) heroin injection. Heroin injection was therefore more likely in London than in either Santos or Toronto, cocaine injection more likely

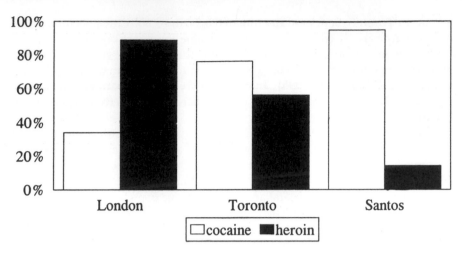

Figure 9.2   Cocaine and heroin injection in previous 6 months

in Santos than in either Toronto or London, and heroin injection more likely and cocaine injection less likely in London than in Toronto.

These differences become more marked as frequency of drug use and injection increases. When considering, for example, the drugs injected on a weekly basis, only 2 per cent (5) of Santos injectors report heroin injection, only 15 per cent (78) of London injectors report cocaine injection and 37 per cent (176) of Toronto injectors report heroin injection while 51 per cent (246) report cocaine injection. Only two Santos respondents reported injecting heroin daily (44 per cent [97] reported daily cocaine injections) and only 34 London respondents reported daily cocaine injections (41 per cent [205] reported daily heroin injections).

Levels of Sexual Activity

The majority of respondents in London (75 per cent, 370/496), Toronto (79 per cent, 379/479) and Santos (77 per cent, 169/220) reported having had vaginal or anal sex with a partner of the opposite sex in the prior six months. A further 10 per cent (35) of male London injectors, 4 per cent (15) of male Toronto injectors and 27 per cent (35) of male Santos injectors reported anal sex with non-paying male partners, of whom 9, 7 and 15 in each respective city reported sex with both men and women. Twenty per cent (100) of the sample in London, 19 per cent (93) in Toronto and 14 per cent (31) in Santos reported no penetrative sex with either (non-paying) men or women in the six months prior to interview.

These findings indicate higher levels of sexual activity among men in the Santos sample (27 per cent) than was the case in London (10 per cent) or Toronto (4 per cent). Among those sexually active (that is who had penetrative sex) with

Table 9.1 Penetrative sex with opposite sex partners in last 6 months

Partner	London (N=505)		Toronto (N=479)		Santos (N=220)	
	n	%	n	%	n	%
Primary	276	55	244	51	106	48
Casual	126	25	222	46	138	63
Client	35	7	53	11	55	25

opposite sex partners (75 per cent London, 79 per cent Toronto, and 77 per cent Santos), there was a higher likelihood of anal sex with partners of the opposite sex in Santos (35 per cent, 59) than in London (17 per cent, 64) or Toronto (14 per cent, 53), as well as a slightly higher reported frequency of vaginal or anal penetrative sex with opposite sex partners. Whereas in Santos 83 per cent (140) of those sexually active with non-paying opposite sex partners reported penetrative sex at least once a week, 60 per cent (223) of respondents in London and 61 per cent (232) in Toronto reported sex this frequently.

Table 9.1 gives the proportions of the total sample reporting penetrative sex (vaginal or anal) with primary and casual 'non-paying' partners of the opposite sex. Findings show that among those sexually active with partners of the opposite sex, higher proportions of injectors in London (75 per cent, 276) and Toronto (64 per cent, 244) reported sex with non-paying primary partners than did so in Santos (56 per cent, 106), but that considerably higher proportions of Santos injectors (79 per cent, 138) reported sex with non-paying casual partners than was the case in either London (34 per cent, 126) or Toronto (59 per cent, 222).

Table 9.1 also shows the proportions of the total sample reporting penetrative sex with 'paying' partners of the opposite sex, where sex was exchanged for money, drugs or other commodities. Findings show higher levels of sex in exchange for money or drugs among injectors (male or female) in Santos (25 per cent, 55/220) than among injectors in London (7 per cent, 35/505) or Toronto (15 per cent, 70/479). Among female injectors who were sexually active in the six months prior to interview in Santos, over half (51 per cent, 47) reported exchanging sex for money or drugs, as did 6 per cent (8) of sexually active men. The proportions in London and Toronto were 17 per cent (28/163) and 30 per cent (32/107) among women and 2 per cent (7) and 10 per cent (38/372) among men.

Number of Sexual Partners

Not only was the frequency of reported penetrative sex with casual partners higher in Santos than in London or Toronto, but Santos injectors also reported a higher mean number of opposite sex partners. Of those sexually active with opposite sex partners (75 per cent London, 79 per cent Toronto, and 77 per cent Santos), a total of 656 non-paying opposite sex partners were reported in London, 1415 in Toronto and 1031 in Santos. Excluding those in each city who had sex with paying partners only, this gives an overall mean of 1.8 different sexual partners per sexually active respondent in London, 3.7 in Toronto and 6.1 in Santos. Injectors in Santos thus reported a considerably higher mean number of opposite sex partners in the six-month study period than injectors in London or Toronto.

These differences were particularly emphasized in the reported number of casual partners. Among injectors who reported sex with primary partners in the six-month study period, there was little difference in the mean number of primary partners of the opposite sex reported in London (1.2, SD=0.5, range 1–4), Toronto (1.2, SD=0.8, range 1–10) and Santos (1.5, SD=3.69, range 1–4). However, whereas injectors reported a mean number of 3.0 (SD=3.9, range 1–20) casual partners in London, and 5.0 (SD=6.8, range 1–50) in Toronto, a mean number of 10.6 (SD=23.76, range 1–52) casual partners was reported in Santos.

These findings point to relatively high rates of sexual partner change in each of these three cities, but especially in Santos. Not only are injectors in each city having, on average, more than one opposite sex partner in a six-month period, but there is a significant minority reporting vaginal sex with both primary *and* casual partners. While in London and Toronto, 12 per cent (46) and 22 per cent (87) of those sexually active reported sex with both primary and casual partners of the opposite sex, in Santos the figure was as high as 79 per cent (133). Of these, the mean number of sexual partners (primary or casual) was 4.2 (SD=4.6, range 1–24) in London, 6.7 (SD=8.2, range 1–50) in Toronto and 10.6 (SD=23.7, range 1–52) in Santos.

The majority of those in London and Toronto who were sexually active with both primary and casual partners were having at least one non-commercial sexual encounter a week (76 per cent [35/46] London; 87 per cent Toronto [76/87]), while 9 per cent in London and 53 per cent in Toronto were having at least one sexual encounter a day. In Santos, 31 per cent of those sexually active with both primary and casual partners were having at least one sexual encounter a week, while 16 per cent were doing so at least once a day. This points to high rates of primary and casual partner change and sexual activity among a significant minority of injectors in London and Toronto, yet higher rates of partner change among drug injectors in Santos as a whole. Whereas sex with both primary and casual partners among London and Toronto injectors is the exception rather than the rule, it is more likely to be the norm among injectors in Santos.

Add to these findings the estimated number of 'paying' sexual partners among those exchanging sex for money or drugs, and it becomes clear that in some cities some injectors are having high levels of penetrative sex. Female injectors who exchanged sex for money or drugs in London (28) and Toronto (32) estimated a mean number of 33.0 (SD=35.4, range 1–120) and 68.2 (SD=156.9, range 1–888) paying partners a month. The median number of paying partners was 24 in London and 20 in Toronto. In Santos, where a higher proportion of female injectors exchanged sex for money or drugs (51 per cent, 47), the mean number of paying partners in a typical month was 41. This points to a higher average number of sex for money exchanges reported among female injectors involved in sex work in Toronto than in Santos or London, yet a greater likelihood of involvement in sex for money exchanges *per se* among female injectors in Santos.

Condom use

If sex is safe, high levels of sexual mixing need not be associated with an increased likelihood of sexually transmitted disease or HIV-1 transmission. Table 9.2 shows that a significant proportion of injectors in each of the three cities reported never using condoms when having penetrative sex, although they were more likely to do so with casual partners and paying partners than with primary partners.

In each city injectors were more likely to report 'never' using condoms with primary partners than with casual partners of the opposite sex (57 per cent vs. 25 per cent in London; 62 per cent vs. 35 per cent in Toronto; and 69 per cent vs. 46 per cent in Santos). While there were no marked differences between the cities in the proportions of injectors who never used condoms with primary partners, Santos injectors were more likely to report never using condoms with casual partners (see Table 9.2).

Of those reporting penetrative sex with more than one non-paying sexual partner in the six months prior to interview (28 per cent [103/370] London; 56 per cent [214/379] Toronto; 71 per cent [96/135] Santos), 15 per cent (London), 16 per cent (Toronto) and 11 per cent (Santos) reported 'always' using condoms with primary partners and 38 per cent (London), 32 per cent (Toronto) and 22 per cent (Santos) reported 'always' using condoms with casual partners. These figures point to a relatively high irregularity of condom use even among injectors who report more than one sexual partner in a six-month period, particularly among injectors in Santos.

Among female injectors who exchanged sex for money or drugs (n=28 London; n=32 Toronto; n=47 Santos), frequency of condom use was much

Table 9.2 Condom use with opposite sex partners in last 6 months

| | Primary partners | | | | | | Casual partners | | | | | |
| | London (N=269) | | Toronto (N=244) | | Santos (N=106) | | London (N=115) | | Toronto (N=220) | | Santos (N=78) | |
	n	%	n	%	n	%	n	%	n	%	n	%
Always	50	19	31	13	12	11	45	39	77	35	17	22
Sometimes	63	23	60	25	11	10	38	33	65	30	23	32
Never	156	58	151	62	73	69	32	28	78	36	35	46

higher than that reported with non-paying partners and higher in London and Toronto than in Santos. Whereas 89 per cent (25) and 73 per cent (22) of London and Toronto female injectors respectively 'always' used condoms with paying partners, this figure in Santos was 61 per cent (29).

Sexual Safety in Cities of High and Low HIV-1 Prevalence

High levels of sexual activity and partner change in combination with high levels of unsafe sex clearly encourage a higher likelihood of HIV-1 transmission, particularly in cities where HIV-1 prevalence is high or shows no signs of decreasing. Findings from the WHO study conducted between 1990 and 1991, show 12.8 per cent of London injectors, 4.7 per cent of Toronto injectors and 63.1 per cent of Santos injectors to be HIV-1 positive (Chapter 4). In this 1992 sample of injectors, confirmed antibody test results show 7.0 per cent (30/396) of London injectors, 4.5 per cent (21/471) of Toronto injectors and 60 per cent (81/135) of Santos injectors to be HIV-1 antibody positive. Whereas HIV-1 prevalence among injectors in London and Toronto is 'low' by international standards,[1] and has declined in London (Stimson *et al.*, 1996), HIV-1 prevalence in Santos remains 'high'.

Sexual Safety in London and Toronto

The majority of injectors in London and Toronto reported never using condoms with their primary partners. Between a quarter and a third also reported never using condoms with their casual partners, while in a six-month period each sexually active injector reported an average of almost two partners in London and almost four partners in Toronto. This points to the possibilities for continued HIV-1 transmission via unprotected sex between injectors and their sexual partners. As syringe sharing becomes less indiscriminate and less the norm in these cities, sexual transmission is likely to become more important in shaping future HIV-1 spread than parenteral transmission routes. Current estimates of HIV-1 prevalence among injecting drug users in these two cities may be low by international rates, but the irregular use of condoms and the average rate of partner change may be sufficient to introduce and sustain HIV-1 spread within and among injectors' sexual networks. Future epidemiological studies in these cities might consider the sexual network as a unit of analysis for mapping and predicting the spread of HIV-1 infection and sexually transmitted diseases.

Sexual Safety in Santos

The potential for the sexual transmission of HIV among IDUs and their sexual partners is higher in Santos than in London or Toronto (Barbosa *et al.*, 1996).

The majority of injectors there reported never using condoms with their primary partners. In addition, greater proportions than in London or Toronto reported never using condoms with casual partners and on average each sexually active injector reported 6.1 partners in a six-month period. In cities like Santos, with a high HIV-1 prevalence among injectors, sexual transmission is likely to be of increasing significance in determining the dynamics of HIV-1 spread both within drug injectors' networks, and between drug injectors and non-injecting sexual partners. In circumstances where at least one in every two injectors is HIV-1 positive, where almost two-thirds never use condoms with primary partners and where almost half never use condoms with casual partners, there exist, by international standards, relatively high chances for the creation of sexual transmission networks. The need for sexual behaviour change is apparent in London as in Toronto, but the need for such change in Santos takes on an added public health urgency and policy importance.

These points are reinforced by our finding that among the three cities, rates of casual sexual partner change were highest where rates of condom use with casual partners were lowest. Such a combination, particularly in cities where there is a high HIV-1 prevalence among injectors, emphasizes the need for recognizing on a global scale the importance of sexually transmitted HIV-1 infection among drug injecting populations. Not only did the majority of injectors (79 per cent) in Santos have sex with *both* primary and casual partners in the study period, a third (33 per cent) reported over five casual partners, and over half of women (58 per cent) reported exchanging sex for money or drugs, but these behaviours may continue in unsafe circumstances. If future health interventions among drug injectors are to be effective in creating and sustaining the conditions necessary for sexual behaviour change, then not only is it important to recognize the *epidemiological* significance of sexual transmission, but it is equally, if not more, important to understand why it is that many injectors continue to have unprotected sex, despite high HIV-1 prevalence and the changes they have made in their drug use behaviour.

Towards a Social Epidemiology of Sexual Risk

A preliminary cross-national comparison such as this cannot adequately describe the social dynamics and contexts which give rise to, and sustain, differences in sexual behaviour among drug injectors in different cities. Data do, however, suggest important sexual behavioural differences between drug injectors in the three cities, for example the pattern of sexual behaviour which is common to Santos injectors is uncommon to London and Toronto injectors. Findings indicate the considerably higher rate of sexual partner change reported by Santos injectors, the higher levels of sex between men, and of anal sex between women and men, the higher levels of involvement in sex for money or drug exchanges, and the lower levels of condom use in primary and casual sexual relationships.

These differences in risk behaviour may correspond to a 'social etiquette' which 'strutures' sexual behaviour differently in Santos than in London or Toronto. In short, the social organization of sexual behaviour may be different. While in Santos, the norm is for drug injectors to report having had penetrative sex with both primary and casual sexual partners within a six-month period, this is relatively uncommon in London and Toronto. It is less common in Santos for injectors to report having had sex with primary or regular partners than it is for them to report having had sex with casual partners. The reverse is true in London and Toronto. These comparisons may not only suggest that casual sex and a high frequency of sexual partner change (even when in relationship with a 'primary' partner) may be more common among Santos injectors than among London or Toronto injectors, but they may also indicate cross-national, indeed cross-*cultural*, differences in sexual norms.

If cultural differences in sexual norms do exist between Santos and the city contexts of London and Toronto, then it is the job of the social epidemiologist to determine why this is the case and how such norms contribute to producing different levels of sexual risk and health behaviour. Do different cultural norms exist between London and Santos, for example, in the extent to which anal sex is perceived by injectors to be socially acceptable behaviour? Are Santos injectors more likely than Toronto injectors, for example, to view commerical sexual encounters as not only socially legitimate but also economically necessary? Is non-use of condoms more likely to be viewed as a socially acceptable risk in both casual and primary sexual encounters by injectors in Santos than by injectors in London or Toronto?

On the basis of our findings we observe that important cross-national sexual behavioural differences exist between injectors in Santos and those in London and Toronto. While this provides crude pointers to whether or not public health interventions are needed, and in which city contexts they are sorely missed, our data cannot provide the descriptions necessary to outline precisely *how* such interventions should respond. There is therefore a need to understand the *social* and *material* factors which encourage and constrain individual attempts at condom use and sexual behaviour change.

We emphasize the need for a social epidemiology of injecting drug use and associated risk behaviour. This social epidemiology of risk behaviour should aim to delineate the factors which encourage and sustain behaviour change at the level of the individual and his or her community, city and socio-political environment. If future cross-national studies are to gain practical insights from observed behavioural differences in IDUs of distinct cities and countries, then it is important to highlight not only how these differences shape HIV-1 transmission, but also why these differences exist and whether there should be national differences in how interventions respond.

Interventions in a Cross-national Context

If sexual risk and safety are context dependent, then it follows that the effectiveness of public health interventions are also, to some extent, dependent on social context. The perceived costs and benefits associated with wearing a condom among Toronto injectors may, for example, be 'worlds apart' from their perceived costs and benefits among Santos injectors. In an economic climate where an individual's consideration of condom use may rest as much on the purchase price as the potential for avoiding the transmission of disease or unwanted pregnancy, Santos injectors' perceptions of risk and safety may be 'situated' in areas that are uncommon to the deliberations and perceptions of injectors in London or Toronto. Interventions will need to take account of such differences in how they determine what kind of solutions are most likely to bring about a lasting change in individuals' condom use. What works in London or Toronto may be inappropriate or ineffectual in Santos.

If they are to be efficient and effective in different social, cultural and political environments, interventions need to be based not only on cross-national survey comparisons of risk epidemiology but on local expertise, knowledge and research. Current research clearly favours an intervention approach which is 'community-oriented' wherein changes in individual behaviour and the social environment are simultaneously targeted (Rhodes and Hartnoll, 1996; Tawil, Verster and O'Reilly, 1995). Evidence shows peer group and social network norms, for example, to be an important determinant of condom use among drug injectors (Jose *et al.*, 1996). Research also shows that drug injectors' perceptions of expectations and norms about condom use influence whether and how interpersonal condom negotiations proceed (Rhodes and Quirk, 1996).

The task of changing sexual norms — through peer education, community action and other group behaviour change strategies — presents interventions targeting drug users with an array of practical and theoretical difficulties, and to date, with few demonstration examples to follow (Rhodes and Quirk, 1995). However, research indicates that such interventions are possible and that they can be effective, particularly if undertaken at the same time as interventions which target concomitant changes in restrictive political infrastructures and punitive health and legal policies.

If on the basis of a social epidemiology of sexual risk behaviour it is possible to delineate the social and behavioural factors which encourage or constrain condom use in different social contexts, it becomes practically possible to develop experimental interventions designed to bring about community-wide changes in sexual risk perception and behaviour. This demands more than an intervention approach which targets individuals with exhortations to change their behaviour. At the outset, it requires a community action approach which aims to bring about changes in the social norms and etiquette of risk behaviours as well as in the wider political and policy environment (Myers *et al.*, 1995b; Rhodes and Hartnoll, 1996).

That individuals' beliefs and behaviours are often constrained by the actions of their communities serves as a reminder that the actions of communities are in turn influenced by the actions of politicians and policy makers. An effective HIV prevention strategy, whether targeting change in developed or developing country contexts, needs to target change in individual and community as well as political behaviour. This is as much the case when targeting changes in sexual behaviour as changes in injecting drug use. In each of the cities of London, Toronto and Santos, sexual behaviours are an everyday part of the social, material and political economy of city life. Perhaps the most useful pointer to successful HIV prevention is to recognize that individuals — and individual beliefs and behaviours — are only a small part of the picture that makes up 'public health'. If the 'public health' is to remain protected then it is towards bigger systems — such as policy, political and resource infrastructures — that interventionists must turn. Changes at the community level may facilitate further changes in individual behaviours, but they are no substitute for changes in the wider social and political environment.

Note

1 The World Health Organization Multi-City Study on Drug Injecting and the Risk of HIV Infection previously categorized HIV-1 prevalence among drug injectors in London as 'medium' by international standards (WHO, 1994). This categorization was based on data collected in 1990 which found HIV-1 prevalence, as reported above, to be 12.8 per cent. A decline and subsequent levelling-off in HIV-1 prevalence has been observed among London drug injectors since this time (9.8 in 1991, 7.0 per cent in 1992 and 6.9 per cent in 1993; see Stimson *et al.*, 1996). Current estimates therefore suggest HIV-1 prevalence among drug injectors to be 'low' by international standards.

References

BARBOSA, H., MESQUITA, F., BUENO, R. *et al.* (1996) 'HIV and infections of similar transmission patterns in an IDU community of Santos, Brazil', *Journal of AIDS*.

BATTJES, R.J., PICKENS, R.W., AMSEL, Z. and BROWN, L.S. (1990) 'Heterosexual transmission of human immunodeficiency virus among intravenous drug users', *Journal of Infectious Diseases*, **162**, pp. 1007–11.

BATTJES, R.J., PICKENS, R.W., HAVERKOS, H.W. and SLOBODA, Z. (1994) 'HIV risk factors among injecting drug users in five US cities', *AIDS*, **8**, pp. 681–7.

CHAISSON, M.A., STONEBURNER, R.L., HILDERBRANDT, W.E. *et al.* (1991) 'Heterosexual transmission of HIV-1 associated with the use of smokable freebase cocaine (crack)', *AIDS*, **5**, pp. 1121–6.

CHIRWIN, K., DEHOVITZ, J.A., DILLON, A. and McCORMACK, W.M. (1991) 'HIV infection, genital ulcer disease and crack cocaine use among patients attending a clinic for sexually transmitted diseases', *American Journal of Public Health*, **81**, pp. 1576–9.

CHITWOOD, D. and COMERFORD, M. (1990) 'Drugs, sex and AIDS risk', *American Behavioural Scientist*, **33**, pp. 465–77.

DES JARLAIS, D.C. (1992) 'The first and second decade of AIDS among injecting drug users', *British Journal of Addiction*, **87**, pp. 347–53.

DES JARLAIS, D.C., FRIEDMAN, S.R., CHOOPANYA, K. *et al.* (1992) 'International epidemiology of HIV and AIDS among injecting drug users', *AIDS*, **6**, pp. 1053–68.

EVANS, B.G., NOONE, A., MORTIMER, J. *et al.* (1992) 'Heterosexually acquired HIV-1 infection: cases reported in England, Wales and Northern Ireland, 1985–1991', *PHLS Communicable Disease Reports*, **2** (April).

FRIEDMAN, S.R., JOSE, B., NEAIGUS, A. *et al.* (1994) 'Consistent condom use in relationships between seropositive drug users and sex partners who do not inject drugs', *AIDS*, **8**, pp. 357–61.

JOSE, B., FRIEDMAN, S.R., NEAIGUS, A. *et al.* (1996) 'Collective organisation of injecting drug users and the struggle against AIDS', in RHODES, T. and HARTNOLL, R. (Eds) *AIDS, Drugs and Prevention: Perspectives on Individual and Community Action*, London: Routledge.

LEWIS, D.K. and WATTERS, J.K. (1991) 'Sexual risk behaviour among heterosexual intravenous drug users: Ethnic and gender variations', *AIDS*, **5**, pp. 77–83.

LIMA, E.S., FRIEDMAN, S.R., BASTOS, F.I. *et al.* (1994) 'Risk factors for HIV-1 seroprevalence among drug injectors in the cocaine-using environment of Rio de Janeiro', *Addiction*, **89**, pp. 689–98.

MILLSON, P., MYERS, T., RANKIN, J. *et al.* (1995) 'Prevalence of human immunodeficiency virus and associated risk behaviour in injecting drug users in Toronto', *Canadian Journal of Public Health*, **86**, pp. 176–80.

MIRIN, S.M., MEYER, R.E., MENDLESON, J. and ELLINGBOE, J. (1980) 'Opiate use and sexual function', *American Journal of Psychiatry*, **137**, pp. 909–15.

MOSS, A. (1987) 'AIDS and intravenous drug use: The real heterosexual epidemic', *British Medical Journal*, **294**, pp. 389–90.

MOSS, A., VRANIZAN, K., BACCHETTI, P. *et al.* (1990) 'Seroconversion for HIV in intravenous drug users in treatment, San Francisco 1985–1900', *Sixth International Conference on AIDS*, San Francisco.

MYERS, T., MILLSON, P., RIGBY, J. *et al.* (1994) 'Biographical characteristics of injection drug users and behavioural predispositions related to HIV prevention and drug use', *Canadian Journal of Public Health*, **85**, pp. 264–8.

MYERS, T., MILLSON, P., RIGBY, J. *et al.* (1995a) 'A comparison of the determinants of safe injecting and condom use among injecting drug users', *Addiction*, **90**, pp. 217–26.

MYERS, T., COCKERILL, R., MILLSON, P. *et al.* (1995b) *Canadian Community Pharmacies HIV/ AIDS Prevention and Health Promotion: Results of a National Survey*, Toronto: University of Toronto.

RHODES, T. and QUIRK, A. (1995) 'Where is the sex in harm reduction?', *International Journal of Drug Policy*, **6**, pp. 76–82.

RHODES, T. and QUIRK, A. (1996) 'Heroin, risk and sexual safety: some problems for interventions encouraging community change', in RHODES, T. and HARTNOLL, R. (Eds) *AIDS, Drugs and Prevention: Perspectives on Individual and Community Action*, London: Routledge.

RHODES, T., STIMSON, G.V. and QUIRK, A. (1996) 'Sex, drugs, intervention and research: From the individual to the social', *International Journal of the Addictions*, **31**, pp. 375–407.

RHODES, T., DONOGHOE, M.C., HUNTER, G.M. and STIMSON, G.V. (1993) 'Continued risk behaviour among HIV positive drug injectors in London: Implications for inter-verntion', *Addiction*, **88**, pp. 1553–60.

RHODES, T. and HARTNOLL, R. (Eds) (1996) *AIDS, Drugs and Prevention: Perspectives on Individual and Community Action*, London: Routledge.

ROBERTSON, J.R. and BUCKNALL, A.B.V. (1986) 'Pregnancy and HTLVIII/LAV transmission in heroin users', *Health Bulletin*, **4**, pp. 364–6.

ROSS, M.W., GOLD, J., WODAK, A. and MILLER, M.E. (1991) 'Sexually transmissable diseases in injecting drug users', *Genito-urinary Medicine*, **67**, pp. 32–6.

SANTOS, N.J.S., KALICHMAN, A., GRANJEIRO, A. *et al.* (1994) 'Heterosexual transmission in women in São Paulo, Brasil', paper presented at Tenth International Conference on AIDS, Yokohama, Japan.

SIDTHORPE, B. (1992) 'The social construction of relationships as a determinant of HIV risk perception and condom use among injection drug users', *Medical Anthropological Quarterly*, **6**, pp. 255–70.

SOLOMAN, L., ASTEMBORSKI, J., WARREN, D. *et al.* (1993) 'Differences in risk factors for human immunodeficiency virus type 1 seroconversion among male and female intravenous drug users', *American Journal of Epidemiology*, **137**, pp. 892–8.

STIMSON, G.V. (1993) 'The global diffusion of injecting drug use: implications for human immunodeficiency virus infection', *Bulletin on Narcotics*, **1**, pp. 3–17.

STIMSON, G.V. (1995) 'AIDS and injecting drug use in the United Kingdom, 1987–1993: The policy response and the prevention of the epidemic', *Social Science and Medicine*, **41**, 5, pp. 699–716.

STIMSON, G.V., HUNTER, G.M., DONOGHOE, M.C. *et al.* (1996) 'HIV-1 prevalence in community-wide samples of injecting drug users in London (1990–1993)', *AIDS*, **10**, 6, pp. 657–66.

TAWIL, O., VERSTER, A. and O'REILLY, K.R. (1995) 'Enabling approaches for HIV/AIDS prevention: Can we modify the environment and minimize the risk?', *AIDS*, **9**, pp. 1299–1306.

VAN AMEIJDEN, E.J., VAN DEN HOEK, J.A.R., VAN HAASTRECHT, H.J. and COUTINHO, R.A. (1994) 'Trends in sexual behaviour and the incidence of sexually transmitted diseases and HIV among drug-using prostitutes, Amsterdam 1986–1992', *AIDS*, **8**, pp. 213–21.

VAN DEN HOEK, J.A.R., VAN HAASTRECHT, H.J.A. and COUTINHO, R.A. (1992) 'Little change in sexual behaviour in injecting drug users in Amsterdam', *Journal of Acquired Immune Deficiency Syndromes*, **5**, pp. 518–22.

WATTERS, J.K. (1996) 'The Americans and syringe exchange: roots of resistance', in RHODES, T. and HARTNOLL, R. (Eds) *AIDS, Drugs and Prevention: Perspectives on Individual and Community Action*, London: Routledge.

WORLD HEALTH ORGANIZATION INTERNATIONAL COLLABORATIVE GROUP (1994) *Multi-City Study on Drug Injecting and Risk of HIV Infection* (WHO/PSA/94.4), Geneva: World Health Organization.

Chapter 10

Cities Responding to HIV-1 Epidemics among Injecting Drug Users

Francisco Bastos, Gerry V. Stimson, Paulo Telles and Christovam Barcellos

This chapter utilizes information about the patterns of spread of HIV/AIDS and the public health responses to the epidemic in the cities involved in the World Health Organization Multi-City Study on Drug Injecting and Risk of HIV Infection. The emphasis here concerns the responses the different cities gave (and are giving) to the crisis evoked by the spread of HIV-1 among injecting drug users (IDUs) and their acquaintances (see also Appendix 2). The chapter contrasts positive and problematic responses from a range of cities clustered in terms of epidemic status using the classification by Des Jarlais (1994): prevented epidemics, intermediate patterns and established epidemics. It deals mainly with the period from 1990 onwards. Very powerful differences were observed. Significant is the difference between those cities which had early and vigorous implementation of prevention measures (and mainly low HIV-1 prevalence) and those cities with a lesser commitment to HIV-1 prevention and a greater commitment to law enforcement as a strategy for drug policy (often with higher prevalence).

A case study of the spread of HIV/AIDs in Brazil will be developed using techniques of geo-processing of the registered AIDS cases in the period between 1982 and 1993.

The Multiple Determinants of the HIV/AIDS Epidemic

The HIV/AIDS epidemic is a multifaceted crisis that has evolved around the world across different cultures and socio-economic structures. Contrary to early forecasts, the HIV/AIDS epidemic among IDUs and their partners is a global problem involving today over 80 countries in the developed and developing world.

Although the HIV/AIDS epidemic depends directly on the intimate interaction of individuals transmitting HIV-1 through needle and syringe sharing, sexual intercourse or blood transfusion, it is too simplistic to understand its different dimensions on the basis of individual activity. This is due to several factors. First, the strong differences in the dynamics of the epidemic in distinct countries and regions can only be understood considering the shaping of the epidemic by macro-social forces and by public health responses to the HIV/ AIDS crisis. Second, the greatest spread of the epidemic occurred in situations characterized by multiple, sometimes anonymous interactions between people from different cultural, ethnic, social or geographic backgrounds. In the specific case of HIV/AIDS among IDUs, interaction occurred in the common use of needles and syringes in the penitentiary system (Dolan, 1993), in the shooting galleries of New York City or through the common use of dealer's needles and syringes (Des Jarlais, 1994), and by the use of professional injectors in South-east Asia (Stimson, 1995) determining an epidemiologically efficient mixing pattern.

Third, the idea that there are different individual and social vulnerabilities to HIV-1 infection, and variation in access to treatment, is an essential tool for an adequate understanding of different national and regional patterns of the epidemic. One of the axes proposed by Mann *et al.* (1992) concerns individual vulnerability, and is labelled the *behavioural* axis. It emphasizes the need for the development of self-confidence and assertiveness in order to adopt safer injecting and sexual behaviours. It is deeply influenced by the social climate, prejudice and impoverishment of IDUs and their acquaintances. In turn it is helped by initiatives of community development, outreach preventive strategies, and self-organization of IDUs whose self-help groups, advocacy groups and other grass-root associations have proved to be perhaps the most efficient 'channels' in the diffusion of safer behavioural patterns. With particular concern to stigmatized and prejudiced groups of people like the IDUs, it is necessary to identify the social patterns of interaction and to encourage such groups to locate and engage in preventive actions using these networks (Friedman, de Jong and Wodak,

Table 10.1 Attitudes of the general public towards IDUs, and engagement of IDUs in preventive strategies (*Source*: WHO Collaborative Study Group, 1994)

Cities	Public attitudes towards IDUs	Engagement of IDUs in the implementation of preventive strategies
Athens	negative	rare
Bangkok	NAI	no
Berlin	negative	high
Glasgow	compassionate	no
London	indifferent	low to moderate
Madrid	negative	NAI
New York	highly stigmatized	rare
Rio de Janeiro	highly stigmatized	no
Rome	hostile	NAI
Santos	stigmatized	no
Sydney	changing to more comprehensive	high
Toronto	negative	moderate

NAI — no available information

1993). Table 10.1 gives for each of the cities in the study an indication of public attitudes towards IDUs, and an indication of the extent to which IDUs were engaged in the implementation of preventive strategies. The most vigorous preventive actions directed towards the epidemic were often observed in communities that utilized their own resources and developed culturally sensitive strategies against it, following the paradigm of the homosexual communities of developed countries (Friedman, 1993) and, on a lesser scale, the middle-class homosexuals of the major cities of developing countries like Brazil (Parker, 1994).

Prevention Strategy and the Development of the HIV-1 Epidemic

As analyzed by Pollak and Schiltz (1994), early and appropriate responses to the HIV/AIDS epidemic in the beginning of the 1980s occurred in countries with a long established tradition of public health policies. Often a network of existing resources was used in the prevention of the epidemic, in a co-operative work with non-governmental organizations (NGOs) and the civil society. The prevention of HIV-1 spread among IDUs in the province of Skane in the South of Sweden would be one such example (Ljunberg *et al.*, 1991; Des Jarlais *et al.*, 1995). In the town of Lund, in the province of Skane, an integrated programme delivering free condoms, exchanging syringes and needles, and providing easy contact with a well established network of treatment facilities, instituted in November 1986, seems to have prevented a local epidemic among IDUs, with consistent low levels ($\sim$ 1–2 per cent) of HIV-1, as observed through a continued assessment.

A wide range of preventive activities have been developed to help drug injectors reduce their risk of HIV-1 infection or of transmitting it to others. These include the expansion of drug treatment programmes and improving access to treatment, and its acceptability to clients. Drug treatment programmes include methadone substitution, pharmacologically assisted abstinence programmes, residential facilities (often operating on therapeutic community concepts), and self-help groups such as Narcotics Anonymous. Probably the most significant HIV-1 prevention activity has been the distribution of sterile needles and syringes to current injectors, commonly through needle exchange programmes, through pharmacy sales, through shops and vending machines and through outreach. Needle exchange programmes were first developed in Amsterdam and then adopted in other European and Australian cities. Table 10.2 gives the date of introduction of needle exchange programmes in cities involved in the Multi-City Study, and some indication of the scale of development. In the UK, for example, after the introduction of pilot programmes in many cities including London, there was a rapid expansion so that by the beginning of the 1990s two out of three of all drug agencies were involved in some kind of needle distribution programme. Elsewhere (and sometimes concomitantly with needle and syringe distribution) there has been the distribution of bleach to decontaminate syringes.

Table 10.2 Implementation of needle exchange programmes and bleach distribution (*Source*: WHO Collaborative Study Group, 1994)

Cities	Estimated level of NEP activity vis-à-vis demand	NEPs functioning since	Level of regular bleach distribution	Bleach distribution since
Athens	0	–	0	–
Bangkok	0	–	+++	1988
Berlin	+++	1989	0	–
Glasgow	+++	1988	0	–
London	+++	1987	+	1988
Madrid	+++	1991	+	NAI
New York	++	1992*	+++	1987
Rio de Janeiro	0	–	+**	1994
Rome	++	1992	0	–
Santos	0	–***	+**	1992
Sydney	+++	1987	+++	1988
Toronto	++	1989	+++	1988

NEP — needle exchange programme
NAI — no available information
* does not include underground initiatives
** distributed in only one site
*** does not include aborted pilot programme (see text)

Such programmes first commenced in San Francisco, Chicago and other North American cities around 1987. Bleach distribution has often been used for HIV-1 prevention in contexts where there are legal or resource contraints against the distribution of needles and syringes. Many HIV-1 prevention programmes were supported by local or mass media campaigns. Of particular relevance have been targeted information campaigns which involve drug injectors in the production of appropriate posters, leaflets and comics with health and harm reduction information.

A variety of methods have been tried for reaching and involving drug injectors. Outreach, as a community-based prevention strategy, has aimed to reach individuals or groups who do not come into contact with conventional health or educational services. In some cities (for example Zurich and Berlin) outreach services were delivered directly to open drug scenes (known as *tolerance zones*). Outreach has used a number of different strategies including straightforward service delivery in venues used by injectors, and peer education, utilizing injectors as AIDS prevention advocates.

There is considerable evidence of AIDS-related behavioural change by drug injectors in many parts of the world. There are methodological difficulties in making links between public policy, HIV-1 behavioural changes and the course of HIV epidemics. However, the data from the WHO Multi-City Study is contributing to an understanding of these interactions.

Prevented Epidemics

Among the countries who participated in the WHO Multi-City Study, Australia could be considered the best model of an HIV/AIDS prevented epidemic among IDUs. Its responses to the crisis posed by the dissemination of HIV-1 among IDUs could be described as one of an enlightened pragmatism (ANCA, 1988).

Epidemiological data point to the fact that in Australia, in the beginning of the 1980s there were the conditions for a rapid and extensive dissemination of HIV-1 among IDUs through bridging from homo- or bisexual IDUs, since relatively high levels of seroprevalence were found among men who have sex with men in this period (Arachne and Ball, 1986). Higher rates of seroprevalence continued to be observed among homo- and bisexual men who were also injecting drugs (generally around 5 per cent) during the first half of the 1990s (Wodak, 1994).

An integrated set of diverse preventive strategies was put into practice in Australia, when levels of seroprevalence were incipient among IDUs. These efforts continued during the whole period, with strategies ranging from needle exchange programmes (NEPs) to methadone clinics. A particular feature of the Australian experience, also observed in the Federal Republic of Germany (Pieper, 1993), is the support of advocacy groups of IDUs by federal funds to develop preventive campaigns. In Australia, this included funds to run NEPs by the IDUs themselves. The continued achievements of the Australian experience show that it is possible to integrate services and strategies despite different philosophies.

The Sydney 'tribes' campaign, that took place in the beginning of the 1990s, was paradigmatic in its engagement of different subgroups of IDUs to implement preventive actions for themselves (Herkt, 1993). By avoiding the common stereotype of IDUs as dysfunctional, it was possible to identify and contact persons who did not fit the 'typical' IDU profile ('functional' or successful drug users), and thus promote safe behavioural patterns, through peer education.

As recently stated by Des Jarlais *et al.* (1995) (see also Chapter 12), Sydney has characteristics in common with other cities that have maintained low HIV-1 seroprevalences among their IDUs (Glasgow, Scotland; Tacoma, USA; Toronto, Canada; and Lund, Sweden). These include: early introduction of preventive measures, expanded access to sterile equipment and development of community outreach. All these cities benefited in their preventive efforts from structural advantages: an invariable population of IDUs and a stable drug use scene (steady prices of the drugs consumed and the absence of new injectable drugs), good media coverage of local preventive strategies and significant spontaneous behavioural changes by local IDUs. Mutable drug scenes as commonly observed in decayed neighbourhoods both in developing and developed countries, frequently with a high turnover of IDU population (secondary to the 'entering' of new injectors or migrations), probably would represent additional difficulties even to preventive strategies as comprehensive and extensive as those mentioned here.

Major Trends of HIV/AIDS Epidemic in Contemporary Brazil

The first wave of HIV/AIDS diffusion in Brazil, as shown through the register of AIDS cases in the first half of the 1980s, was largely restricted to major cities and surrounding areas on the south-east coast (Figure 10.1). This pattern was replaced by extensive diffusion through hierarchical networks of regional urban centres. The epidemic is spreading not only in its primary locations — big cities of the industrialized south-east such as São Paulo and Rio de Janeiro — but also in all the other states of the federation, including far counties in centre-west and northern regions (the tropical forest) (Figure 10.2). The initial epidemic mostly affected men who have sex with men, but this is changing and Brazil now has an epidemic with an important participation of IDUs and heterosexual transmission.

The proportion of IDUs among the registered AIDS cases in Brazil increased from around 4 per cent in 1986 to around 25 per cent in the beginning of the 1990s. The magnitude of heterosexual transmission can be deduced by the

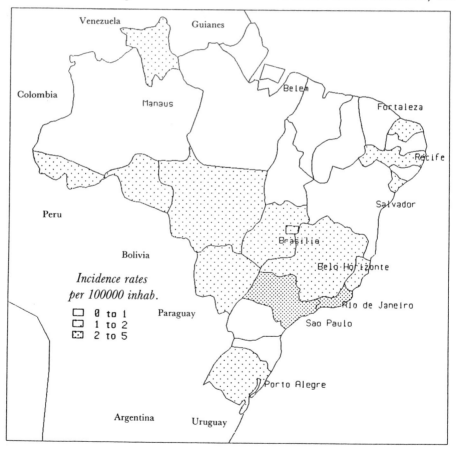

Figure 10.1 AIDS incidence rates in Brazilian states, 1987

difference in the proportions of men and women with AIDS at the beginning of the epidemic compared with today — an increase from 80 males for each female case in the beginning of the 1980s to the current proportion of three males for each female case.

Initially the epidemic affected mostly the Brazilian élite and middle class, but we can observe a continuous trend towards the 'impoverishment' of the epidemic that is affecting mainly the poorest segments of Brazilian society (after the necessary correction for demographic variables). This can be observed in the registered AIDS cases where new cases are mainly unskilled workers or unemployed people and individuals with only primary levels of education. Geographical analysis shows that new cases are being registered at a faster pace in the destitute surroundings of Brazilian big cities (Grangeiro, 1994). Analysis has also shown a trend of 'interiorization' and spread of the epidemic towards middle-sized cities, especially in the State of São Paulo (Bastos and Barcellos, 1995). In this process IDUs play a central role.

As shown in Figure 10.3, AIDS cases registered among IDUs are distributed

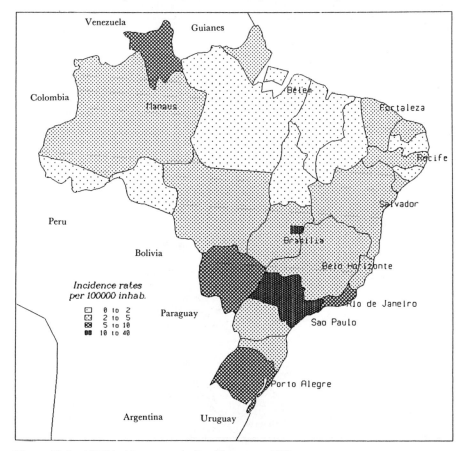

Figure 10.2 AIDS incidence rates in Brazilian states, 1992

along a corridor that connects the centre-west of the country with the main ports and airports of the industrialized south-east. This path coincides with the primary routes of cocaine traffic and passes through the main middle-sized cities of the richest state of Brazil — São Paulo. Contrasting with this pattern, the cases registered among men who have sex with men exhibit a patchwork pattern all around the country without any definite geo-political orientation other than the concentration in the biggest cities and their surroundings (Figure 10.4).

The episodes of two malaria outbreaks among HIV-1 infected IDUs in areas of São Paulo that are free of primary transmission of malaria (through mosquitoes) and distant from malarigenic areas (located in the centre-west, and in the tropical forest in the north) attest to the role of IDUs in the geographical diffusion of HIV-1, and perhaps both types of infection in contemporary Brazil (Bastos *et al.*, 1995).

Data from recent research in HIV-1 molecular epidemiology in Brazil reinforce former geographical analyses, both showing that Brazil has a complex, although interactive, pattern of multiple sub-epidemics, as described by Cantoni

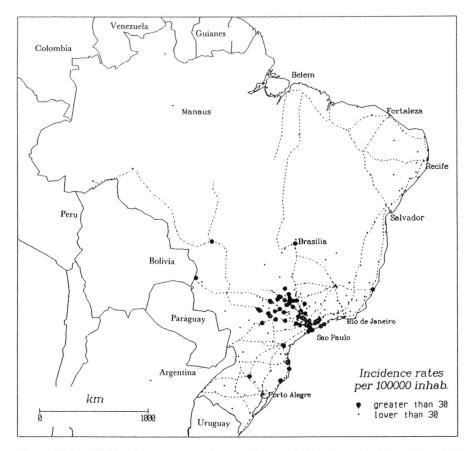

Figure 10.3 AIDS incidence rates related to drug injecting in Brazilian main cities, 1983 to 1992

et al. (1995) respecting Italy, but with a greater diversity, probably due to its continental size and social heterogeneity. It seems that the pattern described by Weniger *et al.* (1994) for Thailand, of partial segregation of epidemics among the different exposure categories and distribution of HIV-1 subtypes, is somewhat, although to a lesser extent, observed in São Paulo, with a higher proportion of F subtypes being identified among IDUs, concerning other exposure categories (Sabino, 1995; Rossini *et al.*, 1995). Conversely, a more mixed and non-segregated pattern is being disclosed from Rio de Janeiro's data (Guimarães *et al.* 1995).

It seems that the initial hypothesis (Lima *et al.*, 1992) of a bridging effect from men who have sex with men to IDUs, through the activity of homo- and bisexual IDUs, is perhaps incomplete as an explanation for the epidemics among IDUs in the different regions of Brazil. Instead a more complex epidemic pattern emerges with different 'gateways' of introduction of HIV-1 (Morgado, 1995), and a more 'autonomous' role of the epidemic among IDUs.

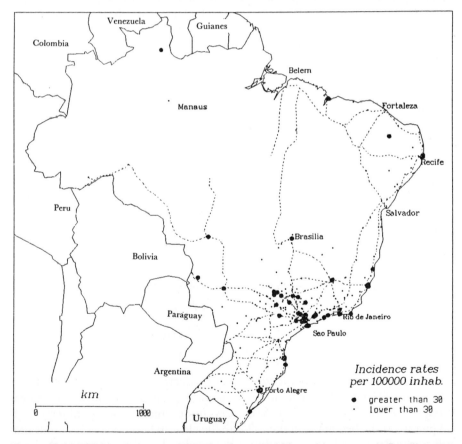

Figure 10.4 AIDS incidence rates related to homo- and bisexual intercourse in Brazilian main cities, 1983 to 1992

F. Bastos, G. V. Stimson, P. Telles and C. Barcellos

The Brazilian Contemporary Drug Scene and the Main Limitations of Preventive Strategies in the First Decade (1982–1992)

Harm reduction is an expression seldom heard in the Brazilian academic or government milieus, except perhaps among AIDS researchers who have had personal experience of these strategies while studying abroad.

Years of legal enforcement, and paucity of preventive and treatment alternatives (or to quote Henman (1993), the influence of 'harm aggravation' policies), combined with a long period of high inflation and recession of the 1980s, changed both the socio-economic standards of the country and the patterns of drug use and traffic. Over the last decade a growing number of people in Brazil have lost their positions in the formal employment market and have moved to informal part-time occupations that include dealing in small amounts of illicit drugs (Carlini, 1993). The main cities, and especially the slums (*favelas*) have become overcrowded and homeless people, including an increasing number of children, are living and sleeping on the streets. Brazil today has a real and multifarious drug problem, that combines challenges characteristic of the developed world, such as strong cocaine distribution networks, with other more typically third world drug problems, such as psychotropic drugs diverted from the legal market or bought over the counter (Carlini, 1983, 1993), and glue/solvent sniffing by street children (Carlini-Cotrim and Carlini, 1988).

The 1980s were a time of vigorous increase in cocaine traffic through Brazil, and the register of AIDS cases shows a gradual increase in the number of cases attributed to needle sharing. At the end of the 1980s and beginning of the 1990s the first seroprevalence surveys undertaken in the state of São Paulo and Rio de Janeiro disclosed high levels of seroprevalence for HIV-1 among IDUs (Bastos *et al.*, 1995).

This situation has become a demanding problem for public health professionals working in the main areas affected by HIV/AIDS epidemic, but control initiatives have remained, until recently, restricted to unco-ordinated local efforts depending on the limited amount of local funds of the Municipal Departments or Universities (Mesquita, 1992), who are traditionally dependent on federal support.

Until recently, very few NGOs and self-help organizations (excluding the ones strictly connected with the promotion of abstinence), and no advocacy groups are involved in the development of prevention activities among IDUs. The only exception has been the rare HIV-1 infected IDUs who belonged to broader organizations concerned with the support and advocacy of HIV-1 infected people and patients with AIDS.

The fight for a harm reduction strategy directed to IDUs received a boost only after 1992, when the Federal Government requested financial and technical support from the World Bank for AIDs prevention. Analysis of the epidemiological picture at the beginning of the 1990s made clear to both the World Bank staff and to the Brazilian health authorities the need to highlight the central role of programmes specifically directed to IDUs and their partners in halting the spread of the epidemic. This awakening of interest endeavoured to put an end to a long period of neglect, but took place at a time when HIV-1 seroprevalence levels among IDUs had already reached high plateaux.

Despite the fact that Brazil is a federation, there is very little opportunity for implementing regionally independent initiatives possible in other federations such as the USA (for example the Point Defiance needle-exchange programme in Tacoma, Washington) or Germany (Stöver and Schuller, 1992), where local funding and regional juridicial arrangements can support such initiatives. In Brazil the fate of harm reduction strategies is strongly dependent on centralized decisions. The actual commitment of the National AIDS Programme is very important, but the political situation in Brazil is unstable, and changes can occur at any time.

Another major limitation is posed by the present legislation that perceives some initiatives as condoning (or even promoting) drug use. This can encompass almost any harm reduction strategy such as bleach-and-teach programmes, every kind of outreach activity, and the activity of self-help groups that are not abstinence orientated. Criticism of the present legislation has grown in recent years; the issue is being debated more openly by Brazilian society and deserves a greater media coverage. At the time of writing, alternatives to the present legislation are being examined by the Brazilian Congress towards a more liberal juridical environment respecting public health initiatives.

The present preventive initiatives are basically supported by public health professionals and researchers in the 'front line' of AIDS prevention programmes, in the states more strongly affected by the epidemic. Other influential public opinion makers are scarcely aware of harm reduction approaches, which receive no support from public authorities or social leaders not directly concerned with the AIDS epidemic. In this respect, it becomes essential to educate members of the judiciary, which will be required to ensure the implementation and the development of the different harm reduction programmes across the whole country, in very different regional contexts but under the same federal law.

It will similarly be important to redefine harm reduction philosophy as a human rights issue, enrolling the support of the general community and of NGOs who are currently involved in similar efforts to support people living with AIDS, street children, and other minority and stigmatized groups.

In all these activities, the roles of the media, international experts, political leaders and opinion makers are essential in creating a strong coalition of interest necessary for their further development.

Acknowledgments

Ongoing field research in Rio de Janeiro, Brazil are being sponsored by the National Coordination of STD/AIDS, Brazilian Ministry of Health and by Oswaldo Cruz Foundation. Rio de Janeiro's State Foundation for the Development of Science (FAPERJ) sponsored Drs Bastos and Barcellos' work at

Oswaldo Cruz Foundation. Dr Bastos benefited from a short-stay as visiting-researcher at the Department of Criminology of the University of Hamburg, sponsored by DAAD. We would also like to acknowledge the help of Sam Friedman, Don Des Jarlais, Patricia Friedmann and Professors Klaus Püschel and Sebastian Scheerer (University of Hamburg).

References

ADES, A.E. (1995) 'Serial HIV seroprevalence surveys: interpretation, design, and role in HIV/AIDS prediction', *Journal of Acquired Immune Deficiency Syndromes and Human Retrovirology*, **9**, 5, pp. 490–9.

ALBOTA, M., KOOPS, A. and LEWERENZ, J. *et al.* (1995) 'HIV-Praevalenz intravenoes Drogenabhaengiger im Hamburger Strafvollzug im Jahresvergleich 1992–1993', *AIDS-Forschung*, **10**, 3, pp. 127–32.

ANCA (1988) AIDS IVDU working group, 'Containing the spread of HIV infection in IVDU', mimeo pp. 20.

ANCHUELA, O.T., CATALÁN, J.C. and DÍAZ, M.F.S. (1994) 'Evolución dels patrón epidemiológico del SIDA en España', *Publicacion Oficial de la Sociedade Española Interdisciplinaria de SIDA*, **5**, 3, pp. 80–1.

ARACHNE, J. and BALL, A. (1986) 'AIDS and IV drug users: the situation in Australia', *Drug and Alcohol Review*, **5**, pp. 175–85.

BASTOS, F.I. and BARCELLOS, C. (1995) 'A geografia social da AIDS no Brasil', *Revista de Saúde Pública*, **29**, 1, pp. 52–62.

BASTOS, F.I., TELLES, P.R., CASTILHO, E.A. and BARCELLOS, C. (1995) 'A epidemia de AIDs no Brasil', in MINAYO, C. (Ed.) *Os muitos brasis: Saúde e População na década de 80*, pp. 245–68, São Paulo/Rio de Janeiro: Hucitec & ABRASCO.

CANTONI, M., LEPRI, A.C., GROSSI, P. *et al.*. (1995) 'Use of AIDS surveillance data to describe subepidemic dynamics', *International Journal of Epidemiology*, **24**, 4, pp. 804–12.

CARLINI, E.A. (1983) 'O uso e a propaganda de medicamentos. Exemplos com psicotrópicos', *Revista da Associação Brasileira de Psiquiatria*, **5**, pp. 152–8.

CARLINI, E.A. (1993) 'Uso ilícito de drogas lícitas pela nossa juventude. É um problema solúvel?, in BASTOS, F.I. and GONÇALVES, O.D. (Eds) *Drogas é legal? Um debate autorizado*, pp. 51–66, Rio de Janeiro: Ed. Imago and Goethe Institute.

CARLINI-COTRIM, B. and CARLINI, E.A. (1988) 'The use of solvents and other drugs among homeless and destitute children living in the city streets of Sao Paulo, Brazil', *Social Pharmacology*, **2**, pp. 51–62.

CARVALHO, H., MESQUITA, F.C., MASSAD, E. *et al.* (1996) 'HIV and infections of similar transmission patterns in an IDU community of Santos, Brazil', *Journal of Acquired Immune Deficiency Syndromes and Human Retrovirology*, **12**, pp.84–92.

CHOOPANYA, K., VANICHSENI, S., DES JARLAIS, D. *et al.* (1991) 'Risk factors and HIV seropositivity among injecting drug users in Bangkok', *AIDS*, **5**, 12, pp. 1509–13.

DAVIES, A.G., DOMINY, N.J., PETERS, A. *et al.* (1995) 'HIV in injecting drug users in Edinburgh: Prevalence and correlates', *Journal of Acquired Immune Deficiency Syndromes and Human Retrovirology*, **8**, 4, pp. 399–405.

DE LA FUENTE, L., BARRIO, G., VICENTE, J. *et al.* (1994) 'Intravenous administration among heroin users having treatment in Spain', *International Journal of Epidemiology*, **23**, 4, pp. 805–11.

Des Jarlais, D.C. (1989) 'Le VIH à New York', in Charles-Nicolas, A. (Ed.) *Sida et Toxicomanie Répondre*, pp. 99–113, Paris: Frison-Roche.

Des Jarlais, D.C. (1994) 'Cross-national studies of AIDS among injecting users', *Addiction*, **89**, pp. 383–92.

Des Jarlais, D.C., Casriel, C., Friedman, S.R. and Rosenblum, A. (1992) 'AIDS and the transition to illicit drug injection: Results of a randomized trial prevention program', *British Journal of Addiction*, **87**, 6, pp. 493–8.

Des Jarlais, D.C., Hagan, H., Friedman, S.R. *et al.* (1995) 'Maintaining low HIV seroprevalence in populations of injecting drug users', *Journal of the American Medical Association*, **274**, 15, pp. 1226–31.

Dolan, K. (1993) 'Drug injectors in prison and the community in England', *International Journal of Drug Policy*, **4**, 4, pp. 179–83.

Friedman, S. (1993) 'AIDS as a sociohistorical phenomenon', in Albrecht, G.L. and Zimmerman, R.S. (Eds) *Advances in Medical Sociology*, pp. 19–36, Greenwich: JAI Press.

Friedman, S.R., De Jong, W. and Wodak, A. (1993) 'Community development as a response to HIV among drug injectors', *AIDS*, **7**, (suppl. 1), pp. 263–9.

Friedman, S.R., Stepherson, B., Woods, J. *et al.* (1992) 'Society, drug injectors, and AIDS', *Journal of Health Care for the Poor and Underserved*, **3**, 1, pp. 73–89.

Friedman, S.R., Curtis, R, Ward, T.P. *et al.* (1995) 'Drogenabhaengigkeit und Tuberkulose in den USA', in Göltz, J. (Ed.) *Der drogenabhaengige Patient*, pp. 229–36, München, Wien and Baltimore: Urban und Schwarzenberg.

Grangeiro, A. (1994) 'O perfil sócio-econômico da AIDS no Brasil', in Parker, R. *et al.* (Eds) *A AIDS no Brasil*, pp. 91–128, Rio de Janeiro: ABIA/UERJ & Relume-Dumará.

Guimarães, M.L., Gripp, C.B.G., Costa , C.I. *et al.* (1995) 'HIV-1 diversity in patients from Rio de Janeiro, BR', Poster presented at 'I Simpósio Brasileiro de Pesquisa Básica em HIV/AIDS', Abstract book, p. 22, Rio de Janeiro: Angra dos Reis.

Hamouda, O., Schwartländer, B., Koch, M.A. *et al.* (1993) 'AIDS/HIV 1992 — Bericht zur epidemiologischen Situation in der Bundesrepublik Deutschland zum 31.12.1992', *AZ Hefte*, Berlin: AIDS-Zentrum in Bundesgesundheitsamt.

Heckman, W., Püschel, K., Schmoldt, A. *et al.* (Eds) (1993) *Drogennot- und -todesfaelle — Eine differentielle Untersuchung der Praevalenz und Aetiologie der Drogenmortalitaet*, Baden-Baden: Nomos Verl.-Ges.

Henman, A. (1993) 'Harm reduction or harm aggravation? The impact of the developed countries' drug policies in the developing world', in Heather, N. *et al.* (Eds) *Psychoactive Drugs and Harm Reduction: From Faith to Science*, pp. 247–56, London: Whurr Publishers.

Herkt, D. (1993) 'Peer-based user groups: The Australian experience', in Heather, N. *et al.*. (Eds) *Psychoactive Drug and Harm Reduction: From Faith to Science*, pp. 320–30, London: Whurr Publishers.

Lima, E.S., Telles, P.R., Bastos, F.I. *et al.* (1992) 'Homosexual and bisexual male drug injectors as a potential bridge for HIV to reach other drug injectors in Rio de Janeiro', Poster (PoC 4258) presented at the VII International Conference on AIDS, Amsterdam. The Netherlands.

Ljunberg, B., Christensson, B., Tunving, K. *et al.* (1991) 'HIV prevention among injecting drug users: Three years of experience from a syringe exchange programme in Sweden', *Journal of Acquired Immune Deficiency Syndromes*, **4**, pp. 890–5.

MANN, J. *et al.* (Eds) (1992) *AIDS in the World*, Cambridge: Harvard University Press.

MESQUITA, F.C. (1992) 'Drogas injetáveis e AIDS', in PAIVA, V. (Ed.) *Em tempos de AIDS*, pp. 187–92, São Paulo: Summus.

MORGADO, M.G. (1995) 'Polymorphisme de la région V3 de la GP 120 des échantillons brésiliens du VIH-1', *Annales du Seminaire 'Proces de developpement de vaccins anti-VIH-SIDA: Problèmes et bénéfices'*, pp. 101–4. Ministère de la Santé.

NATIONAL RESEARCH COUNCIL (1993) *The social impact of AIDS in the United States*, Washington: National Academy Press.

PANT, A. and KLEIBER, D. (1993) 'Explaining decline and stabilization of HIV seroprevalence in Berlin between 1989 and 1993', oral presentation (WS-C09-5) in the IX International Conference on AIDS, Berlin.

PARKER, R. (1994) 'Sexo entre homens: Consciência da AIDS e comportamento sexual entre homens homossexuais e bissexuais no Brasil', in PARKER, R. *et al.* (Eds) *A AIDS no Brasil*, pp. 129–50, Rio de Janeiro: ABIA/UERJ & Relume-Dumará.

PIEPER, K. (1993) 'On the history of the AIDS-Hilfe', AIDS Forum D.A.H.- Band XII, *Aspects of AIDS and AIDS-Hilfe in Germany*, pp. 9–18, Berlin: Deutsche AIDS-Hilfe.

POLLAK, M. and SCHILTZ, M-A. (1994) 'L'état des recherches universitaires sur la population des bi- et homosexuels masculins en Europe', Brazilian version in LOYOLA, M.A. (Ed.) *AIDS e sexualidade*, pp. 183–208, Rio de Janeiro: Relume-Dumará.

PÜSCHEL, K. and MOHSENIAN, F. (1991) 'HIV-1 prevalence among drug deaths in Germany', in LOIMER, N. *et al.* (Eds) *Drug Addiction and AIDS*, pp. 89–96, Vienna: Springer-Verlag.

REZZA, G., NICOLOSI, A., ZACCARELLI, M. *et al.* (1994) 'Understanding the dynamics of the HIV epidemic among Italian intravenous drug users: A cross-sectional versus a longitudinal approach', *Journal of Acquired Immune Deficiency Syndromes and Human Retrovirology*, **7**, 5, pp. 500–3.

ROBERTSON, R. (1990) 'The Edinburgh epidemic: A case study', in STRANG, J. and STIMSON, G. (Ed) *AIDS and Drug Misuse*, pp. 95–107, London: Routledge.

ROSSINI, M., TURQUATO, G., ACETTURI, C. *et al.* (1995) 'Subtipos de HIV-1 em usuários de droga na cidade de São Paulo', poster presented at 'I Simpósio Brasileiro de Pesquisa Básica em HIV/AIDS', Abstract book, p. 13, Rio de Janeiro: Angra dos Reis.

SABINO, E. (1995) 'Sous-typage du VIH-1 à travers l'éssai de mobilité des rubans hétheroduplexes de DNA en gel d'acrilamide', *Annales du Séminaire 'Proces de developpement de vaccins anti-VIH/SIDA: problèmes et bénéfices'*, pp. 143. Ministère de la Santé.

STEFFEN, M. (1993) 'AIDS policies in France', in BERRIDGE, V. and STRONG, P. (Eds) *AIDS and Contemporary History*, pp. 240–64, Cambridge: Cambridge University Press.

STIMSON, G.V. (1995) 'AIDS and injecting drug use in the United Kingdom, 1987–1993: The policy response and the prevention of the epidemic', *Social Science and Medicine*, **41**, 5, pp. 699–716.

STIMSON, G.V. (1996) 'Drug injecting and the spread of HIV infection in south-east Asia', in SHERR, L., CATALAN, J. and HEDGE, B. (Eds) *The Impacts of AIDS: Psychological and Social Aspects of HIV Infection*, Reading: Harwood Academic Publishers.

STÖVER, H. and SCHULLER, K. (1992) 'AIDS prevention with injecting drug users in the former West Germany: A user-friendly approach on a municipal level', in O'HARE, P. *et al.* (Eds) *The Reduction of Drug-Related Harm*, pp. 186–94, London: Routledge.

STRANG, J., DES JARLAIS, D.C., GRIFFITHS, P. and GOSSOP, M. (1992) 'The study of transitions in the route of drug use: The route from one route to another', *British Journal of Addictions*, **87**, 6, pp. 473–84.

VERDECCHIA, A., MARIOTTO, A., CAPOCACCIA, R. and MARIOTTI, S. (1994) 'An age and period reconstruction of the HIV epidemic in Italy', *International Journal of Epidemiology*, **23**, 5, pp. 1027–39.

WALLACE, R. (1993) 'Social disintegration and the spread of AIDS', *Social Science and Medicine*, **38**, 7, pp. 887–96.

WALLACE, R., FULLILOVE, M., FULLILOVE, R. *et al.* (1994) 'Will AIDS be contained within U.S. minority urban populations', *Social Science and Medicine*, **39**, 8, pp. 1051–62.

WENIGER, B.G., LIMPAKARNJANARAT, K., UNGCHUSAK, K. *et al.* (1991) 'The epidemiology of HIV infection and AIDS in Thailand', *AIDS*, **5**, 2, pp. 571–85.

WENIGER, B.G., TAKEBE, Y., OU, C-Y. and YAMAZAKI, S. (1994) 'The molecular epidemiology of HIV in Asia', *AIDS*, **8**, 2, pp. 513–28.

WODAK, A. (1994) 'Needle exchange and bleach distribution programmes in Australia: A review of the first eight years', oral presentation (Session B2, Abstract book p. 86) at the Vth International Conference on Reduction of Drug Related Harm, Toronto.

WODAK, A., FISHER, R. and CROFTS, N. (1993) 'An evolving public health crisis: HIV infection among injecting drug users in developing countries', in HEATHER, N. *et al.* (Eds) *Psychoactive Drugs and Harm Reduction: From Faith to Science*, pp. 280–96, London: Whurr Pubishers.

WORLD HEALTH ORGANIZATION INTERNATIONAL COLLABORATIVE GROUP (1994) *Multi-City Study on Drug Injecting and Risk of HIV Infection* (WHO/PSA/94.4), Geneva: WHO.

Chapter 11

Prison and HIV-1 Infection among Drug Injectors

Damiano Abeni, Carlo A. Perucci, Kate Dolan and Massimo Sangalli

HIV-1 and AIDS are major public health concerns for prisons. The problem has been fuelled mainly by two phenomena: the rapidly increasing numbers of prisoners in many countries, for example a 300 per cent increase in the number of prisoners in the USA over the last 15 years (Dolan, Wodak and Penny, 1995), and the increasing proportion of inmates who are injecting drug users. Prisons are 'selectively enriched' (Bird and Gore, 1994) with injecting drug users (IDUs): in Italy, for instance, IDUs accounted for 19 per cent of the total prison population in 1986, increasing to 31 per cent in 1992 (and over 50 per cent in some metropolitan areas) (Presidenza del Consiglio dei Ministri, 1993). AIDS became the leading cause of death among inmates in New York prisons in 1985 (Vlahov *et al.*, 1989) and in Maryland (USA) prisons in 1987 (Salive, Smith and Dolan, 1990).

The Centers for Disease Control (CDC, 1986), the Council of Europe (Harding, 1987), and the World Health Organization (WHO, 1987) have authoritatively highlighted the key aspects of the problem of HIV-1 infection in prisons: the relevance of the proportion of IDUs among AIDS cases, the high prevalence of HIV-1 infection among some populations of IDUs, and the high and increasing proportion of IDUs in prison populations. Within custodial settings, the often wide supply of drugs together with limited availability of sterile injecting equipment (Turnbull, Stimson and Stillwell, 1994), and the incidence of sexual behaviours (that is mainly homosexual contacts – Harding, 1987) have a tremendous potential for transmission of HIV-1 and other blood-borne and/or sexually transmitted infections.

Various studies, mainly in developing countries (Gaughwin, Douglas and Wodak, 1991), indicate that approximately one in ten male inmates have sex with another person while in prison and that penetrative sex is as common as non-penetrative (Turnbull, Dolan and Stimson, 1991; Turnbull and Stimson, 1993). There are also indications that sexual assault occurs in prison (Crofts, Webb-Pullman and Dolan, 1996).

The potential contribution of prisons to the spread of HIV-1 infection has been seriously underestimated. In Bangkok, the epidemic of HIV-1 infection among IDUs is thought to have begun in prison (Choopanya, 1989). Even more worrying is the lack of prevention measures and evaluation of such measures in the prison environment. Only a handful of countries provide condoms, bleach for disinfecting needles and syringes (Dolan, Wodak and Penny, 1995) and methadone maintenance (Dolan and Wodak, 1996) or other treatments for drug problems to inmates. One Australian study which monitored the ease of access to bleach in prison found that even after several years of such a programme being set up prisoners in New South Wales still found bleach difficult to obtain (Dolan, Hall and Wodak, 1994). A follow-up study found access to bleach had improved (Dolan *et al.*, 1995), but serious concerns have been raised about the efficacy of bleach to destroy HIV-1 (Shapshank *et al.*, 1993). Only Switzerland operates a syringe exchange scheme for inmates (Federal Office of Public Health, 1993; Nelles and Harding, 1995). However, an exploratory study found that syringe exchange is feasible in a prison setting if strict guidelines are followed (Rutter *et al.*, 1995).

An outbreak of HIV-1 infection among prisoners in Scotland (see below) resulted in the total number of known infected inmates in Scotland doubling within a matter of months (Scottish Affairs Committee, 1994). The potential for an outbreak of infection in the prison to contribute to the spread of HIV-1 infection in other prisons and in the community can be best appreciated by this example. There had been 636 inmates in Glenochil prison in Glasgow at the time of the outbreak between January and June 1993, but only 378 were still there in June. Of the 258 absent prisoners, nearly three quarters had been transferred to other prisons, with the remainder being released to the community (Taylor *et al.*, 1995).

AIDS was first reported among prisoners in 1983 by Wormser *et al.* (1983). Between September 1981 and June 1982 seven cases of AIDS were diagnosed in previously healthy males incarcerated in New York correctional facilities. None of these inmates were homosexual, but all had been IDUs prior to incarceration and it was concluded therefore that a significant segment of the prison population was at high risk of developing AIDS.

Since then, many studies have investigated drug injectors in prison. This chapter briefly reviews reports on prevalence and incidence of HIV-1 infection, and prevalence of risk behaviours, and considers the available evidence from the data collected within the framework of the World Health Organization Multi-City Study on Drug Injecting and Risk of HIV Infection.

Prevalence of HIV-1 Infection in Prisons

United States and Canada

In the USA, many state correctional systems have instituted either mass screening programmes or large-scale, blinded serologic surveys for HIV-1 infection. The Federal Bureau of Prisons tests a 10 per cent sample of federal prisoners. Other jurisdictions conduct screening or testing programmes for selected groups of prisoners, such as known IDUs and others thought to be at particularly high risk (homosexuals, sex workers) (Hammett, 1988). The Centers for Disease Control (CDC, 1989) reported the results of surveys and studies on HIV-1 antibody prevalence in prisoners, conducted in 29 different states or areas for the period 1985–7. Most routine screening programmes yielded seroprevalence rates higher than those estimated for the general population, but much lower than those seen in groups composed of persons at increased risk. A geographic variation in seroprevalence was observed, ranging from low rates (0 per cent in Iowa and Idaho, 0.3 per cent in Wisconsin) to appreciably high rates (7.0 per cent in Maryland and 17.4 per cent in New York).

Subsequent studies were conducted to identify temporal trends and update prevalence estimates, mainly in Wisconsin, Maryland and New York City. In Wisconsin, voluntary and blinded HIV-1 testing was conducted among newly incarcerated male inmates in 1986, 1987 and 1988. HIV-1 seroprevalence remained stable here over the three-year periods (0.30 per cent, 0.53 per cent and 0.56 per cent respectively), without difference between voluntary and blinded samples (Hoxie *et al.*, 1990). In Maryland, results of serosurveys of HIV-1 infection using excess sera from male inmates (Vlahov *et al.*, 1990) showed stability of prevalence: 7.0 per cent, 7.7 per cent, 7.0 per cent and 8.0 per cent during four years of surveillance in the 1985–8 period. A blinded seroprevalence survey conducted among all individuals entering New York City prisons in 1989 provided an overall rate of 18.5 per cent, with a significantly lower value for males as compared with females (16.1 per cent vs. 25.8 per cent) (Weisfuse *et al.*, 1991).

While all these serosurveys focused on individual correctional systems, the study by Vlahov *et al.* (1991) included 10 distinct systems within the United States in order to account for geographical diversity. HIV-1 seroprevalence was assessed among 10 994 consecutive male and female inmates, from 1988 to 1989. Overall prevalence was 4.3 per cent, ranging from 2.1 per cent to 7.6 per cent for men and 2.5 per cent to 14.7 per cent for women. Seroprevalence among women was higher than among men across nine of the 10 systems.

During 1989 to 1992, the CDC, in collaboration with state and local health departments, conducted anonymous unlinked HIV-1 seroprevalence surveys in 46 correctional facilities in 19 metropolitan areas (Withum *et al.*, 1993). Of 69 407 specimens tested for HIV-1, 4.2 per cent were positive. Females had higher rates than males in 10 of the 16 metropolitan areas where both female and male entrants were surveyed. Gellert *et al.* (1993) reported a prevalence of 2.5 per cent in 1985 and 2.7 per cent in 1991 in the women's jail of Orange County, California.

In Canada, Hankins *et al.* (1994) observed during 1988–9 a prevalence of 13.0 per cent among a self-selected sample of IDU women in prison, compared to 1.0 per cent among non-IDU women in the same setting.

Europe

Early in 1987, a survey of the extent to which the AIDS epidemic was affecting prisons with inmate populations totalling about 270 000 in 17 European countries, was conducted on behalf of the Council of Europe (Harding, 1987). The estimates for the rate of HIV-1 seropositivity ranged from low (0 per cent in Portugal, 1.3 per cent in Belgium, 2.1 per cent in Luxembourg) to high values (11 per cent in Switzerland, 12.6 per cent in France, 16.8 per cent in Italy). An extremely low figure was reported from England and Wales (<0.1 per cent). Even if these results are not strictly comparable since data were collected in different ways, it seemed reasonable to estimate an overall prevalence of seropositivity in prisons of member states of the Council of Europe to be in excess of 10 per cent. Subsequently, available data on HIV-1 seroprevalence for prison populations have remarkably increased.

In 1989 and 1990, studies of female prisoners in Spain (Granados, Miranda and Martin, 1990) and France (Clavel *et al.*, 1992) showed HIV-1 seroprevalence levels of 26 per cent and 1.8 per cent respectively.

In the United Kingdom, the study conducted among male inmates of Saughton Prison (Edinburgh) in 1991 was the first attempt to establish HIV-1 prevalence with risk-factor elicitation in a UK prison (Bird *et al.*, 1992). Seventy-five per cent of the available inmates (378/499) volunteered to participate in this anonymous surveillance study, which involved giving a saliva sample for anonymous testing for HIV-1 antibodies and completing an anonymous risk-factor questionnaire. Documented HIV-1 prevalence was 4.5 per cent, which — assuming no volunteer bias (as supported by questionnaire returns) — suggested that actual prevalence was 25 per cent greater than that known or revealed to the prison medical service.

Incidence of HIV-1 Infection

Studies of HIV-1 incidence in correctional facilities are rare. Kelley *et al.* (1986) in their study of a maximum-security prison in the USA failed to document evidence for intra-prison transmission of HTLV-III. Follow-up serum samples were initially screened for HTLV-III antibody during 1983 to 1984 and later retested in July 1985. Among 542 inmates representing 685 person-years of incarceration, the annual incidence was 0.0 per cent. Data representing an additional 641 person-years of follow-up were obtained by pairing 199 specimens collected in July 1985 with samples collected in May 1982. None of these pairs showed evidence of HTLV-III infection.

In Nevada (Horsburgh *et al.*, 1990), all incoming inmates to the State Prison System beginning in August 1985 routinely received HIV-1 antibody testing, and, starting from August 1987, also received testing at the time of their release. A total of 1105 inmates had samples obtained on entry, and again on leaving, the prison system; 1069 inmates whose initial test was negative were followed by a total of 1207 person-years. Two definite cases of seroconversion to HIV-1 were detected: the seroconversion rate was therefore 2/1069 or 0.19 per cent of those susceptible.

In the Orange County study (Gellert *et al.*, 1993), of 865 women with two or more tests during the 1985–91 period, 29 seroconverted. The overall incidence rate was 1.6 per 100 person-years, with yearly incidences of 5.7, 0.0, and 1.4 per 100 person-years in 1985, 1989, and 1991 respectively. The extent of the presence of risk behaviours and the circumstances in which transmission might have occurred were not explored or discussed in this study.

The first report of an outbreak of HIV-1 infection occurring within a prison in Glenochil, Scotland (Taylor *et al.*, 1995) documented, on the basis of sequential test results and time of entry, that eight cases of transmission of HIV-1 definitely occurred within that prison in the period between 1 January 1993 and 30 June 1993.

Risk Behaviours for HIV-1 Transmission

During the early 1980s in the USA some studies documented transmission of hepatitis B between inmates (Hull *et al.*, 1985; Decker *et al.*, 1985) and the consistent association between the prevalence of hepatitis serological markers, and risk behaviours prior and during incarceration. For example 26 per cent of inmates in Tennessee reported injecting drug use and 17 per cent reported homosexual activity while in prisons (Decker *et al.*, 1984). Since HIV-1 is transmitted by the same routes as hepatitis B virus, it was reasonable to conclude that transmission of HIV-1 within prisons may occur. As prevalence of infection in correctional settings increases, so too does risk of transmission. Therefore, data on prevalence of risk behaviours for HIV-1 transmission within prisons are critical to assess whether imprisonment is an independent risk factor for acquiring HIV-1 infection. Several studies have provided evidence that significant rates of high risk behaviour (injecting drug use, sharing of needles and syringes, and sexual activity) occur in correctional settings.

Carvell and Hart (1990) undertook a study at two drug agencies in central London. Fifty self-selected IDUs, all of whom had been held in custody at some time since 1982, completed an anonymous self-administered questionnaire about their use of drugs while in custody, and their injecting and sexual risk behaviours for HIV-1 infection. Just over half of the sample had not only injected drugs while in prison, but also shared equipment (66 per cent and 52 per cent respectively). At particularly high risk were those who had been held on remand. Some of the male prisoners compounded their risk of HIV-1 infection by engaging in sexual activity with multiple partners and some of them had female partners subsequent to their release. Those serving shorter sentences were more likely to have engaged in sexual activity.

In the same year, a study using an indirect method of estimating the prevalence of risk behaviours was conducted among 373 male prisoners at all of

South Australia's prisons (Gaughwin *et al.*, 1991). Prisoner respondents estimated that 36 per cent of all prisoners injected drugs at some stage during their incarceration, and that 12 per cent engaged in anal intercourse at least once.

Estimates of the prevalence of injecting behaviour and sexual activity in prison, obtained by subsequent studies, vary widely. In 1990, a study among 81 IDUs at two Glasgow needle exchanges showed that 25 per cent of those who had served at least one term in custody had injected drugs in prison, and 43 per cent of those who admitted injecting, also shared needles (Kennedy *et al.*, 1991). In 1991, a Scottish study found that of the 123 inmates interviewed, 24 per cent (two-thirds of the injectors) had injected drugs in prison (Dye and Isaacs, 1991). In two samples of English prisoners, one found no evidence of injecting in prison (Maden, Swinton and Gunn, 1991), while the other reported that 27 per cent of injectors continued injecting once in prison (Turnbull, Dolan and Stimson, 1991). Of those who injected in prison, as documented by these studies, three-quarters shared injecting equipment (Dye and Isaacs, 1991; Turnbull, Dolan and Stimson, 1991). The study in Saughton prison (Bird *et al.*, 1992), found that 47 per cent of individuals who reported drug injecting behaviour also admitted injecting in prison.

Sexual activity was reported by 10 per cent of the 451 prisoners in England who received a structured interview within three months of release (Dolan, Turnbull and Stimson, 1991). By contrast Power *et al.*'s (1991) study of Scottish prisons reported a 'low rate' of homosexual activity in prison: 'only one male inmate reported being sexually active during a period of incarceration'. The total number of male inmates was not specified.

Among drug users who had recently been released from a custodial setting, Turnbull, Stimson and Stillwell (1994) found that 16/44 (36.4 per cent) had injected the last time they were in prison, and that extensive awareness that injecting occurred in prison was present also among those who did not have actual contact with needles and syringes or those using them. In the study conducted after the outbreak of HIV-1 infection in Glenochil prison in Scotland (Gore *et al.*, 1995) the prevalence of injecting behaviour among IDU inmates was 59 per cent. Gore, Bird and Ross (1995) and Gore *et al.* (1995) also found that 25 per cent of Glenochil's and 6 per cent of Barlinnie prison's IDU inmates had started injecting inside a prison.

A study conducted in Austria (Pont *et al.*, 1994) in the years 1989, 1990, and 1992, found that 31 of 371 (8.4 per cent) imprisoned male IDUs reported needle sharing while in prison. Prevalence of HIV-1 infection was 35.5 per cent among IDUs who shared needles in prison, and 12.4 per cent among those who did not.

Evidence from the WHO Multi-City Study

The WHO Multi-City Study did not collect specific information on drug injectors and their behaviours in prison. However, one of the survey questions asked 'How many times have you been in prison or jail overnight or longer since you first injected drugs?' This section of the chapter summarizes the observations from the complete dataset of the Multi-City Study, and reports results from a specific analysis of the data collected in Rome in 1990 and in 1992, conducted to assess whether an association exists between frequency of incarceration and HIV-1 infection among drug injectors.

All Centres

The complete dataset from the study includes 6437 subjects: of these, one has to be excluded from all analysis because of missing information. Information on frequency of incarceration is available in all but 142 (2.2 per cent) of the 6436 valid records. Among the 6294 subjects with adequate information, 70.7 per cent had been in prison at least once. Prison experience is widespread among IDUs from all the participating centres: Table 11.1 shows that in only three centres (Madrid, Rome, Sydney) less than 70 per cent of the study participants were incarcerated at least once, while in Santos as many as 96 per cent of subjects had already experienced imprisonment. In Toronto, New York and Glasgow over 30 per cent of the participants had been to prison more than five times since first injecting drugs. In the same centres, 5 per cent of the participants were incarcerated 25 times or more, and in Athens, London and Santos the same proportion of subjects were incarcerated 20 times or more.

Table 11.2 summarizes the prevalence of HIV-1 infection in the different centres according to the levels of frequency of incarceration for the 4575 subjects with available information both on HIV-1 testing and on number of times in prison. Overall, prevalence of HIV-1 infection increases from 15.9 per cent among those who report never having been in prison, to 21.5 per cent among those who were imprisoned only once, to over 25 per cent among those who were in prison two or more times. This pattern is strikingly consistent across centres, and most evident in New York, Rome and Rio de Janeiro. The only two notable exceptions are London and Sydney, with observed prevalences that actually decrease as frequency of incarceration increases.

The Rome Data

Nine hundred and thirty-seven drug injectors were recruited in the two years of the survey. Of these, 846 (90.3 per cent) had already been tested for anti-HIV-1 antibodies and knew their test results: 268 (31.7 per cent) were HIV-1 positive. The study conducted testing for HIV-1 on saliva samples, and valid results were available for 399 subjects (26.1 per cent HIV-1 positive). The following analysis considers separately the two sets of 846 ('self-reported' group) and 399 ('saliva' group) subjects.

Three hundred and fifty subjects (41.1 per cent) in the 'self-reported' group and 182 (45.6 per cent) in the 'saliva' group had never been in prison. The

Table 11.1 Frequency of imprisonment among participants in the WHO Multi-City Study

Cities	Total	Times in prison or jail overnight since first injected												
		0		1		2–5		6–10		>10		mi	
	n	n	%	n	%	n	%	n	%	n	%	n	%
Athens	(400)	(85)	21.3	(86)	21.5	(130)	32.5	(47)	11.8	(51)	12.8	(1)	0.3
Bangkok	(601)	(175)	29.1	(139)	23.1	(225)	37.4	(41)	6.8	(12)	2.0	(9)	1.5
Berlin	(380)	(127)	33.4	(87)	22.9	(135)	35.5	(24)	6.3	(4)	1.1	(3)	0.8
Glasgow	(503)	(111)	22.1	(47)	9.3	(120)	23.9	(91)	18.1	(101)	20.1	(33)	6.6
London	(534)	(156)	29.2	(96)	18.0	(162)	30.4	(58)	10.9	(59)	11.0	(3)	0.6
Madrid	(472)	(225)	47.7	(79)	16.7	(119)	25.2	(32)	6.8	(15)	3.2	(2)	0.4
New York	(1470)	(238)	16.1	(203)	13.7	(538)	36.4	(239)	16.2	(241)	16.3	(19)	1.3
Rio	(479)	(188)	39.2	(61)	12.7	(187)	39.0	(33)	6.9	(8)	1.7	(2)	0.4
Rome	(487)	(226)	46.4	(65)	13.3	(141)	29.0	(41)	8.4	(14)	2.9	(0)	0.0
Santos	(220)	(7)	3.2	(55)	25.0	(76)	34.5	(18)	8.2	(20)	9.1	(44)	20.0
Sydney	(424)	(198)	46.7	(77)	18.2	(104)	24.5	(32)	7.5	(12)	2.8	(1)	0.2
Toronto	(458)	(106)	23.1	(60)	13.1	(123)	26.9	(87)	19.8	(57)	12.4	(25)	5.5
Total	(6436)	(1842)	28.6	(1055)	16.4	(2060)	32.0	(743)	11.5	(594)	9.2	(142)	2.2

mi = missing information. Percentage calculated on total n

Table 11.2 Prevalence of HIV-1 infection among IDUs who underwent HIV-1 testing in the WHO Multi-City Study (n=4695), by frequency of imprisonment

Cities	Times in prison or jail overnight since first injected*							
	0		1		2–5		>5	
	n	%HIV+	n	%HIV+	n	%HIV+	n	%HIV+
Athens	(85)	1.2	(86)	0.0	(130)	0.0	(98)	1.0
Bangkok	(173)	23.1	(139)	40.3	(225)	35.6	(53)	49.1
Berlin	(115)	8.7	(80)	10.0	(128)	23.4	(28)	21.4
Glasgow	(99)	0.0	(45)	0.0	(101)	1.0	(181)	2.2
London	(143)	18.9	(87)	5.7	(148)	16.2	(111)	6.3
Madrid	(74)	58.1	(23)	39.1	(38)	71.1	(10)	80.0
New York	(134)	32.8	(115)	40.9	(295)	50.2	(295)	54.6
Rio	(47)	27.7	(18)	27.8	(45)	35.6	(20)	50.0
Rome	(95)	13.7	(21)	19.0	(51)	25.5	(19)	42.1
Santos	(6)	50.0	(53)	67.9	(75)	66.7	(38)	68.4
Sydney	(198)	2.0	(77)	2.6	(104)	1.9	(44)	0.0
Toronto	(105)	4.8	(60)	1.7	(119)	2.5	(141)	8.5
Total	(1274)	15.9	(804)	21.5	(1459)	27.0	(1038)	25.9

Subjects with a result from HIV-1 testing but with missing information on the frequency of imprisonment (n=120) are not considered here.

univariate analysis shows a strong association between HIV-1 infection and frequency of incarceration. The prevalence rate ratio (PRR) for HIV-1 infection in subjects who reported having been incarcerated ranged from 1.4 (95 per cent confidence interval [CI], 1.03–1.8) to 3.0 (95 per cent CI, 2.2–4.3) in the four exposed levels for the 'self-reported' group, and from 1.8 (95 per cent CI, 1.1–2.7) to 3.3 (95 per cent CI, 1.8–6.0) in the 'saliva' group, with a strong statistically significant trend ($p<0.001$).

Among several variables associated with imprisonment, the highest risks of imprisonment were seen for males, older injecting drug users, injecting drug users with longer drug injecting experience, those with lower educational level, and those unemployed. None of the variables related to sexual practices were associated with imprisonment. Of the variables that in univariate analysis appeared to be associated with incarceration, some were also associated with HIV-1 infection. Statistically significant associations with HIV-1 infection were observed for older age, lower educational level, being in drug treatment programmes, longer drug injecting experience, and needle/syringe borrowing. Females were more likely, although not significantly, to be HIV seropositive than males. No statistically significant association with HIV-1 infection was observed for variables related to sexual practices.

Table 11.3 summarizes the results of the logistic regression analysis. Frequency of incarceration remained associated with HIV-1 infection after adjusting for the potential confounders listed above. Also associated with HIV-1 infection, in the final model, were duration of drug use, gender, educational level, occupational status, and needle borrowing. When fitted as a continuous varible, frequency of incarceration was significantly associated with HIV-1

Table 11.3 Factors associated with HIV-1 positivity among injecting drug users, Rome 1990–2 (Final logistic regression models)

		HIV-1 Saliva Tested Group		HIV-1 Self-reported Group	
		OR	95% CI	OR	95% CI
Frequency of	0	1.0	–	1.0	–
imprisonment	1–2	1.8	0.97–3.3	1.2	0.8–1.9
	3–5	1.6	0.7–3.4	2.5	1.5–4.1
	6–10	2.9	1.2–7.0	3.0	1.6–5.5
	>10	4.4*	1.2–16.1	3.4**	1.5–8.1
Gender	Men	–	–	1.0	–
	Women	–	–	1.5	1.04–2.3
Education	<9	1.0	–	1.0	–
(years)	9–13	0.4	0.2–0.7	0.7	0.5–1.01
	>13	0.9	0.4–2.0	0.9	0.5–1.6
Occupation	Employed	–	–	1.0	–
	Unemployed	–	–	1.4	0.97–1.9
Duration of	≤5	1.0	–	1.0	–
drug use	6–10	2.7	1.1–6.7	2.6	1.5–4.5
(years)	11–15	6.0	2.4–15.0	4.9	2.9–8.6
	>15	4.8	1.8–12.8	3.0	1.6–5.8
Needle	No	1.0	–	1.0	–
borrowing	Yes	2.1	1.1–3.8	3.4	2.3–5.0

OR = Odds Ratio (adjusted)
CI = Confidence Interval
*Adjusted Chi square for trend = 7.77, p<0.005
**Adjusted Chi square for trend = 21.88, p<0.001

infection (OR 1.07, 95 per cent CI 1.02–1.12 in the 'self-reported' group and OR 1.07, 95 per cent CI 1.01–1.15 in the 'saliva' group, for a unit increase in the frequency of incarceration). Transformations (that is quadratic, log) failed to add information to the model.

Discussion

A high proportion of IDUs is characteristic of prison populations. The preliminary analysis of the data from the WHO Multi-City Study confirms the high burden of incarceration suffered by IDUs, and shows how widespread and consistent this is in different countries from four continents, and in developed as well as developing nations.

Serosurveys of HIV-1 infection among inmates entering prison serve to estimate the extent and scope of infection, to identify the reservoir from which intra-prison transmission might occur, to provide an empirical foundation for the development and refinement of policy and prevention programmes, and to supplement information from other sources on the extent and scope of HIV-1 infection in the community from which the inmates originate and to which they return. HIV-1 serosurveillance studies within prisons in the United States and

Europe have shown widely different HIV-1 prevalence; even if methodological and temporal differences among these studies limit strict comparisons of the results, the possible effects of sampling variation or selection bias should be taken into account. The overall rate of seropositives in prisons appears to be closely related to that of the local population of drug injectors, mainly depending upon prevalence of IDUs among inmates. The possible effects of selection bias are even more relevant as regards the results of studies on risk behaviours for HIV-1 transmission. In most of these surveys, sample size was small and the respondents were self-selected because of the voluntary nature of the studies, so therefore the samples were unlikely to be representative of all prisons.

Further research on a much wider scale and in a larger number of countries is required to document the extent of risk activity within prisons. However, even with these limitations, the existing data provide consistent evidence that significant rates of high risk behaviour do occur in correctional settings, and occurrence of HIV-1 transmission in prison has been documented. This highlights the need for prison systems to take a responsible and active role in addressing the issues surrounding risk behaviours in appropriate, effective, ethical and accountable ways in order to avoid HIV-1 transmission among inmates.

Consistent across participating centres in the WHO Multi-City Study is the evident pattern of an association between frequency of incarceration and presence of HIV-1 infection, with the exception of London and Sydney. The analysis of the Roman data show that this association is independent from other known risk factors for HIV-1 infection, and that a 'dose-response' effect seems to be present. The cross-sectional nature of the study does not allow inference to be made that a direct causal relationship exists between incarceration and HIV-1 infection. In fact, it could be that IDUs who engage in very high risk behaviours are more likely to go to prison. This would suggest that IDUs in prison are more likely to be at higher risk, and are therefore more in need of support, preventive action, and harm reduction intervention.

The growing evidence on the role of prisons in the spread of HIV-1 infection, and the realization of the huge potential for prevention and harm reduction programmes in the prison setting, should urge intervention in prisons. In most countries, programmes are rare or absent, and need urgently to be introduced. In some the emphasis has been placed mainly on HIV-1 testing and counselling, rather than on risk reduction programmes (for example in the USA the CDC reported 378 HIV-1 counselling and testing programmes in correctional facilities of 41 states, compared with 56 HIV-1 health education/ risk reduction programmes in 22 states — CDC, 1992): this balance needs to be redressed.

The WHO Global Programme on AIDS has released guidelines for HIV-1 prevention in prisons (WHO, 1993) that have been ignored in most prison systems worldwide. The first general principle of such guidelines, that 'All prisoners have the right to receive health care, including preventive measures, equivalent to that available in the community without discrimination', has been commonly disregarded. Effective preventive measures such as methadone maintenance, syringe exchange and condom distribution, now implemented in the community in many nations, are still much needed in the correctional setting.

Since the time spent in prison by drug injectors offers a definite and valuable setting for programmes aimed at preventing sexual transmission of HIV-1 to non-drug-using heterosexuals outside of prisons, failure to provide prison populations with adequate interventions will result in reduced possibilities to control the HIV-1 epidemic in the wider community, and in a more rapid and extensive spread of infection to the so-called 'general population'.

References

BIRD, A.G. and GORE, S.M. (1994) 'Inside methodology: HIV surveillance in prisons', *AIDS*, **8**, pp. 1345–6.

BIRD, A.G., GORE, S.M., JOLLIFFE, D.W. and BURNS, S.M. (1992) 'Anonymous HIV surveillance in Saughton Prison, Edinburgh', *AIDS*, **6**, pp. 725–33.

BREWER, T.F., VLAHOV, D., TAYLOR, E., HALL, D., MUÑOZ, A. and POLK, F. (1988) 'Transmission of HIV-1 within a statewide prison system', *AIDS*, **2**, pp. 363–7.

CARVELL, A.L.M. and HART, G.J. (1990) 'Risk behaviours for HIV infection among drug users in prisons', *British Medical Journal*, **300**, pp. 1383–4.

CASTRO, K., SHANSKY, R., SCARDINO, V., NARKUNAS, J. and HAMMETT, T. (1991) 'HIV transmission in correctional facilities', 16–21 June, p. 314. Paper presented at the VIIth International Conference on AIDS, Florence.

CENTERS FOR DISEASE CONTROL (1986) 'Acquired immunodeficiency syndrome in correctional facilities: A report of the National Institute of Justice and the American Correctional Association', *Morbidity and Mortality Weekly Report*, **35**, pp. 195–9.

CENTERS FOR DISEASE CONTROL (1989) 'AIDS and human immunodeficiency virus infection in the United States: 1988 update', *Morbidity and Mortality Weekly Report*, **38**, (S–4), pp. 1–38.

CENTERS FOR DISEASE CONTROL (1992) 'HIV prevention in the U.S. correctional system, 1991', *Morbidity and Mortality Weekly Report*, **41**, pp. 389–97.

CHOOPANYA, K. (1989) *AIDS and Drug Addicts in Thailand*, Bangkok: Bangkok Metropolitan Authority Department of Health.

CHRISTIE, B. (1993) 'HIV outbreak investigated in Scottish jail', *British Medical Journal*, **307**, pp. 151–2.

CLAVEL, T., LECOURT, J.F., DEMAIN, A., ROUSSEAU, I. and THOMAS, P. (1992) 'HIV seroprevalence and risk factors among female inmates in a French prison', *Journal of the Acquired Immune Deficiency Syndromes*, **5**, pp. 428–30.

CROFTS, N., WEBB-PULLMAN, J. and DOLAN, K. (1996) *An analysis of trends over time in social and behavioural factors related to the transmission of HIV among IDUs and prison inmates*, Canberra: AGPS.

DECKER, M.D., VAUGHN, W.K., BRODIE, J.S., HUTCHESON, R.H. and SCHAFFNER, W. (1984) 'Seroepidemiology of hepatitis B in Tennessee prisoners', *Journal of Infectious Diseases*, **150**, pp. 450–59.

DECKER, M.D., VAUGHN, W.K., BRODIE, J.S., HUTCHESON, R.H. and SCHAFFNER, W.

(1985) 'Incidence of hepatitis B in Tennessee prisoners', *Journal of Infectious Diseases*, **152**, pp. 214–17.

DOLAN, K. and WODAK, A. (1996) 'An international review of methadone provision in prisons', *Addictions Research*, **4** (1), pp. 85–97.

DOLAN, K., HALL, W. and WODAK, A. (1994) 'Bleach availability and risk behaviour in prison in New South Wales', Technical Report, 22, Sydney: National Drug and Alcohol Research Centre.

DOLAN, K.A., TURNBULL, P.J. and STIMSON, G.V. (1991) 'HIV prevalence and risk behaviour of 452 prisoners in England', Abstract W.C. 3321, VII International Conference on AIDS. Florence.

DOLAN, K., WODAK, A. and PENNY, R. (1995) 'AIDS behind bars: Preventing HIV spread among incarcerated drug injectors', AIDS, **9**, pp. 825–32.

DOLAN K., SHEARER, J., HALL, W. and WODAK, A. (1995) 'Bleach easier to obtain but inmates still risk infection in New South Wales prisons', Technical Report, Sydney: National Drug and Alcohol Research Centre.

DYE, S. and ISAACS, C. (1991) 'Intravenous drug misuse among prison inmates: Implications for spread of HIV', *British Medical Journal*, **302**, p. 1506.

FEDERAL OFFICE OF PUBLIC HEALTH (1993) 'HIV prevention in Switzerland: Targets, strategies, interventions', Bern: National AIDS Commission.

GAUGHWIN, M.D., DOUGLAS, R.M. and WODAK, A.D. (1991) 'Behind bars — risk behaviours for HIV transmission in prisons, a review', in NORBERRY, J., GERULL, S.A. and GAUGHWIN, M.D. (Eds) *HIV/AIDS and Prisons Conference Proceedings*. Canberra: Australian Institute of Criminology.

GAUGHWIN, M.D., DOUGLAS, R.M., LIEW, C., DAVIES, L., MYLVAGANAM, A., TREFFKE, H., EDWARDS, J. and ALI, R. (1991) 'HIV prevalence and risk behaviours for HIV transmission in South Australian prisons', *AIDS*, **5**, pp. 845–51.

GELLERT, G.A., MAXWELL, R.M., HIGGINS, K.V., PENDERGAST, T. and WILKER, N. (1993) 'HIV infection in the Women's jail, Orange County, California, 1985 through 1991', *American Journal of Public Health*, **83**, pp. 1454–6.

GORE, S.M. and BIRD, A.G. (1993) 'No escape: HIV transmission in jail', *British Medical Journal*, **307**, pp. 147–8.

GORE, S.M., BIRD, A.G. and ROSS, A.J. (1995) 'Prison rites: Starting to inject inside', *British Medical Journal*, **311**, pp. 1135–6.

GORE, S.M., BIRD, A.G., BURNS, S.M., GOLDBERG, D.J., ROSS, A. J. and MACGREGOR, J. (1995) 'Drug injection and HIV prevalence in inmates of Glenochil prison', *British Medical Journal*, **310**, pp. 293–6.

GRANADOS, A., MIRANDA, M.J. and MARTIN, L. (1990) 'HIV seropositivity in Spanish prisons'. Abstract Th.D.116, VI International Conference on AIDS, San Francisco.

HAMMETT, T. (1988) 'AIDS in correctional facilities: Issues and options', Washington, DC: US Department of Justice, National Institute of Justice.

HANKINS, C.A., GENDRON, S., HANDLEY, M.A., RICHARD, C., LAI TUNG, M.T. and O'SHAUGHNESSY, M. (1994) 'HIV infection among women in prison: An assessment of risk factors using a nonnominal methodology', *American Journal of Public Health*, **84**, pp. 1637–40.

HARDING, T.W. (1987) 'AIDS in prison', *The Lancet*, **ii**, pp. 1260–3.

HORSBURGH, C.R., JARVIS, J.Q., McARTHUR, T., IGNACIO, T. and STOCK, P. (1990) 'Seroconversion to human immunodeficiency virus in prison inmates', *American Journal of Public Health*, **80**, pp. 209–10.

HOXIE, N.J., VERGERONT, J.M., FRISBY, H.R., PFISTER, J.R., GOLUBJATNIKOV, R. and

DAVIS, J.P. (1990) 'HIV seroprevalence and the acceptance of voluntary HIV testing among newly incarcerated male prison inmates in Wisconsin', *American Journal of Public Health*, **80**, pp. 1129–31.

HULL, H.F., LYONS, L.H., MANN, J.M., HADLER, S.C., STEECE, R. and SKEELS, M.R. (1985) 'Incidence of Hepatitis B in the penitentiary of New Mexico', *American Journal of Public Health*, **75**, pp. 1213–14.

KELLEY, P.W., REDFIELD, R.R., WARD, D.L., BURKE, D.S. and MILLER, R.N. (1986) 'Prevalence and incidence of HTLV-III infection in a prison', *Journal of the American Medical Association*, **256**, pp. 2198–9.

KENNEDY, D.H., NAIR, G., ELLIOTT, L. and DITTON, J. (1991) 'Drug misuse and sharing of needles in Scottish prisons', *British Medical Journal*, **302**, p. 1507.

MADEN, A., SWINTON, M. and GUNN, J. (1991) 'Drug dependence in prisoners', *British Medical Journal*, **302**, p. 880.

MUTTER, R.C., GRIMES, R.M. and LABARTHE, D. (1994) 'Evidence of intraprison spread of HIV infection', *Archives of Internal Medicine*, **154**, pp. 793–5.

NELLES, J. and HARDING, T. (1995) 'Preventing HIV transmission in prison: A tale of medical disobedience and Swiss pragmatism', *The Lancet*, **346**, pp. 1507–8.

PONT, J., STRUTZ, H., KAHL, W. and SALZNER, G. (1994) 'HIV epidemiology and risk behavior promoting HIV transmission in Austrian prisons', *European Journal of Epidemiology*, **10**, pp. 285–9.

POWER, K.G., MARKOVA, I., ROWLANDS, A., McKEE, K.J., ANSLOW, P.J. and KILFEDDER, C. (1991) 'Sexual behaviour in Scottish prisons', *British Medical Journal*, **302**, pp. 1507–8.

PRESIDENZA DEL CONSIGLIO DEI MINISTRI-DIPARTIMENTO PER GLI AFFARI SOCIALI, (1993) 'Relazione sui dati relativi allo stato delle tossicodipendenze in Italia, sulle strategie adottate e sugli obiettivi raggiunti nel 1992', Roma.

RUTTER, S., DOLAN, K., WODAK, A., HALL, W., MAHER, L. and DIXON, D. (1995) 'Is syringe exchange feasible in a prison setting? An exploratory study of the issues', Technical Report, Sydney: National Drug and Alcohol Research Centre.

SALIVE, M.E., SMITH, G.S. and DOLAN, K.A. (1990) 'Death in prison: Changing mortality patterns among male prisoners in Maryland 1979–87', *American Journal of Public Health*, **80**, pp. 1479–80.

SCOTTISH AFFAIRS COMMITTEE (1994) 'Drug Abuse in Scotland, Report', London: HMSO.

SHAPSHANK, P., McCOY, C.B., RIVERS, J.E., CHITWOOD, D.D., MASH, D.C., WEATHERBY, N.L., INCIARDI, J.A., SHAH, S.M. and BROWN, B.S. (1993) 'Inactivation of human immunodeficiency virus–1 at short time intervals using undiluted bleach', *Journal of the Acquired Immune Deficiency Syndromes*, **6**, pp. 218–19.

TAYLOR, A., GOLDBERG, D., EMSLIE, J., WRENCH, J., GRUER, L., CAMERSON, S., BLACK, J., DAVIS, B., McGREGOR, J., FOLLETT, E., HARVEY, J., BASSON, J. and McGAVIGAN, J. (1995) 'Outbreak of HIV infection in a Scottish prison', *British Medical Journal*, **310**, pp. 289–92.

TURNBULL, P.J. and STIMSON, G.V. (1993) 'Prisons: Heterosexuals in a risk environment', in SHERR (Ed.), *AIDS and the heterosexual population*, Reading: Harwood.

TURNBULL, P.J., DOLAN, K.A. and STIMSON, G.V. (1991) *Prisons, HIV and AIDS: Risk and Experiences in Custodial Care*, Horsham: Avert.

TURNBULL, P.J., STIMSON, G.V. and DOLAN, K.A. (1992) 'Prevalence of HIV infection among ex-prisoners in England', *British Medical Journal*, **304**, pp. 90–1.

TURNBULL, P.J., STIMSON, G.V. and STILLWELL, G. (1994) *Drug use in prison*, Horsham: Avert.

VLAHOV, D., BREWER, F., MUÑOZ, A., HALL, D., TAYLOR, E. and POLK, B.F. (1989) 'Temporal trends of human immunodeficiency virus type 1 (HIV–1) infection among inmates entering a statewide prison system, 1985–1987', *Journal of the Acquired Immune Deficiency Syndromes*, **2**, pp. 283–90.

VLAHOV, D., MUÑOZ, A., BREWER, F., TAYLOR, E., CANNER, C. and POLK, B.F. (1990) 'Seasonal and annual variation of anitbody to HIV-1 among male inmates entering Maryland prisons: Update', *AIDS*, **4**, pp. 345–50.

VLAHOV, D., BREWER, T.F., CASTRO, K.G., NARKUNAS, J.P., SALIVE, M.E., ULLRICH, J. and MUÑOZ, A. (1991) 'Prevalence of antibody to HIV-1 among entrants to US correctional facilities', *Journal of the American Medical Association*, **265**, pp. 1129–32.

WEISFUSE, I.B., GREENBERG, B., BACK, S.D., MAKKI, H.A., THOMAS, P., ROONEY, W.C. and RAUTENBERG, E. L. (1991) 'HIV-1 infection among New York city inmates', *AIDS*, **5**, pp. 1133–8.

WHO (1987) World Health Organization, 'WHO consultation on prevention and control of AIDS in prisons', *The Lancet*, **ii**, pp. 1263–4.

WHO (1993) World Health Organization, Global Programme on AIDS, 'WHO guidelines on HIV infection and AIDS in prisons', Geneva: World Health Organization.

WITHUM, D.G., GÜEREÑA-BURGUEÑO, F., GWINN, M., STAN LEHMAN, J. and PETERSEN, L.R. (1993) 'High HIV prevalence among female and male prisoners in the United States (1989–1992): Implications for prevention and treatment strategies,' Abstract PO-C21-3115, IX International Conference on AIDS, Berlin.

WORMSER, G.P., KRUPP, L.B., HANRAHAN, J.P., GAVIS, G., SPIRA, T.J. and CUNNINGHAM-RUNDLES, S. (1983) 'Acquired immunodeficiency syndrome in male prisoners', *Annals of Internal Medicine*, **98**, pp. 297–303.

Chapter 12

Preventing Epidemics of HIV-1 among Injecting Drug Users

Don C. Des Jarlais, Holly Hagan, Samuel R. Friedman,
Patricia Friedmann, David Goldberg, Martin Frischer,
Steven Green, Kerstin Tunving, Bengt Ljungberg, Alex
Wodak, Michael Ross, David Purchase, Peggy Millson and
Ted Myers

In many areas, the spread of HIV-1 among injecting drug users (IDUs) due to the multi-person use of drug injection equipment has occurred with extreme rapidity. In New York City, for example, HIV-1 seroprevalence among IDUs increased from under 10 per cent to over 50 per cent in a period of five years (Des Jarlais *et al.*, 1989); in Edinburgh, HIV-1 seroprevalence among IDUs increased from zero to over 40 per cent in one year (Robertson *et al.*, 1986); in Bangkok, HIV-1 seroprevalence increased from 2 per cent to over 40 per cent in two years (Vanichseni and Sakuntanaga, 1990); and in the state of Manipur, India, levels increased from zero to approximately 50 per cent in one year (Naik *et al.*, 1991). HIV-1 has spread rapidly among populations where there has been a lack of awareness of AIDS as a local threat and mechanisms such as 'shooting galleries', 'dealer's works' and professional injectors that provide rapid and efficient mixing among large numbers of IDUs (Friedman and Des Jarlais, 1991).

There is also considerable evidence, mostly from developed countries, that most IDUs will change their behaviour in response to the threat of AIDS, given the opportunity to do so. Indeed, the great majority of subjects in the World Health Organization Multi-City Study on Drug Injecting and Risk of HIV infection reported changing their behaviour in order to avoid getting AIDS (see Chapter 4). The fact that extremely rapid spread of HIV-1 has occurred under certain circumstances, and the demonstrated capacity of many IDUs to modify their HIV-1 risk behaviour, lead to the question of whether it is possible to prevent epidemics of HIV-1 transmission among injecting drug users. The WHO Study formed the basis of the first examination of 'prevented HIV epidemics' among IDUs.

This chapter presents case histories of five cities in which HIV-1 has been introduced into a heterosexual IDU community, but where HIV-1 seroprevalence has remained low and stable. Operationally, we defined 'introduction of HIV' into a local population as an HIV-1 seroprevalence rate of at least 1 per cent, and 'stable low seroprevalence' as a seroprevalence rate of less than 5 per cent with no increasing trend for a period of at least five years. The 5 per cent HIV-1 seroprevalence level was selected because it is well below the 10 per cent level from which rapid, epidemic-scale increases in HIV-1 seroprevalence among IDUs have frequently been observed (Friedman and Des Jarlais, 1991). Moreover, because HIV-1 seroprevalence is often higher among IDUs not in drug treatment (Lamothe, Bruneau and Soto, 1992; Lampinen *et al.*, 1992), we also required seroprevalence data from at least one non-treatment sample of IDUs.

Several methods were utilized to identify geographic areas with stable low seroprevalence among IDUs. Searches were made of published literature reviews (Stimson, 1990, 1995; Lurie *et al.*, 1993), the abstracts of the most recent International Conferences on AIDS (Florence 1991, Amsterdam 1992, Berlin 1993, Yokohama 1994), and computerized bibliographical databases. Unpublished seroprevalence studies and personal communications with other researchers in the field were also used. The search was initiated in 1992 and conducted through the first quarter of 1995.

The Low Prevalence Cities

Five cities were identified that met the aforementioned operational definition for stable low HIV-1 seroprevalence: Glasgow, Scotland; Lund, Sweden; Sydney, Australia; Tacoma (Washington), USA; and Toronto, Canada. Serial cross-sectional seroprevalence data were available from studies conducted in Glasgow (Frischer *et al.*, 1992a, 1992b, 1993), in Tacoma (Hagan and Hale, 1993), in Toronto (Millson *et al.*, 1993), and from multiple studies in Sydney (reviewed by Kaldor *et al.*, 1993). In each of these five cities there were at least two studies of HIV-1 prevalence among IDUs not in treatment. The minimum sample size for determining seroprevalence for a given year in these studies was at least 95 subjects in each of the treatment and non-treatment samples.

In Lund (and the surrounding Skane province), there has been extensive voluntary HIV-1 counselling and testing of IDUs, with individually coded reports for all HIV-seropositives (as described in Ljungberg *et al.*, 1991). Each positive case is investigated to determine where the person was living when the seroconversion occurred. There is also post-mortem HIV-1 testing for all known IDUs in Skane, and there have been no cases of deceased HIV-positive IDUs who had not been previously reported. (For full details on the seroprevalence studies in each of the sites, see Frischer *et al.*, 1992a, 1992b, 1993; Hagan and Hale, 1993; Millson *et al.*, 1993; Kaldor *et al.*, 1993; Ljungberg *et al.*, 1991).

Three of these cities (Glasgow, Sydney, Toronto) had participated in the WHO Multi-City Study, so that risk behaviour data were already available from IDUs in those cities. The European Community Multi-Site Study questionnaire

(Papaevangelou, Ancelle-Park and Seyrer, 1991) was administered to a sample of IDUs in Lund, while a questionnaire developed for a syringe-exchange evaluation study was used in Tacoma (Hagan *et al.*, 1993). The interview data were collected between 1990 and 1993 in the different cities. Sample sizes were 919 for Glasgow, 112 for Lund, 424 for Sydney, 874 for Tacoma, and 582 for Toronto.

Local experts (including co-authors of this report) completed questionnaires describing the characteristics of the local drug-injection situation and the local AIDS prevention activities for IDUs. All of these local experts have been conducting research on HIV-1 infection among IDUs in their communities over the last five or more years. The descriptions of the local IDU situations included available data on the size of the IDU population, availability of drug use treatment, and 'informed judgements' on characteristics such as the geographic concentration of the local IDU population, the quality of public transportation, police tactics, and access to health care for IDUs. The description of prevention activities included recording when they were first initiated ('early' prevention was defined as beginning when HIV-1 seroprevalence was <5 per cent), and assessing the extent to which ready access to sterile injection equipment, community outreach, bleach distribution, drug treatment programmes, and HIV-1 counselling and testing were used as prevention methods.

The Injecting Drug Use Population in the Five Cities

Table 12.1 presents descriptive information about the local IDU population and available health care for IDUs in each of the five cities. According to the local experts, the IDU population was rated as somewhat concentrated in all cities except Lund, where it was highly concentrated; public transportation was good in all cities except Tacoma, where it was poor; local police did not make it difficult to carry syringes in Glasgow, Lund, or Sydney, but made it somewhat difficult to carry syringes in Tacoma and Toronto. All cities except Tacoma had universal health insurance; discrimination against IDUs in health-care settings was rated as moderate in Glasgow, Lund and Sydney, and severe in Tacoma and Toronto. These descriptions are as of early 1994, and thus reflect the historical impact of some HIV-1 prevention efforts, such as expansion of drug treatment programmes (described below).

It is also important to note that the IDU population was relatively stable over time in these five cities. There were no major changes in the size of the IDU population; in particular, there were no increases in the numbers of new injectors and no appreciable in-migration of IDUs from other areas. Street prices for injectable drugs remained fairly constant, and no new types of injectable drugs were introduced in any of the cities. The demographic and social characteristics of the IDU populations in these cities also did not change appreciably over the time period of stable low seroprevalence.

Table 12.1 Characteristics of the injecting drug user populations in five cities with stable low HIV seroprevalence

Cities	Estimated IDUs	City population	Drugs injected	Drug treatment
Glasgow	8500	700 000	buprenorphine heroin	1000 methadone 100 detoxification 2500 outpatient 30 residential
Lund (Skane province)	500 city (3000 province)	90 000	amphetamine heroin	60 methadone 12 detoxification 6 residential 500 outpatient
Sydney	8–10 000	3 100 000	heroin amphetamine	6000 methadone 200 detoxification 700 residential 900 outpatient
Tacoma (Pierce county)	500 city (3000 county)	177 000	heroin cocaine	240 methadone 12 detoxification 700 outpatient
Toronto	8–10 000	635 000	heroin cocaine	200 methadone 128 detoxification 329 residential

Number of IDUs in a community is estimated by: capture/recapture in Glasgow; multiple methods in Lund and Sydney; synthetic area analysis in Tacoma. Data on 'drug treatment' include treatment provided to non-injecting drug users. City population is from most recent census data for each city.

HIV-1 Infection in the IDU Population

How HIV-1 was first introduced into a local population of IDUs usually cannot be known with certainty, but there is some evidence as to probable means of virus entry for the five cities described here. In Glasgow, HIV-1 was probably introduced by travellers to and from Edinburgh, less than 80 km distant, where HIV-1 seroprevalence among IDUs has been high since the mid-1980s (Robertson *et al.*, 1986). In Lund, HIV-1 was almost certainly introduced by immigration of HIV-positive IDUs from other parts of Sweden and by travellers to and from nearby Copenhagen, Denmark (Ljungberg *et al.*, 1991). In Sydney (Ross *et al.*, 1992, in press), Tacoma (Hagan and Hale, 1993), and Toronto (Millson *et al.*, 1992), HIV-1 probably entered through IDUs who were initially infected through male-with-male sex, as these cities have substantially higher HIV-1 seroprevalence rates among IDUs reporting male-with-male sex than among other IDUs.

Seroprevalence studies in the five cities are presented in Table 12.2. In the four cities where seroprevalence was studied through serial cross-sectional designs (Glasgow, Sydney, Tacoma and Toronto), the observed rates were all within narrow ranges, with no increasing trend over time in any city. In Lund, where HIV-1 counselling and testing of IDUs is conducted on a continuous basis, the HIV-1 infection level has remained low and stable.

Table 12.2 Injecting drug users in five cities with stable low HIV seroprevalence

Cities	Studies	Subjects tested	Sites	Years	Seroprevalence
Glasgow	7	2300	hospital outreach	1986–92	3%, 5%, 4%, 1%, 2%, 1%, 1%
Lund	continuous	>90% at least once >80% more than once	syringe-exchange	1986–92	<2% cumulative
Sydney	7	2700	drug treatment STD clinics outreach	1984–91	among heterosexual IDUs: 4%, 5%, 0.5%, 1%, 1%, 3%, 2%, 4%
Tacoma	7	1000	drug treatment syringe exchange outreach	1988–93	0.4%, 3%, 3%, 4%, 3%, 4%, 3%
Toronto	7	1300	drug treatment outreach syringe exchange	1988–93	among heterosexual IDUs: 0%, 2%, 3%, 3%, 1%, 3%, 2%

Number of study subjects is estimated by adding subjects from individual studies, reducing by one-third for possible multiple participation, and rounding to the nearest 100. Seroprevalence results are presented in order of the first year of data collection in different studies in each city, except that there are data from two concurrent 1992 studies in Tacoma, and Sydney results are from studies conducted in the following periods: 1984–8; 85–9; 85; 86–8; 86–8; 87; 87–91; 89–90. In Glasgow, testing from 1986–9 was done on a voluntary, named basis, and thus persons suspecting they were HIV-positive may have been more likely to volunteer; Glasgow data from 1990–2 were collected as part of anonymous studies, and may thus be less susceptible to volunteer bias. In Lund, there have been approximately 50 cases of HIV-seropositive IDUs who have moved into the province, and there have been eight local seroconversions. In Sydney, seroprevalence was notably higher among IDUs also reporting male-with-male sex, varying from 13 per cent to 44 per cent across different studies (see review by Kaldor *et al.*, 1993). For seroprevalence estimates in this table, IDUs reporting male-with-male sex were excluded in Sydney and Toronto, but were included in the other cities.

HIV-1 Prevention Activities

There have been a variety of HIV-1 prevention efforts in each of the five cities. Only brief comparative summaries are provided here (for more detailed descriptions of the HIV-1 prevention activities in these cities, see Ljungberg *et al.*, 1991; Hagan *et al.*, 1991; Frischer and Elliot, 1993; Friedman, de Jong and Wodak, 1993; Des Jarlais and Friedman, 1992; Millson *et al.*, 1991).

The first two common characteristics across the five cities were that prevention efforts were initiated relatively early and that they included large-scale provision of sterile injection equipment. In Glasgow, a syringe exchange and a programme to sell sterile needles and syringes in pharmacies to IDUs were both begun in 1987; in Lund, a syringe exchange programme was begun in 1986; in Sydney, the law requiring prescriptions for the purchase of needles and syringes was repealed, and a programme of over-the-counter sales and syringe exchange was begun in 1987 — indeed, an educational campaign to 'Never share needles' was launched by the wife of the Australian prime minister in 1987. In Tacoma, a syringe exchange programme was begun in 1988; and in Toronto, a street outreach/bleach-distribution programme for IDUs was begun in 1987, followed by a syringe exchange programme initiated in 1989. As indicated in Table 12.2, seroprevalence was <5 per cent among IDUs in each of these cities at the time these prevention efforts were initiated.

In each of the five cities, an estimated one-fifth to one-third of the IDUs were regular users of the local syringe exchanges. Moreover, many of these regular participants also exchanged injection equipment on behalf of others who did not directly participate in the exchanges. The exchanges in Sydney, Tacoma, and Toronto did not place limits on the number of needles and syringes that could be exchanged at one visit, which enhanced the likelihood that IDUs coming to exchange would also provide sterile injection equipment to others. In addition, while it was not possible to generate numerical estimates of the percentage of IDUs who regularly obtained sterile injection equipment from pharmacies in these five cities, legal pharmacy sales were also, in the assessment of the local experts, an important source of sterile injection equipment in all of the cities except Lund. (Pharmacy sales of equipment for injecting illicit drugs are illegal in Lund, and IDUs would have to take a half-hour ferry ride to Copenhagen to purchase injection equipment from a pharmacy).

The third common characteristic of the prevention programmes in the five cities was that they all involved community outreach to IDUs to disseminate AIDS information and risk-reduction supplies, and to build trust between healthcare workers and IDUs. All outreach programmes also provided referrals to other services, such as drug abuse treatment and HIV-1 counselling and testing. Several outreach programmes also provided some services 'on-site'. In Glasgow, outreach was conducted both in association with the original pharmacy sale programme and concurrent with the expansion of the syringe exchange programme, and 'drop-in centres' were established for female sex workers (many of whom were IDUs) (Taylor *et al.*, 1993; Carr *et al.*, 1992). In

Lund, health-care workers went out into the community to recruit participants for the syringe exchange (Christensson and Ljungberg, 1991); and in Sydney, 'drug users' groups' were supported with government funding to advise the design of AIDS prevention efforts and to operate some of the services (including syringe exchanges) (Friedman, de Jong and Wodak, 1993). In Tacoma, the syringe exchange programme was initiated in a high-drug-use area by a former drug use treatment programme staff person who had developed ongoing good relationships with IDUs (Hagan *et al.*, 1991); and in Toronto, among other efforts, the outreach included an 'ambassador' component, in which active drug users were trained to serve as outreach workers to their peers (Millson *et al.*, 1991). Moreover, in each of these cities, the information imparted by community outreach workers, and the resulting climates of trust, were further disseminated throughout the oral communication networks of IDUs themselves, thus reaching persons who were not in direct contact with the outreach workers (Hagan *et al.*, 1991; Friedman, de Jong and Wodak, 1993; Neaigus *et al.*, 1994).

Large-scale expansion of drug treatment programmes as a method of preventing HIV-1 infection among IDUs was utilized only in Sydney. Expansion of methadone maintenance treatment was begun there in 1985 (when there were only 840 persons in methadone programmes in the state of New South Wales), and increased until 5829 persons (out of an extimated total of 8000 IDUs) were in methadone treatment in 1991. In the other four cities, there has been modest (Glasgow, Lund, Toronto) or no (Tacoma) expansion of drug treatment. The community outreach efforts did, however, led to increased demand for pre-existing drug treatment slots among IDUs in all five cities. Indeed, in several cities, the outreach programmes became very important sources of referral to drug treatment.

The distribution of bleach for disinfecting injection equipment was an HIV-1 prevention strategy used extensively in Sydney, Tacoma and Toronto. In Sydney and Tacoma, bleach distribution was primarily in conjunction with syringe exchange, while Toronto had begun conducting a bleach-distribution outreach programme prior to initiating its syringe exchange programme.

Extensive voluntary HIV-1 counselling and testing as a principal method of AIDS prevention was utilized only in Lund, where the syringe exchange/ outreach greatly increased the numbers of IDUs who received voluntary HIV-1 counselling and testing. All the other cities did provide some HIV-1 counselling and testing to IDUs, often through referral from the outreach efforts and as part of research studies. (In Tacoma, some co-ordination difficulties occurred between the syringe exchange/outreach programme and the local counselling and testing site, so that this city probably had the least amount of voluntary HIV-1 counselling and testing among IDUs.)

The prevention activities for IDUs in these cities received substantial coverage in the local mass media. Even though some of the prevention activities — such as syringe exchanges — were controversial, the news coverage was generally favourable.

Of the six different aspects of prevention programming outlined here, three

— beginning early, community outreach, and ready access to sterile injection equipment — were present in all five cities; bleach distribution was present in three cities; and large-scale expansion of drug treatment and extensive HIV-1 counselling/testing were each present in only one city. While the number of cities in this report is modest, it is large enough to assess the likelihood of observing this pattern of prevention activities against a no-association null hypothesis that a particular prevention component is equally likely to be present or absent (p = 0.5) in a set of stable low-seroprevalence cities.

Under this null hypothesis, the probability that any one prevention component would be found in all five cities is $(0.5)^5 = .03125$. The probability of any three prevention components occurring in all five cities under the null hypothesis stated above is $.00016$.[1] The null hypothesis that the three common prevention components are equally likely to be present or absent in these cities can therefore be rejected.

HIV Risk Behaviour among IDUs

Table 12.3 shows selected demographic characteristics, as well as selected drug-use and sexual HIV-1 risk behaviours of the IDU respondents. In all five studies, a large majority of the subjects reported that they had changed their behaviour because of concern about AIDS. Complete elimination of HIV-1 risk behaviour did not occur in any of the cities; moderate-to-large percentages of the subjects reported that they had recently injected at least once with needle and syringes previously used by others. Much smaller proportions reported having recently engaged in the particularly high-risk behaviour of injecting in 'shooting galleries'

Table 12.3 Selected demographic characteristics and HIV-related risk behaviours of IDUs in five cities

Cities	Drugs commonly injected	Male %	Mean age (years)	Injection with previously used n/s*	Shooting gallery use* %	Unsafe sex with casual partners* %	Change in behaviour because of AIDS %	n
Glasgow	Buprenorphine Heroin	73	25	36	3	22	84	(919)
Lund	Amphetamine Heroin	71	30	58	3	35	82	(112)
Sydney	Heroin Amphetamine	78	27	41	1	13	84	(424)
Tacoma	Heroin Cocaine	70	37	30	9	53	73	(874)
Toronto	Heroin Cocaine	86	28.3	46	9	21	87	(582)

Risk behaviour in the six months prior to interview for Glasgow, Lund, Sydney and Toronto; for the one month prior to interview in Tacoma

Table 12.4 Prevention components and injecting drug user responses to AIDS in five cities with stable low HIV seroprevalence

Cities	Began early	Provided sterile equipment	Community outreach	Greatly expanded drug treatment	Extensive HIV testing	Bleach distribution	Self-reported behaviour change among IDUs	Residual risk behaviour
Glasgow	X	X	X				X	X
Lund	X	X	X		X		X	X
Sydney	X	X	X	X		X	X	X
Tacoma	X	X	X			X	X	X
Toronto	X	X	X			X	X	X

— places where injection equipment is rented to an IDU, used, returned to the gallery operator, and then rented to other IDUs.

Fully comparable data on detailed specifics of risk behaviour were not available from the different questionnaires. In general, however, it appears that much of this continued 'needle sharing' was infrequent and usually confined to small social networks. For example, in Lund, where a majority of the subjects reported at least one unsafe injection in the six months preceding the interview, only 28 per cent of the total sample reported more than two unsafe injections during that time period and, for the 52 per cent of persons reporting repeated unsafe injection, this risk practice was confined to 'sharing' with sexual partners only. In Tacoma, 30 per cent of the subjects reported some injecting with needles and syringes used by others, but only 8 per cent reported that half or more of their injections were with used needles and syringes. Moreover, while 9 per cent reported injecting in shooting galleries, only 3 per cent reported that half or more of their injections took place in shooting galleries.

Table 12.4 summarizes the prevention activities and response to concerns about AIDS among IDUs in these five cities. Again, it is worth noting that the prevention activities and response among IDUs occurred while the IDU population in these cities were basically stable — that is without any notable increases in the size of the population, in-migration from other areas, frequencies of drug injected, or types of drugs injected.

Limitations

No search for areas of stable low HIV-1 seroprevalence that attempts to include all unpublished data is likely to be fully comprehensive. Nevertheless, the search conducted for this study was relatively extensive and, as far as we could determine, was biased neither towards any geographic region nor towards the presence/absence of any specific type of AIDS prevention programming. The most likely source of bias is that cities conducting sufficient research to permit a determination of stable low seroprevalence by our criteria might also be more likely to be those which were sufficiently concerned about HIV-1 infection among IDUs to have implemented at least some type of prevention programme.

Stable low HIV-1 seroprevalence in a population of injecting drug users, however, does not imply an absence of new HIV-1 infections or guarantee against all future outbreaks of HIV-1 transmission in these cities. There have been reports of relapses to unsafe sexual behaviour among men who have sex with men in San Francisco, despite the considerable HIV-1 prevention activities in that city (Stall *et al.*, 1990; Ekstrand and Coates, 1990; Osmond *et al.*, 1993). In at least three of these five cities (Tacoma, Toronto, Sydney), HIV-1 seroprevalence is substantially higher among IDUs who also engage in male-with-male sex. Relapses from either sexual or injection risk reduction among IDUs who also engage in male-with-male sex could, therefore, lead to increased HIV-1 transmission for the local IDU population as a whole. Also, as noted above, the

IDU populations in these five cities were essentially 'stable' during the time periods of the study, without any notable in-migrations or changes in drugs injected or in frequencies of injection. Some types of large-scale changes in the characteristics of an IDU population might facilitate outbreaks of HIV-1 transmission. If an outbreak of increased HIV-1 transmission should occur in a low-seroprevalence area, it will be important to ensure that the public-health system can react quickly enough to contain such an outbreak.

The five case histories presented here, however, demonstrate that rapid transmission of HIV-1 is not inevitable among IDUs. Stable low HIV-1 seroprevalence can be maintained even with a substantial proportion of IDUs still engaging in some injection risk behaviour. This finding in itself has important policy implications. It clearly contradicts the opinion expressed by some public officials that the only way to prevent HIV-1 infection among IDUs is to stop their drug injection (ONDCP, 1992).

There are also data indicating low and possibly stable HIV-1 seroprevalence among IDUs in other cities in Australia (Kaldor *et al.*, 1993), in the United Kingdom (Stimson, 1995; Dolan *et al.*, 1993) and in New Zealand (Baker, Tobias and Brady, 1991). Preliminary analyses of data collected through the Centres for Disease Control blinded seroprevalence surveys at drug treatment programmes suggest that low seroprevalence may also exist in a number of other US cities (Lehman, personal communication, 1994). A major limitation in identifying other cities with stable low seroprevalence was the lack of comparable data from non-treatment samples which, as noted above, is an important limitation. It is also important to note that, to the best of our knowledge, at least some of the three common prevention components identified here had been implemented in all of these other cities in which stable low seroprevalence appears to be occurring.

Possible Causation

While it is important in itself to demonstrate that stable low seroprevalence is possible among populations of IDUs, it is also important to consider whether the specific AIDS prevention components identified here were responsible for the observed stable low seroprevalence. Did the prevention activities implemented in these cities prevent epidemics of HIV-1 infection in the local IDU populations?

With full recognition of the limits of relying upon case histories, we believe that it is possible at least to outline the elements of a causal analysis and note the major limitations. The descriptions of the IDU populations and health care for IDUs in these five cities (Table 12.1 and accompanying text) did not identify any obvious reason why HIV-1 would not have spread rapidly in these cities in the absence of the prevention activities that were implemented.

Given the existing research literature on community outreach to IDUs (Brown and Beschner, 1993; DiClemente and Peterson, 1994) and availability of sterile injection equipment (Lurie *et al.*, 1993; Ljungberg *et al.*, 1991; Tunving, Nyholm and Andersson, 1992; Hagan *et al.*, 1991), it is certainly plausible that these two components could help prevent rapid transmission of HIV-1 in a population of IDUs. Mathematical analyses of HIV-1 transmission would also suggest that initiating behaviour change/risk reduction when HIV-1 seroprevalence is low would also be effective in limiting HIV-1 transmission (Anderson *et al.*, 1991). Thus, it is possible to 'rule in' these three components as potential causes of stable low HIV-1 seroprevalence among IDUs (Cordray, 1986).

The prevention activities that were undertaken in some of the five cities examined here might also have contributed to reducing HIV-1 transmission among the local populations of IDUs. The media coverage of AIDS among IDUs in these cities — which often focused on the local prevention programmes — might also have contributed to awareness of AIDS and behaviour change.

As noted above, very large percentages of IDUs in each of these five cities reported behaviour change in response to AIDS. Other analyses of self-reported AIDS behaviour change among IDUs — with the same question used here — have shown that self-reported behaviour change is associated with avoiding HIV-1 infection among IDUs (Des Jarlais *et al.*, 1994a, 1994b; Chitwood, 1994). This suggests that the self-reports of behaviour changes are valid and that these behaviour changes substantially lessen the likelihood of becoming infected with HIV-1.

The related research literature thus suggests that the HIV-1 prevention activities implemented in these five cities did greatly limit HIV-1 transmission in the local IDU populations.

Making causal inferences also requires some form of comparison for the five city case histories. We constructed an illustrative case control analysis for testing an association between the presence of stable low seroprevalence and the presence of all three common prevention components. To identify 'control' cities, we operationally defined a 'lack of stable low seroprevalence' as a seroprevalence rate of 10 per cent or greater for two or more consecutive years or a rate of 20 per cent for one year. Use of this operational definition meant that there would be cities which could not be classified as having or not having stable low seroprevalence, but this was considered preferable to the misclassification that would occur if cities with seroprevalence of approximately 5 per cent but limited available data were included in the case-control analysis.

Using the same search procedures that were used for identifying stable low-seroprevalence cities, we then attempted to identify cities where all three prevention components were present and yet stable low seroprevalence was not present. We were able to identify *no* cases where all three components were clearly present and yet stable seroprevalence was clearly absent.

To identify areas that lacked one or more of the hypothesized critical prevention components, and that lacked stable low seroprevalence, we used only a subset of our search techniques, a single review article that contains serial seroprevalence data for a total of 17 cities (Friedman and Des Jarlais, 1991). This article was chosen because it contained more serial seroprevalence data than any other source we were able to locate, and it is publicly accessible. We are reasonably confident that further searching would only have produced still more cities that lacked one or more of the prevention components and did not have stable low seroprevalence. Table 12.5 presents the results and statistical significance for this case-control analysis.

This case–control analysis is meant to be illustrative rather than definitive. The 'controls' were selected on a convenience basis rather than on any 'matched' basis. Indeed, it would be a very difficult task to determine appropriate epidemiological criteria for selecting 'matched' control cities. The case–control data do show, however, that a strong association between the three common prevention components and stable low HIV-1 seroprevalence among IDUs will be very likely unless one can locate a moderate number of cities with stable low seroprevalence but without the common prevention components, or a very large number of cities with the common prevention components but without stable low seroprevalence.

Perhaps the most important issue in making causal inferences about 'preventing' epidemics of HIV-1 spread among IDUs is the current lack of specificity in the frequencies and types of risk behaviour that 'cause' such epidemics. The data presented here show that it is possible to maintain stable low HIV-1 seroprevalence in a population of IDUs with at least occasional injection risk behaviour in a substantial proportion of the population. We would

Table 12.5 Case-control analysis of prevention components and stable low HIV seroprevalence in 22 cities

Prevention components	Stable low seroprevalence	
	present	absent
present	5	0
absent	0	17

$p < .001$ by Fisher's exact test

HIV 'prevention components' are here considered 'present' if prevention efforts began to be implemented when seroprevalence was <5 per cent among samples of local in-treatment and out-of-treatment IDUs, *and* if the prevention strategy locally implemented included both community outreach/development of trust and legal access to sterile injection equipment. Otherwise, 'prevention components' are considered 'absent'.

Stable low seroprevalence is considered 'present' only in localities where seroprevalence among IDUs remained between >1 per cent and <5 per cent over a four-year period, with no increasing trend among data from both in-treatment and out-of-treatment samples of IDUs. Stable low seroprevalence is considered 'absent' if a locality experienced two consecutive years with seroprevalence among IDUs at 10 per cent or greater, or else one year with seroprevalence at 20 per cent or greater.

This restrictive operational definition means that there could be many cities that could not be classified as clearly having or clearly lacking stable low seroprevalence. However, this seemed appropriate, given the difficulties in distinguishing 'stable low' from 'low to increasing' seroprevalence.

Both 'prevention components' and 'stable low seroprevalence' were present in five localities — Glasgow, Lund, Sydney, Tacoma and Toronto — while both were absent in 17 localities — New York, Sardinia, San Francisco, Rio de Janeiro, Bangkok, Bologna, Milan, Padua, Rome, Geneva, Berlin, Hamburg, Vienna, Edinburgh, Bilbao, Manipur and Detroit.

suggest that variables reflecting 'rapid and efficient mixing' of persons engaging in risk behaviours, or 'high rates of unsafe partner change' (Anderson *et al.*, 1991), are likely to differentiate stable low seroprevalence from rapid increases in seroprevalence rather than 'the proportion of the population with any recent risk behaviour'. With better specification of the patterns of risk behaviour that differentiate rapid transmission (epidemics) from stable low seroprevalence, it would then be possible to search for linkages between prevention activities and changes in the patterns of risk behaviour, and then to make relatively strong inferences about the causal roles of prevention programmes in avoiding epidemics of HIV-1 transmission.

In conclusion, the data from these five cities show: the existence of stable low HIV-1 seroprevalence among some populations of injecting drug users; that low seroprevalence can be maintained despite at least occasional risky injections among a substantial percentage of IDUs in the population; and that stable low seroprevalence was associated with a distinct pattern of AIDS prevention programming, that is, prevention efforts were begun when seroprevalence was low, there was good access to sterile injection equipment, and community outreach was present, including referrals to other services and development of trust between IDUs and health workers.

The data presented here would appear to be the strongest evidence to date that it is possible to prevent epidemics of HIV-1 transmission in the very high-risk group of injecting drug users. Whether the three common prevention components identified here are necessary or sufficient to avert rapid transmission of HIV-1 among IDUs in other areas, remains to be determined. A conceptual explanation of stable low seroprevalence will require additional understanding of the specific risk-behaviour and population-mixing patterns associated with rapid transmission of HIV-1 among populations of IDUs.

Despite the need for additional information and more detailed theory, the potential consequences of permitting rapid transmission of HIV-1 among injecting drug users are such that responsible public health policy would seem to require, at the very least, utilizing the common prevention components wherever possible.

Acknowledgments

This research was supported by grant DA03574 from the US National Institute on Drug Abuse, by the American Foundation for AIDS Research, by the National Research and Development Programme of Health Canada, by the City of Toronto Department of Public Health, and by the World Health Organization's Multi-City Study on Drug Injecting and the Risk of HIV Infection. The views expressed in this paper do not necessarily reflect the positions of the granting agencies or of the institutions by which the authors are employed. The authors would like to thank Dr James Rankin, Ms Carol Major and Dr Margaret Fearon for their contributions, and Thomas P. Ward for editorial expertise. This chapter is adapted from an article by the same authors titled 'Maintaining low HIV seroprevalence among populations of injecting drug users', published in the *Journal of the American Medical Association*, **274**, 15 (1995), pp. 1266–31, and © 1995 by the American Medical Association.

This paper is dedicated to the memory of Dr Kerstin Tunving, who died in 1994.

Note

1 In each of the five case studies, we examined the presence/absence of six prevention components: (1) beginning early, (2) community outreach, (3) legal access to sterile injection equipment, (4) greatly expanded drug abuse treatment, (5) extensive HIV counselling and testing, and (6) bleach distribution. The probability that one city would have at least three of these prevention components present is based on combinations of 6 objects taken 3, 4, 5 and 6 at a time and = 0.6563. The probability that an additional four cities would then also have the same three prevention components = $(0.5)^{3 \times 4}$. The probability under the null hypothesis of all five cities sharing the three prevention components is the product of these two probabilities, = .00016.

References

ANDERSON, R.M., MAY, R.M., BOILY, M.C., GARNETT, G.P. and ROWLEY, J.T. (1991) 'The spread of HIV-1 in Africa: Sexual contact and the predicted demographic impact of AIDS', *Nature*, **352**, pp. 581–9.

BAKER, M., TOBIAS, M. and BRADY, H. (1991) 'Detection of HIV antibodies in used syringes in New Zealand', in Programme and abstracts of the 7th International Conference on AIDS, Abstract W.C. 3364, 16–21 July, Florence, Italy.

BROWN, B. S. and BESCHNER, G. M. (Eds) (1993) *Handbook on Risk of AIDS*, Westport: Greenwood Press.

CARR, S., GREEN, S., GOLDBERG, D. *et al.* (1992) 'HIV prevalence among female street prostitutes attending a health care drop-in centre in Glasgow', *AIDS*, **6**, pp. 1553–4.

CHITWOOD, D.D. (1994) 'Annotation: HIV risk and injection drug users — evidence for behavioural change', *American Journal of Public Health*, **84**, p. 350.

CHRISTENSSON, B. and LJUNGBERG, B. (1991) 'Syringe exchange for prevention of HIV infection in Sweden: practical experiences and community reactions', *International Journal of Addiction*, **26**, pp. 1293–1302.

CORDRAY, D.S. (1986) 'Quasi-experimental analysis: A mixture of methods and judgment', *New Directions in Program Evaluations*, **31**, pp. 9–28.

DES JARLAIS, D.C. and FRIEDMAN, S.R. (1992) 'AIDS prevention programmes for injecting drug users', in WORMSER, G.P. (Ed.) *AIDS and Other Manifestations of HIV Infection*, 2nd Edn., New York: Raven Press.

DES JARLAIS, D.C., FRIEDMAN, S.R., NOVICK, D. *et al.* (1989) 'HIV-1 infection among intravenous drug users in Manhattan', *Journal of the American Medical Association*, **261**, pp. 1008–12.

DES JARLAIS, D.C., FRIEDMAN, S.R., CHOOPANYA, K. *et al.* (1992) 'International epidemiology of HIV and AIDS among injecting drug users', *AIDS*, **6**, pp. 1053–68.

DES JARLAIS, D.C., CHOOPANYA, K., VANICHSENI, S. *et al.* (1994a) 'AIDS risk reduction and reduced HIV seroconversion among injecting drug users in Bangkok', *American Journal of Public Health*, **84**, pp. 452–5.

DES JARLAIS, D.C., HAGAN, H., FRIEDMAN, S.R. *et al.* (1994b) 'Biological validation of self-reported behaviour change among IDUs', Abstract PD0495, in Programme and abstracts of the 10th International Conference on AIDS, 7–12 August, Yokohama, Japan.

DICLEMENTE, R. and PETERSON, J. (Eds) (1994) *Preventing AIDS: Theories and Methods of Behavioural Interventions*, New York: Plenum Press.

DOLAN, K.A., STIMSON, G.V. and DONOGHOE, M.C. (1993) 'Reductions in HIV risk behaviour and stable HIV prevalence in syringe-exchange clients and other injectors in England', *Drug and Alcohol Review*, **12**, pp. 133–42.

EKSTRAND, M.L. and COATES, T.J. (1990) 'Maintenance of safer sexual behaviours and predictors of risky sex: the San Francisco Men's Health Study', *American Journal of Public Health*, **80**, pp. 973–7.

FRIEDMAN, S.R. and DES JARLAIS, D.C. (1991) 'HIV among drug injectors: the epidemic and the response', *AIDS Care*, **3**, pp. 239–50.

FRIEDMAN, S.R., DE JONG, W. and WODAK, A. (1993) 'Community development as a response to HIV among drug injectors', *AIDS*, Suppl. 1, S263–S269.

FRISCHER, M. and ELLIOT, L. (1993) 'Discriminating needle-exchange attenders from non-attenders', *British Journal of Addiction*, **88**, pp. 681–7.

FRISCHER, M., GREEN, S., GOLDBERG, D. *et al.* (1992a) 'Estimates of HIV infection among injecting drug users in Glasgow from 1985–1990', *AIDS*, **6**, pp. 1371–5.

FRISCHER, M., FLOOR, M., GREEN, S. *et al.* (1992b) 'Reduction in needle sharing among community-wide samples of drug injectors', *International Journal of STD & AIDS*, **3**, pp. 288–90.

FRISCHER, M., HAW, S., BLOOR, M. *et al.* (1993) 'Modelling the behaviour and attributes of injecting drug users: A new approach to identifying HIV risk practices', *International Journal of Addiction*, **28**, pp. 129–52.

HAGAN, H, and HALE, C.B. (1993) *HIV-1 Seroprevalence Surveys in Pierce County, June 1988 to December, 1992*, Tacoma: Tacoma-Pierce County Health Department.

HAGAN, H., DES JARLAIS, D.C., PURCHASE, D., REID, T. and FRIEDMAN, S. R. (1991) 'The Tacoma syringe exchange', *Journal of Addictive Disorders*, **10**, pp. 81–8.

HAGAN, H., DES JARLAIS, D.C., PURCHASE, D. *et al.* (1993) 'An interview study of participants in the Tacoma, Washington syringe exchange', *Addiction*, **88**, pp. 1691–7.

KALDOR, J., ELFORD, J., WODAK, A., CROFTS, J.N. and KIDD, S. (1993) 'HIV prevalence among IDUs in Australia: A methodological review', *Drug & Alcohol Review*, **12**, pp. 175–84.

LAMOTHE, F., BRUNEAU, J. and SOTO, J. (1992) 'Progression of prevalence of HIV-1 infection among injection drug users in Montreal, Quebec', *Canada Communicable Diseases Report*, **18**, pp. 98–101.

LAMPINEN, T.M., JOO, E., SEWERYN, S., HERSHOW, R.C. and WEIBEL, W. (1992) 'HIV seropositivity in community-recruited and drug treatment samples of injecting drug users', *AIDS*, **6**, pp. 123–6.

LJUNGBERG, B., CHRISTENSSON, B., TUNVING, K. *et al.* (1991) 'HIV prevention among injecting drug users: Three years of experience from a syringe exchange programme in Sweden', *Journal of AIDS*, **4**, pp. 890–5.

LURIE, P., REINGOLD, A.L., BOWSER, B. *et al.* (1993) *The Public Health Impact of Needle-Exchange Programmes in the United States and Abroad. Volume 1*, Atlanta: Centres for Disease Control and Prevention.

MILLSON, P., COATES, R., RANKIN, J. *et al.* (1991) *Evaluation of a Programme To Prevent Human Immunodeficiency Virus Transmission In Injection Drug Users in Toronto: Final Report to the National Health Research and Development Programme, Health and Welfare Canada*, Ottawa: NHRDP (NHRDP grant #6606–4333-AIDS).

MILLSON, P., MYERS, T., RANKIN, J. *et al.* (1992) 'Descriptive epidemiology of injection drug users in Toronto', oral presentation at the Second Annual Canadian National Conference on HIV/AIDS, May, Vancouver, Canada.

MILLSON, P., MYERS, T., RANKIN, J., MAJOR, C., FEARON, M. and RIGBY, J. (1993) 'Trends in HIV seroprevalence and risk behaviour in IDUs in Toronto, Canada', Abstract PO–C15–2936, in Programme and abstracts of the 9th International Conference on AIDS, 6–11 June Berlin, Germany.

NAIK, T.N., SARKER, S., SINGH, H.L. *et al.* (1991) 'Intravenous drug users — a new high-risk group for HIV infection in India', *AIDS*, **5**, pp. 117–18.

NEAIGUS, A., FRIEDMAN, S.R., CURTIS, R. *et al.* (1994) 'The relevance of drug injectors' social networks and risk networks for understanding and preventing HIV infection', *Social Science & Medicine*, **38**, pp. 67–78.

ONDCP (1992) Office of National Drug Control Policy, *Needle Exchange Programmes: Are They Effective? ONDCP Bulletin No. 7*, Washington: Executive Office of the President, Office of National Drug Control Policy.

OSMOND, D.H., PAGE, K., WILEY, J. *et al.* (1993) 'Human immunodeficiency virus infection in homosexual/bisexual men, ages 18–29: The San Francisco Young Men's Health Study', Abstract WS–C07–3, in Programme and abstracts of the 9th international Conference on AIDS, 6–11 June, Berlin, Germany.

PAPAEVANGELOU, G., ANCELLE-PARK, R. and SEYRER, Y. (1991) 'HIV prevalence and risk factors for infection among intravenous drug users in the European Community', Abstract M.D. 4074, in Programme and abstracts of the 7th International Conference on AIDS, 16–21 June, Florence, Italy.

ROBERTSON, J.R., BUCKNALL, A.B.V., WELSBY, P. *et al.* (1986) 'Epidemic of AIDS-related virus (HTLV-III/LAV) infection among intravenous drug users', *British Medical Journal*, **292**, pp. 527–9.

ROSS, M.W., WODAK, A., GOLD, J. and MILLER, M.E. (1992) 'Differences across sexual orientation on HIV risk behaviours in injecting drug users', *AIDS Care*, **4**, pp. 139–48.

ROSS, M.W., STOWE, A., WODAK, A., MILLER, M.E. and GOLD, J. (in press) 'Predictors of HIV status among injecting drug users, and health promotion', *Journal of the Royal Society of Health*.

STALL, R., EKSTRAND, M.L., POLLACK, L., MCKUSICK, L. and COATES, T.J. (1990) 'Relapse from safer sex: The next challenge for AIDS prevention efforts', *Journal Acquired Immune Deficiency Syndrome*, **3**, pp. 1181–7.

STIMSON, G.V. (1990) 'The prevention of HIV infection in injecting drug users: Recent advances and remaining obstacles', in Programme and abstracts of the 6th International Conference on AIDS, 20–24 June, San Francisco, CA.

STIMSON, G.V. (1995) 'AIDS and injecting drug use in the United Kingdom, 1988 to 1993:

The policy response and the prevention of the epidemic', *Social Science & Medicine*, **41**, pp. 699–716.

STIMSON, G.V., ADELEKAN, M.L. and RHODES, T. (1996) 'The diffusion of drug injecting in developing countries', *International Journal of Drug Policy*, **7** (4), pp. 245–55.

TAYLOR, A., FRISCHER, M., McKEGANEY, N., GOLDBERG, D., GREEN, S. and PLATT, S. (1993) 'HIV risk behaviours among female prostitute drug injectors in Glasgow', *Addiction*, **88**, pp.1560–4.

TUNVING, K., NYHOLM, K. and ANDERSSON, B. (1992) 'Two successful syringe- and needle-exchange programmes in Lund/Malmö, Sweden: Their effects on the help-seeking drug-using communities and the surrounding drug treatment facilities', Abstract PuC 8231, in Programme and abstracts of the 8th International Conference on AIDS, 19–24 July, Amsterdam, the Netherlands.

VANICHSENI, S. and SAKUNTANAGA, P. (1990) 'Results of three seroprevalence surveys for HIV in IVDU in Bangkok', Abstract F.C. 105, in Programme and abstracts of the 6th International Conference on AIDS, 20–23 June, San Francisco, CA.

Chapter 13

Overview: Policies and Interventions to Stem HIV-1 Epidemics associated with Injecting Drug Use

Andrew L. Ball

Few would deny that HIV infection is one of the major international public health crises of this century. The factors which have contributed to the global dissemination of both injecting drug use and associated HIV infection are extremely complex and dynamic. Whereas sexual transmission of HIV remains the most significant route at a global level, injecting drug use has played a critical role in fuelling the epidemic in various regions, particularly in some countries in Asia, certain developed country communities (including in France, Italy, Spain and the United States of America), and more recently in Eastern Europe and parts of the Commonwealth of Independent States. In previous chapters, some of these factors have been discussed, with consideration given to individual, social and environmental determinants. Recognizing the great diversity of injecting drug use patterns, the complex interplay of factors influencing drug use and sexual behaviour, and differing contexts of drug injecting, it is evident that effective strategies to minimize risks and prevent HIV spread need to be comprehensive, multi-faceted, integrated and flexible.

There is a growing body of scientific evidence that the HIV epidemic associated with injecting drug use can be prevented, slowed, stopped and even reversed. The World Health Organization Multi-City Study on Drug Injecting and Risk of HIV Infection (WHO, 1994a), and a review of prevention activities and risk behaviour in five cities with a stable low HIV prevalence among injecting drug users (IDUs) (Des Jarlais *et al.*, 1995), concluded that at least three prevention components were associated with containment of the epidemic. These three components included: early implementation of prevention initiatives while HIV prevalence was low; community outreach to IDUs which provided HIV/AIDS information and helped develop trust between IDUs and health care providers; and widespread provision of sterile injection equipment. Chapters 6, 10 and 12 describe in more detail these intervention components. At an individual level, there is evidence that, given the opportunity, IDUs will reduce their risk of HIV infection by changing drug injecting practices (Celantano *et al.*, 1994), and in certain circumstances by modifying sexual behaviour (van Ameijden *et al.*, 1994a; see also Chapter 9). Further, as an example of effective action at a national level, Stimson (1995) discusses a range of factors, including significant changes in needle sharing behaviour, which have contributed to the prevention of the epidemic in the United Kingdom. Despite the evidence of success in a range of different countries, in many other countries, political inaction continues to obstruct the introduction of effective interventions.

This chapter will examine in more detail possible intervention points and strategies for reducing risk and preventing HIV infection associated with injecting drug use. Although there are multiple health risks associated with injecting drug use, the focus of this chapter will be on HIV infection. Nevertheless, many strategies preventing HIV infection may also reduce other health risks, including overdose and the transmission of other blood-borne infections, such as hepatitis B and C.

Before effective strategies may be designed and appropriate policies and programmes developed for a specific setting, it is essential that a thorough understanding of the situation exists. The first section of this chapter discusses the role of research, and more specifically situation analysis, in the design of interventions. Central to HIV prevention is the concept of individual and group behaviour change to reduce risks. The second section reviews the range of strategies available for influencing behaviour by enabling drug users to make rational choices to reduce health risks. Behaviour change will occur only where opportunities and support exist for such change. The third section considers the siting of specific strategies within a public health context and the creation of supportive environments within which behaviour change may occur and be sustained.

Assessment for Intervention

The advent of the AIDS epidemic has stimulated a dramatic increase in the quantity and quality of research on injecting drug use, an imperative considering the critical role that this behaviour has played in the unfolding of the global epidemic. Whereas much research had previously focused on quantitative methods designed to measure and monitor levels of drug use, there was a need to pay more attention to HIV risk relating to specific behaviours and the context of substance use. This has involved the reorientation of research programmes, with the promotion of qualitative research methods to complement more traditional survey methods (Wiebel, 1996). Greater emphasis has been placed on defining factors and contexts associated with risk behaviours and drug-related harm as opposed to defining indicators of drug use. Considering the complex nature of injecting drug use and the marginalization of IDUs, new research methods needed to be developed and existing methods adapted. Action research, which aims to provide information quickly to inform the development of appropriate interventions, policies and programmes, is now taking priority.

Situation analysis, in preparation for intervention, needs to gather information across a range of areas. This includes understanding individual and group risk behaviours and how they may vary according to context. Injecting drug use practices, sexual practices, and drug using and sexual networks are areas for such investigation. Understanding community structures, attitudes and mixing dynamics is important in designing and locating individual interventions and intervention packages. The effectiveness, cost, feasibility, acceptability and sustainability of specific interventions; integration of interventions within existing health care services and HIV and drug prevention/ treatment programmes; identifying those at greatest risk and how they may be reached; determining appropriate intervention settings and delivery systems; identifying existing and necessary resources; and recognizing opportunities for involving drug users and the community at all levels of intervention design and implementation, all require attention. Understanding the policy, political, legal, and cultural contexts will illuminate what is feasible and the barriers which may need to be tackled, including: political and public opinion on injecting drug use and HIV infection; religious and cultural beliefs; existing laws and policies; and the role of the mass media and other communication systems. Qualitative methods which may be used for situation analysis include unstructured and semi-structured interviews, systematic interviewing techniques, group interviewing and focus groups, observation, social network analysis, narrative reseach, and projective methods (Hudelson, 1994).

Rapid assessment and simple community monitoring methods have already been developed and implemented for use by local communities, in both developed and developing countries, to assist in the planning and implementation of comprehensive intervention programmes (WHO, 1993a).

Strategies Targeting Behaviour Change

Whereas levels of substance use lie on a continuum, from abstinence through intermittent to intensive use, specific drug using behaviours and harms tend to be discrete. Nevertheless, different behaviours may be ranked on a hierarchy according to risk of HIV transmission. Intervention strategies therefore aim to change behaviour such that risks are reduced, the ultimate goal being risk elimination. In the case of injecting drug use, at the top of the risk hierarchy is the indiscriminate sharing of injecting equipment, while at the bottom lies abstinence from all drug use. In moving down the hierarchy, towards lowering risk, behaviour change may include: reducing the frequency of sharing and the number of sharing partners; cleaning injecting equipment; not sharing injecting equipment; using sterile needles and syringes and not sharing other equipment; changing from the injection of illicit drugs to the supervised injection of prescribed drugs; changing from injecting drug use to non-injecting drug use; reducing frequency of non-injecting drug use; and abstinence from all drug use. Rhodes (1994) graphically illustrates this hier-archy of 'harm-reduction choices', which not only considers the goal of HIV prevention, but also the prevention of drug injecting and the prevention of illicit drug use (see Figure 13.1).

One needs to be careful in using this hierarchical model. Typically, individual drug using patterns are dynamic, influenced by specific events, interactions with others, and different settings. For example, although an injecting drug user may almost always use sterile needles and syringes, where they are available, there are those occasions when he or she may share because sterile equipment is not readily available and sharing with a particular person (such as a sexual partner) is not perceived to be risky. Despite its limitations, the model provides a valuable framework for reviewing possible intervention strategies which target individual behaviours.

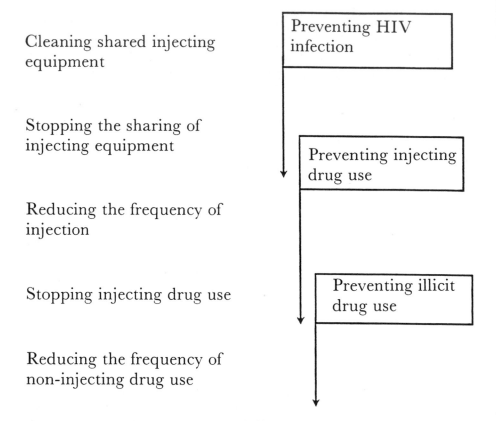

Figure 13.1 Hierarchy of harm reduction choices (*Source*: Rhodes, T. (1994) Risk Intervention and Change, London, Health Education Authority)

Reducing Indiscriminate Sharing, Limiting Sharing Partners and Occasions

The indiscriminate and frequent receptive sharing of injecting equipment by an injecting drug user poses a high risk for HIV infection where HIV infection exists in the network of IDUs. The risk depends on the background prevalence of HIV infection. Where prevalence is high, occasional sharing may be as risky as frequent sharing where prevalence is low. Burt and Stimson (1993) report on a range of strategies used by IDUs to protect themselves, without stopping sharing, including sharing only with selected partners, not sharing where blood is observed to be in the syringe, and assessing the HIV status of potential sharing partners. Limiting sharing partners may have a significant impact on the risk of transmission, particularly in low HIV prevalence areas (Des Jarlais *et al.*, 1995). A reduction in the number of partners gives less opportunity for epidemiological mixing, and discriminate sharing limits the networks within which HIV may spread (see Chapters 2 and 7).

There is evidence that IDUs are changing their sharing behaviour in order to reduce risks, although it is not possible to identify specific factors or interventions which may have influenced these changes (Stimson and Hunter, 1996). Saxon, Calsyn and Jackson (1994) in a longitudinal study of a cohort of IDUs found that sharing with multiple partners declined from 42 per cent to 11 per cent over ten months' follow-up. Laski (1991) reported that in a longitudinal study of San Francisco injecting heroin users the mean number of needle-sharing partners per month declined from 7 to 1.4 over a two-year period.

Limiting sharing to close friends and/or sexual partners is perceived by many IDUs to be of very low risk (Loxley and Ovenden, 1995). In reality, the extent to which such 'risk management' actually reduces risk to an acceptable level will be dependent on the background HIV prevalence among IDUs. The provision of accurate information may increase their awareness of self-risk and individual counselling may reveal those factors influencing risk perception.

Cleaning Injecting Equipment

In most communities around the world, particularly in developing countries, sterile needles and syringes are not readily available or affordable. In such cases, where sharing of equipment is likely, strategies for cleaning equipment need to be implemented. Methods used include boiling of needles and syringes, cleaning with bleach or other decontaminants, and simply rinsing with water. Bleach distribution programmes are most widely implemented in the United States (Broadhead, 1991) where needle and syringe distribution programmes are severely restricted. Information on cleaning techniques and bleach distribution are also major interventions in many prison systems (Correctional Service of Canada, 1994; Dolan, Wodak and Penny, 1995) and in various developing countries, such as Malaysia, Vietnam, India and Thailand (Ball, 1996). In other countries where sterile needles and syringes are readily available, bleach programmes tend to be limited, although information on disinfection techniques is often available through printed materials and outreach services.

Despite evidence of increasing use of bleach programmes and the dissemination of information on disinfection techniques, the effectiveness of such programmes in reducing HIV risk has been questioned (Donoghoe and Power, 1993). Furthermore, bleach programmes are considered to be ineffective in inactivating hepatitis B and C viruses. There are a number of factors which have complicated such programmes. Messages to IDUs have in many cases been confusing, with differing types of decontaminants and concentrations of preparations being proposed (McGeorge, Crofts and Burrows, 1996). IDUs often do not have the time or opportunity to effectively implement recommended bleaching or other sterilization procedures. Boiling often damages or reduces the useful life of the equipment. Many IDUs fear the effect of injecting bleach residue after flushing with bleach. Bleach often is not available in many areas, and IDUs in some communities (including Nepal, India and Thailand) reject its use because of its 'evil' smell. Nevertheless, bleach programmes often provide a link between health-care workers and IDUs which may facilitate other HIV prevention efforts and are desirable in the absence of needle/syringe exchange programmes and pharmacy sales of injection equipment. Efforts should also be made to identify other decontaminants which are acceptable, effective, simple to use and affordable.

Reducing Equipment Sharing

In order to prevent the sharing of needles and syringes, IDUs must have ready and affordable access to sterile supplies. There is strong evidence that increasing the availability of injecting equipment, through such programmes as needle and syringe exchanges (NSEPs) and pharmacy outlets, reduces sharing and the risk of HIV infection (Stimson and Donoghoe, 1996; Des Jarlais *et al.*, 1996). Furthermore, there is no evidence that such programmes reduce the rate of IDUs entering into treatment or increase injecting or non-injecting drug use (Lurie and Reingold, 1993; Normand, Vlahov and Moses, 1995).

Based on extensive evaluation of NSEPs in a range of developed countries, existing programmes are being expanded and new ones are being established in other countries. The focus of research is no longer on whether NSEPs are effective in preventing HIV transmission, but rather on how NSEPs can be made more efficient. In particular, research is focusing on: how to target under-served populations (such as women, ethnic minorities, young IDUs, rural populations, and intermittent users); linking other HIV prevention activities to NSEPs; reducing operational costs; integrating NSEPs into mainstream health and community services; and comparing cost-effectiveness with other HIV prevention and treatment programmes (Lurie and Drucker, 1996).

The feasibility of establishing NSEPs has recently been demonstrated in a number of developing countries, with programmes initiated in Brazil, India, Vietnam (WHO, 1996a), and Thailand (Gray, 1995). Whereas needle and syringe availability have been high in many Western European countries, only recently have NSEPs been established in countries in Central and Eastern Europe, such as the Czech Republic and the Russian Federation.

The risk of HIV transmission also exists when other injecting paraphernalia are shared, such as filters, water for mixing, and 'cookers'. Some practices of sharing drug preparations also pose significant risk of HIV transmission. The practices of 'frontloading' (Jose *et al.*, 1992) and 'backloading' (Vlahov, 1996) have been associated with HIV transmission. Although in the Jose study such practice was reported to be an independent risk factor for HIV infection, in other studies the nature of the relationship is unclear, these practices possibly being markers of other high-risk behaviours. In Vietnam, 'communal injectors' (individuals who are paid to give injections and also usually supply the drugs and injecting equipment) use a common pot for the preparation of opium and heroin solutions, from which used needles and syringes are used to draw up doses for use by large numbers of IDUs. Ethnographic methods can help to identify rituals and other practices associated with drug injection which increase HIV risk, and also to understand the context and meanings of such practices (Koester, 1996). Education campaigns and risk reduction counselling need to take into consideration these issues, and not only target IDUs but others influencing drug use practices, such as 'communal injectors' and dealers. The provision of sterile water and other injecting paraphernalia to IDUs in addition to needles and syringes may help to reduce risks, and is already common practice with many NSEPs.

Injectable Agonist Pharmacotherapy Programmes

Some IDUs who are prepared to enter into drug treatment may not be prepared to stop injecting. A very limited number of programmes exist which provide agonist drugs to IDUs for injection. Such programmes aim to attract more marginalized and vulnerable IDUs into treatment, including those with significant criminal involvement, health damage and a history of failing in other treatment programmes. A commonly stated longer-term goal of these programmes is to encourage clients to move from injectable to oral agonist pharmacotherapy programmes once they are stabilized.

Although the prescribing of injectable heroin in the United Kingdom has a history dating back before its legitimization in 1926, its use as a treatment, along with other injectable opioids (including pethidine and methadone) has been very limited and not stringently evaluated until recently (Strang *et al.*, 1994). The first scientifically evaluated large-scale study of injectable opioid prescribing was initiated by the Swiss National Government in 1991 with clinical trials starting in early 1994 (Rihs-Middel, 1995). The trials include injectable heroin, morphine and methadone. Although final evaluation of the Swiss study has yet to be undertaken, preliminary reports indicate that the trials have managed to engage particularly marginalized IDUs and to maintain them in treatment. Whereas there has been wide acceptability of intravenous heroin by patients, there have been significant drop-out rates for those prescribed intravenous morphine (Uchtenhagen, Dobler-Mikola and Gutzwiller, 1996). Furthermore, research has been undertaken in Australia into the feasibility of implementing clinical trials on the controlled availability of opioids, including injectable heroin (Bammer, 1995).

In India, the use of intramuscular injection of buprenorphine by medical practitioners for the treatment of individuals withdrawing from heroin has triggered an epidemic spread of illicit buprenorphine injecting in some communities (Dorabjee, Samson and Dyalchand, 1996; Kanga, 1996; also see Chapter 1). Large numbers of individuals presented for treatment following a police 'crackdown' on heroin supplies. Whereas prior to this 'crackdown', in these communities, the mode of heroin use was typically by smoking and 'chasing the dragon', buprenorphine treatment introduced users to both a new opioid drug and a new means of drug administration, that being injecting. This undesired effect has implications for the education of medical practitioners and other health-care workers in the use of parenteral treatments and the management of IDUs.

Although a number of small-scale trials and treatment programmes have involved injectable psychostimulants, including cocaine (Strang *et al.*, 1994), and methylamphetamine (Mitcheson *et al.*, 1976), results have been disappointing and such approaches have largely been abandoned.

Transitions between Injecting and Non-Injecting Drug Use

The transition from non-injecting to injecting drug use significantly increases health risks for the user, particularly if sharing of needles and syringes occurs. Research to identify factors influencing a move to injecting is receiving particular attention in order to inform interventions which may prevent such transitions from occurring (Strang *et al.*, 1992; van Ameijden *et al.*, 1994b). Although it is important to understand those factors which influence individual transitions, it would appear more important to understand transitions involving groups and whole populations. Why does injecting drug use become the preferred mode of administration in one community of drug users and not another? The above example of buprenorphine use in India (Dorabjee, Samson and Dyalchand, 1996) demonstrates how a change in the availability of heroin triggered a series of responses resulting in the transition of heroin smokers and chasers into buprenorphine injectors. Focus group discussions in New Delhi among buprenorphine injectors revealed that most made the transition because they believed that buprenorphine injection would assist them in giving up heroin use and also because the cost of buprenorphine was less. An additional factor was that the availability of injectable buprenorphine was greater than the sublingual form in these communities during the period of the drug transition. For each community it is likely that different site-specific factors exist which influence transitions. Stimson and Choopanya (see Chapter 1) discuss in more detail some of the factors which have influenced transitions from non-injecting to injecting drug use in different global regions.

Just as the transition from non-injecting to injecting drug use increases health risks, the reverse is also true. Situations in which there is a natural transition from injecting to non-injecting drug use need careful analysis as they may provide valuable information for the design of interventions. Since the late 1980s there has been a shift of heroin use in New York from injecting to inhalation, with over half of those individuals entering treatment for heroin use reporting inhalation as their primary route of heroin administration. Initial research on inhalation use and transitions suggests that concern about HIV infection is an important factor, but not the only important factor, in increased inhalation use (Des Jarlais *et al.*, 1992; Des Jarlais *et al.*, 1994). The increased purity of heroin in New York in recent years has enabled this transition to occur. Similarly, reports from Australia and Europe suggest that increasing purity of street heroin has made it possible for heroin injectors to change to chasing, smoking or intranasal use (Strang *et al.*, 1992). Also, findings from an unpublished WHO study of cocaine use in Bolivia and Brazil indicate that there has been a dramatic reduction in cocaine hydrochloride injection in Brazil as increased crack smoking and intranasal cocaine use occurs, partly in response to concern about HIV infection among drug users.

Not only is it important to consider transitions with regard to routes of drug administration, but also to consider the factors influencing, and the health implications associated with, changes in types of drugs used, such as the move from cocaine use to heroin use that is being observed in areas of the United States, and from heroin use to amphetamine use in Thailand.

Non-Injecting Agonist Pharmacotherapy Programmes

One strategy for encouraging the transition from injecting to non-injecting drug use is to offer non-injecting agonist pharmacotherapy programmes, such as oral methadone, sublingual buprenorphine, oral morphine sulphate and heroin 'reefers' for opioid users, coca leaf infusions and tablets for cocaine users, and oral dexamphetamine for amphetamine users.

Oral methadone is the most widely used substance for opioid agonist pharmacotherapy. Furthermore, it is one of the most rigorously evaluated forms of all drug treatment, albeit predominantly within developed countries, including Australia, the United States of America and some Western European countries. Since the late 1980s there has been a dramatic expansion of methadone maintenance in Australia (Ward, Mattick and Hall, 1994) and Europe, with all European Union countries now having such programmes (Farrell *et al.*, 1995). The rationale for this expansion has been based on strong evidence that methadone maintenance is effective in the prevention of HIV infection. Studies have demonstrated that methadone maintenance programmes are associated with lower rates of HIV-1 prevalence (Abdul-Quader *et al.*, 1987) and reductions in HIV-1 risk related to injection and sharing behaviours (Ball *et al.*, 1988) for individuals during treatment. Methadone maintenance treatment is also associated with other benefits apart from HIV prevention, including reductions in criminal activity and improved social functioning (Bell, Hall and Blythe, 1992).

Nevertheless, the goals, designs, delivery and effectiveness of methadone maintenance programmes vary considerably. Measures of effectiveness include less illicit opioid use and drug risk practices, reduced criminal activity, greater retention in treatment and improved health status. Comparative studies evaluating the effectiveness of different programmes have identified that more effective programmes are characterized by: the prescription of higher doses of methadone (above 50–60 mg daily); a treatment goal of long-term maintenance as opposed to detoxification to abstinence; better ancillary and supportive services (including counselling, social and medical services); and better staff–client relationships (Ball and Ross, 1991; Farrell *et al.*, 1994; Ward, Mattick and Hall, 1992).

Methadone is not the only opioid used in non-injectable agonist pharmaco-therapy programmes. Other less widely used and evaluated opioid agonist drugs include: levo-alpha-acetylmethadol (LAAM), a long-acting synthetic opioid taken orally; buprenorphine, an opioid agonist and antagonist taken sublingually (Blaine, 1992); tincture of opium, an opium suspension taken orally; ethylmorphine, a morphine analogue taken orally; and pentazocine, an opioid agonist and antagonist taken orally.

Very little research has been undertaken on oral psychostimulant agonist pharmacotherapy programmes (Mattick and Darke, 1995). Trials on the use of coca tea and coca leaf tablets for the treatment of cocaine dependence have been conducted (Llosa, 1994); however, further evaluation is required. A number of small-scale programmes have used dexamphetamine maintenance for the treatment of amphetamine users (Fleming and Roberts, 1994; Sherman, 1990). Further research is required to identify potential agonist drugs for the management of cocaine, amphetamine and other psychostimulant dependence.

The use of anabolic steroids, often by injection, is an increasing phenomenon among both athletes for performance enhancement purposes and others for aesthetic reasons (WHO, 1993c). These two populations are usually very difficult to reach through normal HIV prevention strategies targeting IDUs, primarily because they do not identify themselves as injecting drug users. Initial and limited research on the medical prescribing of oral anabolic steroids to athletes and body builders has been undertaken to determine the feasibility of implementing such programmes to engage these vulnerable groups under medical supervision and reduce health risks (Millar, 1996).

Agonist pharmacotherapy programmes have primarily been located in developed countries, and it has been argued that such treatment approaches are not appropriate, feasible or affordable for developing countries. Despite such beliefs, a range of agonist pharmacotherapy programmes have been established in Asia, Latin America and Eastern Europe. As already discussed, sublingual buprenorphine maintenance programmes have been established in India (Dorabjee, Samson and Dyalchand, 1996). Methadone maintenance programmes are being implemented in Nepal (Shresta, Shresta and Gautam, 1995) and in different regions in Thailand (Vanichseni *et al.*, 1991) and in Latvia, Lithuania, Poland and the former Yugoslav Republic of Macedonia. A small-scale methadone maintenance programme is being piloted in Vietnam. A long-term methadone detoxification programme has been implemented in hill-tribe communities in northern Thailand. Tincture of opium is used for detoxification and substitute maintenance in northern Thailand (WHO, 1996b), while anecdotal reports exist of its informal use in other Mekong countries. There is interest from a number of Asian countries, where opium is readily available, to undertake scientific trials on tincture of opium and methadone pharmacotherapy. An ethylmorphine prescription programme has been established to treat heroin users in the Czech Republic (WHO, 1996c). Agonist pharmacotherapy has also been introduced in Latin America, with coca leaf infusions and tablets being used for the treatment of cocaine dependence in Peru as referred to above (Llosa, 1994).

Most of the Asian agonist pharmacotherapy programmes referred to above have developed in response to dramatic increases in injecting drug use and associated HIV risk practices. Mainstream and traditional drug treatment programmes either did not exist, or were unaffordable or ineffective in preventing relapse to HIV risk practices. These programmes have evolved from within the communities where the drug users live, often without government support or formal approval. The characteristics of these programmes differ markedly from those in developed countries. Principles of community involvement and integration with primary health care services have made these programmes feasible, acceptable and affordable, even in slum communities and remote tribal villages. Nevertheless, there is a need for these programmes to be thoroughly evaluated in order to determine their effectiveness and ways in which they could be better structured.

Despite the benefits of different agonist pharmacotherapy programmes, significant numbers of clients may continue to inject drugs, albeit with less frequency. This has implications for the range of services provided to clients. For the occasions when clients do inject they should still have access to those services that provide them with information and sterile drug injecting equipment in order to minimize their HIV risks. Such services may be provided through the agonist pharmacotherapy programme itself or by referral to other agencies.

Detoxification and Maintaining Abstinence

Many different drug treatment programmes target injecting drug users with abstinence being the goal. It is beyond the scope of this chapter to review all such approaches, although various reviews and reports exist which discuss the effectiveness of various treatment approaches (Heather and Tebutt, 1989; Pickens, Leukefeld and Schuster, 1991; Mattick and Hall, 1993; WHO, 1993d). Nevertheless, it is important to comment on the role of abstinence-orientated drug treatment in HIV prevention.

The HIV epidemic associated with injecting drug use has stimulated a much wider response than just HIV prevention-orientated interventions for IDUs. In some countries this has included the expansion of abstinence-orientated drug treatment programmes. Abstinence not only eliminates HIV risk associated with drug injecting, but may also reduce sexual risk practices associated with sex work, the exchange of sex for drugs, and unprotected sex while intoxicated. It is plausible that strategies aimed at motivating IDUs to enter into such treatment and increasing accessibility to treatment may assist HIV prevention strategies. This is provided that both drug treatment and HIV prevention goals and strategies are compatible. Engaging and retaining IDUs in treatment provide opportunities for HIV education and other preventive interventions. Furthermore, abstinence may be associated with general health improvement and less susceptibility to opportunistic HIV/AIDS related infections. However, acknowledging the high rates of relapse across all drug treatment approaches, specific consideration needs to be given to educating clients in HIV risk management and ensuring access to sterile injection equipment if relapse occurs.

Abstinence-orientated drug treatment may be considered in three phases: preparation for detoxification; detoxification; and maintenance of abstinence. Glaser (1993) describes five broad types of treatment modalities: biophysical (such as acupuncture, massage and electrical stimulation); pharmacological (such as clonidine for detoxification and naltrexone for maintaining abstinence in treatment of opioid dependence); psychological (such as psychodynamic therapies and cognitive-behavioural counselling); socio-cultural (such as thera-peutic communities and mutual help groups); and mixed modalities (using combinations of the four modalities described above). Treatment programmes may be situated in different settings, including specialized alcohol and other drug services, primary health-care settings, the workplace, correctional and criminal justice institutions, educational settings, social welfare programmes and religious settings.

Not all drug users seeking treatment are prepared to stop using drugs immediately. Many treatment approaches in the past have considered detoxifi-cation as the prerequisite for entry into treatment. This principle offered drug users few options in planning for their own treatment and therefore tended to exclude those less motivated to change. Various motivational methods have been developed to encourage drug users to assess their substance use and consider change (Hester, 1993; Miller and Rollnick, 1991). A number of community based drug treatment programmes, particularly in the Asian region, promote 'rehabilitation before detoxification'. This approach recognizes that health risk reduction and improvement in health status and social functioning are valid intermediate goals, with abstinence being a longer-term objective (WHO, 1993e). During this period of 'rehabilitation' individuals and family members are stabilized and prepared for detoxification and the maintenance of abstinence, the dispelling of myths about detoxification being an important component. An important element in many of these programmes is the direct involvement of all, or most, members of the community. Whereas anecdotal reports indicate that some of these programmes are extremely effective, formal evaluation has yet to be undertaken. Less success is reported from those communities where drugs are readily available and other drug using communities exist nearby.

The belief that detoxification is the most critical step in treatment is now being questioned, as the importance of motivation to treatment and relapse prevention are being realized. Often detoxification is the shortest and easiest phase of the treatment process. This phase involves the management of physical and psychological symptoms of acute withdrawal and treatment of medical complications. Withdrawal from most injectable drugs (including opioids, cocaine and amphetamines) rarely results in medical emergencies unless the individual has used combinations of certain depressant drugs (such as alcohol, benzodiazepines or barbiturates) or has a pre-existing medical condition. Therefore, in most cases, detoxification can occur in non-medical settings, thereby reducing costs, increasing accessibility and enabling programmes to be sited within the community. In most detoxification programmes, methods are used to minimize withdrawal symptoms, including pharmacological (such as clonidine, benzodiazepines and methadone for opioid withdrawal, and bromo-criptine and amantadine for cocaine withdrawal) (Kalant, 1993), physical and supportive counselling approaches.

Maintaining abstinence involves three components: continuing care, relapse prevention, and supportive living arrangements (Glaser, 1993). Continuing care involves the provision of ongoing treatment to maintain gains achieved during early stages of treatment. Relapse prevention involves the use of specific methods to minimize the probability of relapse to drug use, such as pharmacological methods to reduce drug effects and cravings (for example naltrexone, an opioid receptor antagonist) (Kalant, 1993), and behavioural methods to avoid high risk situations (for example stress management and assertiveness training). Supportive living arrangements involve interventions which provide supportive and protective environments, particularly for those who are damaged and socially marginalized, such as halfway houses and long-term residential care.

Apart from the three-phase 'Western' model of drug treatment as described above, there are many models of traditional healing for the management of substance use. These models often incorporate significant elements of spiritual healing and symbolic ritual within a framework of holistic care and community involvement (Jilek, 1993). Such approaches are well established in many regions where injecting drug use is common and HIV risk high, but only limited formal evaluation has been undertaken on their effectiveness and suitability for replication in other settings.

Reducing Sexual Risk Practices

There is increasing awareness that sexual transmission plays an important role in the dynamics of HIV infection among IDUs and their non-injecting sexual partners. For various reasons IDUs often have increased risk of both acquiring and transmitting the virus through sexual practices (see Chapters 2 and 9). For example, there is an association between sex work and injecting drug use, particularly for women (McKeganey and Barnard, 1992; Rhodes *et al.*, 1993), and specifically a strong association between HIV-1 infection among female sex workers and injecting drug use (McKeganey *et al.*, 1992). The non-injecting sexual partners of IDUs play an important role in the transmission dynamics of communities, particularly with regard to dissemination to the non-injecting population. The relationship between the use of specific psychoactive substances and sexual behaviour remains unclear. Chapter 2 discusses the association between the use of crack cocaine, exchanging sex for money and HIV infection, and the less clear relationship between the use of alcohol and unsafe sexual practices. Chapter 9 makes comparisons of sexual behaviours among cocaine and opioid injectors.

It is evident that more research is required, particularly in developing countries, to further investigate the different relationships which exist between substance use, sexual behaviour and HIV infection. Areas for further investigation include the role of substance-use-related disinhibition, alcohol and other drug-related expectancies with regard to sexual conduct, the contexts within which both substance use and sex occur, and the influence of substance use on sexual negotiation and the implementation of mechanical protective measures (such as condom use). The dramatic increase in the promotion and consumption of alcohol in developing countries may have significant implications for the sexual transmission of HIV, particularly in regions such as Africa where HIV prevalence in some communities is high. The role of sex and drug tourism, as occurs in parts of Asia, Latin America and some developed countries, also requires special attention.

Chapter 2 reviews the differential response by IDUs, in which drug injecting practices have significantly changed while sexual behaviours have not. Whereas IDUs are able to recognize they are at risk through certain drug injecting practices, most remain unconvinced that they are at risk from sexual transmission of HIV, even in high risk situations. The failure to recognize such sexual risk may in part reflect a reluctance by drug outreach and treatment services to address this issue. The provision of condoms is likely to do little to change sexual risk practices. Therefore, services targeting IDUs also need to better understand the sexual practices of their clients and to offer sexual risk counselling in addition to the provision of condoms.

The Role of Public Health and Health Promotion

Drug injecting and sex do not occur in isolation, free from external influences. Chapter 2 and other chapters have considered those contextual factors which influence both drug use and sexual behaviours and the risk of HIV infection. Rhodes (1994) summarizes current opinion concerning the inadequacies of individualistic models of health behaviour in addressing HIV risk and discusses the need to use social models where the complexities of interpersonal, social and environmental interactions are considered. A health promotion model provides such an integrated appoach, which in turn offers a framework for developing HIV prevention strategies. Nevertheless, it is necessary to be aware of some of the limitations of such a model. Most importantly, not all policy makers and other community members consider injecting drug use to be a public health concern, particularly with regard to non-dependent IDUs.

Ottawa Charter on Health Promotion

Three key documents describe the principles of health promotion and strategies for action within the context of 'health for all': *The Declaration of Alma-Ata on Primary Health Care* (WHO, 1978; WHO, 1994b), *Global Strategy for Health for All by the Year 2000* (WHO, 1981; WHO, 1995a), and *The Ottawa Charter on Health Promotion* (WHO, 1986). The Alma-Ata Declaration recommends a number of areas for action to empower people, including: intersectoral collaboration as a force for health for all; strengthening of district health systems based on primary health care; maximum community participation and control of health; and intensified social and political action for health. The 'Health for All' strategy builds on these principles, calling for equity in health and social justice, emphasis on health promotion, active community participation, multisectoral co-operation, a focus on primary health care, and the need for international co-operation. The Ottawa Charter on Health Promotion outlines five areas for action: building healthy public policy, creating supportive environments, strengthening community action, developing personal skills, and reorientating health services. In the following section of this chapter the Ottawa Charter will be used as a framework for considering a health promotion response to HIV infection associated with injecting drug use.

Building Healthy Public Policy

The Ottawa Charter states:

> Health promotion goes beyond health. It puts health on the agenda of policy makers in all sectors and at all levels, directing them to be aware

of the health consequences of their decisions and to accept their responsibilities for health . . .

Health promotion policy requires the identification of obstacles to the adoption of healthy public policies in non-health sectors, and ways of removing them. The aim must be to make the healthier choice the easier choice for policy makers as well.

The international drug trade is full of intrigues, having a direct impact on national and regional security, global economics and public health. Chapter 1 provides an overview of the global dissemination of injecting drug use and associated HIV infection, and alludes to some of the complex international policy interactions which have influenced this spread. The epidemic has been shaped to a large extent by unintended and unexpected consequences of international policies and actions, often in policy areas which are not considered directly related to health. War and civil unrest, displacement and migration of populations, rapid economic development and political transitions, poverty and exploitation have all contributed to the rapid spread of drug injection and HIV infection. More specifically, efforts to stem the international illicit drugs industry have seen the establishment of new areas of production and routes for trafficking, and subsequently the emergence of new drug use patterns (International Narcotics Control Board, 1996).

Many players influence international drug policy and action. Within the United Nations (UN) system alone there are a number of key players and many minor ones (United Nations, 1995). The United Nations International Drug Control Programme (UNDCP) is mandated to co-ordinate all illicit drug control matters within the UN, which includes assisting Member States to implement a series of four international treaties adopted under the auspices of the UN. These treaties (the 1961 Single Convention on Narcotic Drugs, the 1971 Convention on Psychotropic Substances, the 1972 Protocol Amending the Single Convention, and the 1988 United Nations Convention against Illicit Traffic in Narcotic Drugs and Psychotropic Substances) require that governments exercise control over production and distribution of illicit drugs and psychotropic substances, 'combat' drug abuse and illicit traffic, maintain the necessary administrative machinery, and report to international organs on their actions. The objective of the World Health Organization is 'the attainment by all peoples of the highest possible level of health' (WHO, 1990), which includes HIV prevention and the prevention of health risks and harms associated with substance use. The United Nations Development Programme (UNDP) has as its goal sustainable human development, which includes poverty elimination, environmental regeneration, creation of employment and advancement of women. The goal of the World Bank is to reduce poverty and improve people's living standards by promoting sustainable economic growth and development.

Whereas the objectives of all UN agencies in most circumstances work toward a common goal, the healthy development of all peoples, there are certain areas of conflict. With regard to illicit substance use as discussed above, international drug control in some areas has inadvertently facilitated the global dissemination of injecting drug use through the creation of new trafficking routes (see Chapter 1), thereby hampering public health measures to control the HIV epidemic. On the other hand, irrational prescribing of psychotropic drugs through the health sector can significantly undermine international drug control measures. Furthermore, the various UN agencies have different and competing priorities. Infectious diseases such as tuberculosis and malaria, diarrhoeal diseases, and problems associated with the use of alcohol and tobacco contribute more to the global burden of disease than does injecting drug use, although this may change with the expanding HIV epidemic (WHO, 1996d). Whereas UNDP and the World Bank have focused on development issues, rapid economic development has often increased the vulnerability of certain communities through their exposure to new drug using practices and HIV infection, and has established infrastructures which facilitate drug production and trafficking (such as roads, electronic communication and international banking).

In order to better co-ordinate actions between different UN agencies, various inter-agency mechanisms are being developed. The Joint United Nations Programme on HIV/AIDS (UNAIDS) was established in January 1996. UNAIDS is a co-sponsored programme that brings together six UN agencies: WHO, UNDP, the World Bank, the United Nations Children's Fund (UNICEF), the United Nations Population Fund (UNFPA), and the United Nations Educational, Scientific and Cultural Organization (UNESCO). Its mission is to 'lead, strengthen and support an expanded response aimed at preventing the transmission of HIV, providing care and support, reducing the vulnerability of individuals and communities to HIV/AIDS, and alleviating the impact of the epidemic' (Joint United Nations Programme on HIV/AIDS, 1996). UNAIDS has established a number of inter-agency working groups which aim to develop thematic position papers and frameworks for action. UNDCP has been responsible for co-ordinating the development of the United Nations System-wide Action Plan on Drug Abuse Control (SWAP) (Commission on Narcotic Drugs, 1996), which includes Plans of Action for a number of thematic areas. However, to date, neither the UNAIDS inter-agency working groups nor the SWAP have specifically addressed the issue of injecting drug use and HIV infection through such mechanisms.

Regional policies and actions also have significantly influenced the global epidemic. The critical role of injecting drug use in the dissemination of HIV-1 infection in the Asian region is but only one example. Many factors have contributed to this phenomenon, the complexities of which have been described by various researchers (McCoy, 1991; Stimson, 1994). Of particular importance are border areas and migration, especially in regions of illicit drug production, such as the 'Golden Crescent', the 'Golden Triangle', and the Amazon basin countries. Specific projects have been developed to address regional and cross-border issues (Economic and Social Commission for Asia and the Pacific, 1995).

Just as international policies and strategies need to be multisectoral, so do those at a national level. Certain countries have a tradition of responding to illicit drug use within a public health context and therefore were well positioned to react rapidly to the emergence of HIV infection among IDUs. Such countries, including the United Kingdom (Stimson, 1995), Australia (Blewett, 1987) and Canada (Health and Welfare Canada, 1992), have managed to avert the epidemic among IDUs through their timely action and involvement of all relevant government and non-government sectors. Such countries are in the minority, however, with illicit drug use being viewed by most countries as an internal security or foreign policy matter, where controlling the supply of drugs through law enforcement is the main preoccupation. Gradually, in some countries, both developed and developing, a shift in attitude is being observed, with health ministries taking a greater interest in drug policy. Assistance is being provided to governments by different United Nations agencies in the formulation of national policies and strategies covering areas including health, drug control and HIV/AIDS.

National and sub-national laws exist that present direct obstacles to HIV prevention efforts, particularly with regard to NSEPs, outreach to IDUs, and drug substitution programmes (WHO, 1993b). Other areas where legislation has an impact on HIV prevention efforts among IDUs include restrictive procedures, compulsory treatment, compulsory reporting and registration of drug users, compulsory HIV testing, and exclusion of protection for illegal drug use. WHO has recently completed a survey of 80 countries and two territories in order to review policies and legislation covering these areas (Porter *et al.*, in press).

It is often local policies, their interpretation and enforcement, which have the most impact on IDUs, including those policies on housing, health care, employment and law enforcement. The application of specific policies can vary greatly between different communities depending on political views. For example, within Europe there is increasing polarization between different municipal governments as to the most appropriate response to the problem of illicit drug use and HIV infection. Networks have been established linking together cities which advocate more restrictive drug policies on the one hand (for example European Cities Against Drugs) and those linking together cities promoting a more liberal approach on the other hand (for example European Cities on Drug Policy). At an operational level, municipal authorities can influence the implementation of such programmes as needle/syringe exchanges and the interpretation of drug laws through community policing. A specific example of municipal action in this area is provided by Hartnoll and Hedrich (1996) in their case study on Frankfurt.

It is often argued that many specific HIV prevention strategies targeting IDUs (those frequently referred to as 'harm reduction' strategies) are not feasible or accepted in most of the developing world because of cultural and political sensitivities and prohibitive costs. However, despite competing health and development priorities, in countries where repressive drug policies may exist, there is evidence of growing concern about the public health consequences of injecting drug use. With that concern, increasing numbers of communities are responding with local strategies which may actually challenge national policies.

Creating Supportive Environments

The Ottawa Charter states:

> Our societies are complex and interrelated. Health cannot be separated from other goals. The inextricable links between people and their environment constitutes the basis for a socio-ecological approach to health. The overall guiding principle for the world, nations, regions and communities alike, is the need to encourage reciprocal maintenance — to take care of each other, our communities and our natural environment.
>
> . . . Health promotion generates living and working conditions that are safe, stimulating, satisfying and enjoyable . . .

IDUs are more likely to change their risk behaviours and to sustain any behaviour change if a supportive environment exists. In creating a supportive environment, inequities in health and social injustice should be addressed, ensuring equal access to appropriate health prevention and treatment services. 'Health for all' means health for everybody, including drug users. It is often local and national policies, as discussed above, which determine the living environment of IDUs. In addition to a supportive physical environment (meeting the basic needs of shelter, clothing and food) there is also a need for a supportive psychosocial environment where self-empowerment of IDUs is facilitated. Change is facilitated through community education, leading to community recognition that IDUs are individuals entitled to the same basic rights as all others. This process will assist in overcoming the marginalization of IDUs, which remains the major obstacle to equal access to health services.

Outreach services help to create supportive environments through the delivery of information and services to hard-to-reach populations, and to establish links between IDUs and health services. When considering the developing world, not only are resources limited for implementing outreach programmes, but there are many different vulnerable groups and settings which require different outreach strategies. Particularly vulnerable groups include the urban poor; street children (Ball and Howard, 1995); sex workers; itinerant and guest workers; remote rural communities; refugees and displaced persons from civil conflicts and natural disasters; minority, tribal and indigenous groups; those with physical and mental disabilities; and communities living in drug producing areas. Throughout the world, prisons provide a high risk environment (Dolan, Wodak and Penny, 1995). Despite this, different forms of interventions targeting IDUs have been successfully implemented in prison settings, including peer-led HIV prevention education programmes, bleach distribution, condom distribution, needle/syringe exchange programmes, methadone maintenance programmes, and experimental heroin prescribing.

A supportive environment should include accessible and user-friendly HIV and drug prevention and treatment services. Increasing the range of prevention and treatment options for IDUs is likely to attract greater numbers into intervention. For example, research into, and implementation of, heroin prescribing trials aim to determine whether broadening drug substitution options will attract more marginalized IDUs into treatment (Bammer, 1995; Rihs-Middel, 1995).

Whereas a supportive environment increases the extent of behaviour change, data from at least one city indicate that it does not have to be a prerequisite for change to occur. In New York City, for example, IDUs learned about AIDS through the mass media and large-scale behaviour change occurred among IDUs prior to the implementation of any formal AIDS prevention programmes and prior to any legal access to sterile injection equipment.

Strengthening Community Action

The Ottawa Charter states:

> Health promotion works through concrete and effective community action in setting priorities, making decisions, planning strategies and implementing them to achieve better health. At the heart of this process is the empowerment of communities — their ownership and control of their own endeavours and destinies.
>
> Community development draws on existing human and material resources in the community to enhance self help and social support, and to develop flexible systems for strengthening public participation and direction of health matters. This requires full and continuous access to information, learning opportunities for health, as well as funding support.

Outreach and peer education are key strategies for strengthening community action to reduce HIV risk among IDUs. Various models of outreach exist, including those targeting individual IDUs and those targeting communities or networks of IDUs. Furthermore, outreach may be detached (working off-site on the streets, in locations where IDUs congregate, and so on), domiciliary (visiting IDUs in their homes), or peripatetic (working in different agencies and institutions, such as prisons and needle/syringe exchanges) (Rhodes, 1994). Most outreach programmes provide information and education on HIV risk management related to injecting drug use and sexual practices and offer referral to other services. In addition to education and referral, some programmes provide condoms, injecting equipment, bleach and basic health care (such as the dressing of infected injection sites). Outreach programmes to IDUs are widespread throughout most of the developed world and increasingly they are appearing in developing countries. Needle/syringe exchange or distribution programmes have been established in Santos and Salvador in Brazil (WHO, 1996a), Kathmandu (Maharjan and Singh, 1996) and among Akha hill-tribe communities in northern Thailand (Gray, 1995), while such programmes are being piloted in Vietnam. Programmes providing advice on syringe cleaning techniques and condom and bleach distribution are being implemented in Manipur, north-eastern India (Chatterjee *et al.*, 1996), other areas of India, Malaysia, Vietnam, Thailand and Nepal. Other outreach programmes to IDUs provide HIV prevention information in China, Myanmar, Brazil and Argentina.

Injecting drug users form their own communities and networks. This provides an excellent opportunity for outreach programmes to influence peer group and social norms, resulting in community change. Peer education programmes among drug users have been shown to be effective in reducing both HIV risk behaviour and HIV infection rates (Wiebel *et al.*, 1993), while peer-based needle/syringe exchange programmes have been shown to be more effective in reaching new clients than those conducted by non-peers (Herkt, 1993). The use of ex-IDUs as peer educators also plays an important role in intervention programmes in developing countries such as India (Dorabjee, Samson and Dyalchand, 1996; Chatterjee *et al.*, 1996) and Nepal (Maharjan and Singh, 1996).

In some communities, new models of outreach have been developed which aim to more effectively involve IDUs as outreach workers (Grund *et al.*, 1996). In some countries (notably Australia and many European countries) drug users have self-organized to form drug users' organizations for the purpose of advocating on behalf of IDUs and for implementing HIV prevention programmes (including peer outreach, education and needle/syringe exchange) (Jose *et al.*, 1996). Peers have an opportunity to influence group norms by demonstrating through their own behaviour HIV prevention strategies.

Developing Personal Skills

The Ottawa Charter states:

Health promotion supports personal and social development through providing information, education for health, and enhancing life skills. By so doing, it increases the options available to people to exercise more control over their own health and over their environments, and to make choices conducive to health.

Enabling people to learn, through life, to prepare themselves for all of its stages and to cope with chronic illness and injuries is essential. This has to be facilitated in school, home, work and community settings . . .

There are four main groups which need to be targeted for the development of personal skills in preventing HIV risk associated with injecting drug use, including IDUs themselves, sexual partners and family members, health-care workers (including outreach and peers), and the general community.

IDUs acquire specific knowledge and skills through their own drug using experiences, and those of their peers, which assist them in the assessment and management of risks associated with injecting drug use (Power, 1996). IDUs use risk assessment and management in many situations, for example in preventing overdoses, caring for venous access, regulating the intensity of drug use, and avoiding detection by police. In developing the personal skills of IDUs, particular attention should be given to HIV risk assessment and management, including the provision of accurate information on HIV risk practices, education on needle/syringe cleaning and condom use, information on gaining access to sterile injecting equipment and condoms, and information on referral to drug treatment and HIV services. As already discussed above, the provision of such information, education and counselling is likely to be most effective when delivered by peers.

Sexual partners and significant others of IDUs often require specific attention. For sexual partners this includes the development of risk management skills with regard to sexual behaviour. Some studies have indicated that knowledge of HIV status may increase condom use by IDUs with their primary sexual partners (van den Hoek *et al.*, 1990). This has implications with regard to the use of HIV testing for risk management counselling. In most settings the commonest cause of acute death associated with injecting drug use is overdose. Witnesses, such as drug injecting peers, sexual partners and significant others, can provide life-saving interventions, including resuscitation and calling for medical assistance. It has also been proposed that opioid users be provided with naloxone, an opioid antagonist, for use by witnesses when overdose occurs. Some drug treatment and outreach programmes provide information and training on resuscitation and other first aid to IDUs and their significant others (The Spike Collective, 1995).

Health-care workers and other service providers coming into contact with IDUs need to have sufficient knowledge and skills to offer effective HIV prevention interventions. A number of significant obstacles exist, including negative attitudes towards IDUs and the existence of a wide range of myths about injecting drug use and IDUs. A study of attitudes and skills of medical students and newly registered doctors in Australia revealed that they have a fairly negative perception of intervention outcomes with drug related problems, despite a belief that the doctor has a responsibility to intervene (Britton, Forcier and McKissock, 1986). The same study revealed that as medical training progressed from first year medical school to new registration, the percentage of students expressing disinterest in working with drug users increased from 24 per cent to 55 per cent. It is evident that factors affecting such attitudinal changes need to be addressed through medical education. In the United Kingdom, a number of national surveys have indicated that general practitioners are reluctant to treat drug users (Rhodes *et al.*, 1989) and lack the necessary skills to provide services to this population (Glanz and Taylor, 1986). It is likely that skills-based competence, self-efficacy (confidence in undertaking a particular task) and realistic expectations of response to intervention are more important determinants of effective practice behaviour than level of knowledge and positive attitudes to drug users (Saunders and Roche, 1991). Therefore, medical and other health professional education should focus particular attention on assessment and early intervention skills and exposing trainees to earlier-stage problems and 'success stories'.

The specific training needs of outreach workers and peer educators need to be considered. Apart from developing basic knowledge and skills related to injecting drug use and HIV infection, training should focus on the development of skills for 'streetwork'. Such detached work presents many different challenges to those which typically exist in centre-based programmes. Grey areas exist where such workers may be drawn into criminal situations or placed at physical risk. Special training may include conflict resolution and aggression management, legal and civil rights issues, resuscitation and first aid, community relations, and referral practices. Many of these skills are revelevant for all street outreach workers (WHO, 1995b).

The general population also needs to be addressed through any HIV and drug information and education programme, both because of the need for individuals to understand and minimize their own personal risks and because of the need to dispel community myths which may further marginalize IDUs and compromise the effectiveness of interventions. Such education should enable individuals to accurately assess their own HIV risks and be skilled in reducing any such risks. Certain populations of young people are particularly vulnerable through both drug use and sexual experimentation. New models of drug education are being promoted where the focus is not on the prevention of drug use but rather on reducing risks where drug use may have already been initiated (including experimental and intermittent use) (Cohen, 1993).

Reorientation of Health Services

The Ottawa Charter states:

> The responsibility for health promoting health services is shared among individuals, community groups, health professionals, health service institutions and governments. They must work together towards a health care system which contributes to the pursuit of health.
>
> The role of the health sector must move increasingly in a health promotion direction, beyond its responsibility for providing clinical and curative services. Health services need to embrace an expanded mandate which is sensitive and respects cultural needs. This mandate should support the needs of individuals, and communities for a healthier

life, and open channels between the health sector and broader social, political, economic and physical environment components.

Already in the second section of this chapter, specific intervention strategies were discussed for reducing HIV risk among IDUs. Reorientation of health services involves a careful analysis of how such interventions may be designed, packaged together and delivered in order to achieve maximum reach and impact. Recognizing the diversity among IDUs, the widest possible range of intervention options needs to be offered, with a particular emphasis on the mobilization of primary health care services and injecting drug user networks. The efficacy of such interventions as methadone maintenance, needle/syringe exchange, condom distribution, peer education, and community outreach have already been demonstrated in many communities. Research now needs to move forward to examine the context and design of programmes being delivered and how affordable programmes may be developed for the developing world.

Although methadone maintenance programmes have rapidly spread throughout most of the developed world in response to the HIV epidemic, there are increasing concerns about the cost and sustainability of such programmes. The next generation of research will need to focus on such areas as reducing costs, maximizing reach to and access for the most marginalized IDUs, improving treatment retention, and integration of programmes within other primary health care and outreach services. Furthermore, alternative substitute drugs to methadone need to be considered in order to reduce costs, to attract under-served populations, and to engage those IDUs whose primary drug of use is not an opioid.

The experience of community-based agonist pharmacotherapy programmes in developing countries (such as India, Nepal and Thailand as described above) may help to inform the reorientation of substitution programmes in developed countries. These community-based programmes have been established in response to community-identified needs, designed, implemented and managed by the communities themselves. The settings vary considerably, including a densely populated slum community in Delhi, a group of remote Akha hill-tribe villages in northern Thailand, and a community psychiatric hospital in Katmandu. Costs are very low, with dispensing of drug doses by staff being integrated with a normal day-to-day delivery of other health services in the community. These programmes have mostly been established through the non-government sector, with limited, if any, recognition or support from government. Although they appear to be effective in engaging marginalized and difficult-to-reach IDUs in treatment, and have been accepted within their communities, no formal evaluation has been conducted on these programmes. There is a need to undertake further research on the acceptability and effectiveness of agonist pharmacotherapy programmes in developing countries and the feasibility of expanding such programmes to increase reach. Specific pharmacological research also needs to be undertaken to determine appropriate dosing levels in different populations (particularly where under-nutrition and chronic illness are common); to study the pharmacodynamics of new agonist substitution compounds, such as tincture of opium; and to investigate drug interactions considering the rapid increase in polysubstance use.

As with agonist pharmacotherapy programmes, the effectiveness of needle/syringe exchange programmes in changing risk behaviour and preventing HIV infection has been demonstrated in many developed countries. Despite the growing evidence of effectiveness, due to political concerns, the establishment and support of such programmes have met with considerable resistance in many communities (Watters, 1996). Nevertheless, research is now focusing on increasing the efficiency of these programmes, particularly by increasing reach through broadening the types of outlets available, including the use of outreach and secondary outlets, such as pharmacies (Glanz, Byrne and Jackson, 1989), general practitioners and community health services. The feasibility of implementing needle/syringe exchange programmes has been demonstrated in developing countries as mentioned above, including programmes in Nepal, Brazil, Thailand and Vietnam.

Whereas HIV risk reduction may be the focus for action, consideration must also be given to treatment. The key principle with regard to treatment is equity of access, including the access to drug treatment for HIV positive individuals and access to HIV/AIDS treatment and care for drug users. The current inequities in access to treatment are dramatically portrayed in a presentation by Josef Decosas (1996) where he stated that if the cure for AIDS were a glass of clean water, over half the world's population would not have access to treatment.

Conclusions

In the past 10 years injecting drug use has spread rapidly throughout the world, and associated with this has been the epidemic spread of HIV infection (see Chapter 1). HIV infection is only one of a range of negative health and social consequences of injecting, but it currently poses the greatest public health concern (see Chapter 3). The factors which have contributed to the transition of non-injecting to injecting drug use and the global dissemination of HIV risk practices are multiple and complex (see Chapter 2). In examining the context of injecting drug use and HIV risk, specific issues need to be considered, including: needle/syringe sharing practices; sexual risk behaviours (see Chapter 9); population mixing patterns (see Chapter 7); high risk settings for injecting, such as prisons (see Chapter 11); the vulnerability of new and young injectors (see Chapter 5); and the policy and programme environment of cities where injecting occurs (see Chapter 10).

The WHO Multi-City Study on Drug Injecting and Risk of HIV Infection has contributed much to the global knowledge on the phenomenon of HIV infection and risk behaviour associated with injecting drug use. The study provided a wealth of data from 12 cities around the world (see Chapters 4 and 6, and Appendix 2). It also contributed to the development of standardized research methods, which have been validated across different cultures and settings (see Appendix 1) and the establishment of an international collaborative network of researchers (see Appendix 3). Although the study threw light on many issues, it also raised many new and important questions. A second phase of the study was initiated in late 1995 (WHO, 1996a) with a particular focus on developing countries, rapid assessment methods, the context of injecting drug use, factors influencing transitions between non-injecting and injecting drug use, other health consequences (such as overdose and hepatitis B and C), and prevention interventions.

Substantial evidence now exists from the WHO Study and other research that IDUs do change their behaviour in response to information on HIV risk and if they are given the opportunity to change their behaviours (see Chapter 12). This chapter has discussed the various strategies which may be implemented to prevent HIV infection and its epidemic spread associated with injecting drug use. Although discrete interventions do exist, it is evident that it is the timely implementation of a wide range of strategies combined together within a health promotion framework which will have the greatest impact.

Whereas it is recognized that injecting drug use poses a wide range of health risks, and requires a broad-based response, there are specific intervention components which have been demonstrated to be effective in preventing HIV infection. Increasing the availability of needles, syringes and other injecting equipment, such as through needle/syringe exchange programmes and pharmacies, and encouraging IDUs to use sterile equipment, has been shown to reduce needle and syringe sharing practices and HIV transmission. Such approaches have been demonstrated to be feasible in a range of developed and developing countries. Methadone maintenance programmes reduce HIV risk behaviour and HIV transmission, although there is still need to evaluate other substitute drugs and forms of service delivery. The feasibility of establishing drug substitution programmes in various developing countries has already been demonstrated. Education to increase awareness of HIV risks and skills for HIV risk management, with regard to both drug use and sexual practices, are critical for behaviour change to occur. This requires outreach to marginalized IDUs and a building of trust between IDUs and health and welfare workers. The expansion of drug treatment options and increased accessiblity to treatment services act to attract more IDUs into treatment, where HIV prevention efforts may be implemented. Situation assessment will inform how these specific HIV prevention interventions may be adapted and combined to form a comprehensive and integrated strategy. The vigorous and early implementation of such a stategy, while the prevalence of both injecting drug use and HIV infection is low, will be most effective. This can only occur if there is a supportive policy environment which in turn requires a public health response involving intersectoral co-operation across all areas.

References

ABDUL-QUADER, A.S., FRIEDMAN, S.R., DES JARLAIS, D., MARMOR, M.M., MASLANSKY, R. and BARTELME, S. (1987) 'Methadone maintenance and behavior by intravenous drug users that can transmit HIV', *Contemporary Drug Problems*, **14**, pp. 425–34.

BALL, A. (1996) 'Averting a global epidemic', *Addiction*, **91**, pp. 1095–8.

BALL, A. and HOWARD, J. (1995) 'Psychoactive substance use among street children', HARPHAM, T. and BLUE, I. (Eds) *Urbanization and mental health in developing countries*, pp. 123–49, Aldershot: Avebury.

BALL, J.C. and ROSS, A. (1991) *The Effectiveness of Methadone Maintenance Treatment: Patients, programs, services, and outcome*, New York: Springer-Verlag.

BALL, J.C., LANGE, W.R., MEYERS, C.P. and FRIEDMAN, S.R. (1988) 'Reducing the risk of AIDS through methadone maintenance treatment', *Journal of Health and Social Behaviour*, **29**, pp. 214–26.

BAMMER, G. (1995) *Report and recommendations of Stage 2 Feasibility Research into the Controlled Availability of Opioids*, Canberra: National Centre for Epidemiology and Population Health.

BELL, J., HALL, W. and BLYTHE, K. (1992) 'Changes in criminal activity after entering methadone maintenance', *British Journal of Addiction*, **87**, pp. 251–8.

BLAINE, J.D. (Ed.) (1992) *Buprenorphine: An Alternative Treatment for Opioid Dependence*, Research Monograph Series 121, Rockville: National Institute on Drug Abuse.

BLEWETT, N. (1987) *NCADA: Assumptions, arguments and aspirations*, National Campaign Against Drug Abuse Monograph Series No. 1, Canberra: Australian Government Publishing Service.

BRITTON, A., FORCIER, L. and MCKISSOCK, D. (1986) *Phase I Report of the NSW Medical Education Project: Alcohol and Other Drugs*, Sydney: NSW Medical Education Project: Alcohol and Other Drugs.

BROADHEAD, R.S. (1991) 'Social construction of bleach in combating AIDS among injection drug users', *Journal of Drug Issues*, **21**, pp. 713–37.

BURT, J. and STIMSON, G.V. (1993) *Drug Injectors and HIV Risk Reduction: Strategies for Protection*, London: Health Education Authority.

CELANTANO, D., MUNOZ, A., COHN, S., NELSON, K.E. and VLAHOV, D. (1994) 'Drug-related behaviour for HIV transmission among American injecting drug users', *Addiction*, **89**, pp. 1309–17.

CHATTERJEE, A., HANGZO, C.Z., ABDUL-QUADER, A.S., O'REILLY, K.R., ZOMI, G.T. and SARKAR, S. (1996) 'Evidence of effectiveness of street-based peer outreach intervention to change cleaning behavior among injecting drug users in Manipur, India', Abstract Th.C.422, XI International Conference on AIDS, Vancouver.

COHEN, J. (1993) 'Achieving a reduction in drug-related harm through education', in HEATHER, N., WODAK, A., NADELMANN, E. and O'HARE, P. (Eds) *Psychoactive Drugs and Harm Reduction: From Faith to Science*, London: Wurr Publishers.

COMMISSION ON NARCOTIC DRUGS (1996) *The United Nations System-wide Action Plan on Drug Abuse Control*, E/CN.7/1996/CRP.1, Vienna: CND.

CORRECTIONAL SERVICE OF CANADA (1994) *HIV/AIDS in Prisons: Final Report of The Expert Committee on AIDS and Prisons*, Ottawa.

DECOSAS, J. (1996) 'HIV and Development', Abstract We.13, XI International Conference on AIDs, Vancouver.

DES JARLAIS, D.C., CASRIEL, C., FRIEDMAN, S.R. and ROSENBLUM, A. (1992) 'AIDS and the transition to illicit drug injection: Results of a randomized trial prevention program', *British Journal of Addiction*, **87**, pp. 493–8.

DES JARLAIS, D.C., FRIEDMAN, S.R., SOTHERN, J.L., WENSTON, J., MARMOR, M., YANCOVITZ, S.R., FRANK, B., BEATRICE, S. and MILDVAN, D. (1994) 'Continuity and change within an HIV epidemic: Injecting drug users in New York City, 1984 through 1992', *Journal of the American Medical Association*, **271**, pp. 121–7.

DES JARLAIS, D.C., HAGAN, H., FRIEDMAN, S.R., FRIEDMANN, P., GOLDBERG, D., FRISCHER, M., GREEN, S., TUNVING, K., LJUNGBERG, B., WODAK, A., ROSS, M., PURCHASE, D., MILLSON, M.E. and MYERS, T. (1995) 'Maintaining low HIV seroprevalence in populations of injecting drug users', *Journal of the American Medical Association*, **274**, pp. 1226–31.

DES JARLAIS, D.C., HAGAN, H., PAONE, D. and FRIEDMAN, S.R. (1996) 'HIV incidence among syringe exchange participants: The international data', Abstract Tu.C.322, XI International Conference on AIDS, Vancouver.

DOLAN, K., WODAK, A. and PENNY, R. (1995) 'AIDS behind bars: preventing HIV spread among incarcerated drug injectors', *AIDS*, **9**, pp. 825–32.

DONOGHOE, M.C. and POWER, R. (1993), 'Household bleach is disinfectant for injecting drug users', *Lancet*, **i**, p. 165.

DORABJEE, J., SAMSON, L. and DYALCHAND, R. (1996) 'A community based intervention for injecting drug users (IDUs) in New Delhi slums', unpublished paper available at XI International Conference on AIDS, Vancouver.

ECONOMIC AND SOCIAL COMMISSION FOR ASIA AND THE PACIFIC (1995), *Community-based Drug Demand Reduction: Report on five demonstration projects*, New York: United Nations.

FARRELL, M., WARD, J., MATTICK, R., HALL, W., STIMSON, G.V., DES JARLAIS, D., GOSSOP, M. and STRANG, J. (1994) 'Methadone maintenance treatment in opiate dependence: a review', *British Medical Journal*, **309**, pp. 991–1001.

FARRELL M., NEELEMAN, J., GOSSOP, M., GRIFFITHS, P., BUNING, E., FINCH, E. and STRANG, J. (1995) 'Methadone provision in the European Union', *The International Journal of Drug Policy*, **6**, pp. 168–72.

FLEMING, P.M. and ROBERTS, D. (1994) 'Is the prescription of amphetamine justified as a harm reduction measure?', *Journal of the Royal Society on Health*, pp. 127–31.

GLANZ, A. and TAYLOR, C. (1986) 'Findings of a national survey on the role of general practitioners in the treatment of opiate misuse: extent of contact with opiate misusers', *British Medical Journal*, **293**, pp. 427–30.

GLANZ, A., BYRNE, C. and JACKSON, P. (1989) 'Role of community pharmacists in the prevention of AIDS among injecting drug users: findings of a survey in England and Wales', *British Medical Journal*, **299**, pp. 1076–9.

GLASER, F.B. (1993) 'Descriptors of treatment', in WHO, *Approaches to Treatment of Substance Abuse*, Geneva: Programme on Substance Abuse, World Health Organization.

GRAY, J. (1995) 'Operating needle exchange programmes in the hills of Thailand', *AIDS Care*, **7**, pp. 489–99.

GRUND, J-P. C., BROADHEAD, R.S., HEKATHORN, D.D., STERN, L.S. and ANTHONY, D.L. (1996) 'Peer-driven outreach to combat HIV among IDUs: A basic design and preliminary results', in RHODES, T. and HARTNOLL, R. (Eds) *Aids, Drugs and Prevention: Perspectives on individual and community action*, London: Routledge.

HARTNOLL, R., and HEDRICH, D. (1996) 'AIDS prevention and drug policy: Dilemmas in the local environment', in RHODES, T. and HARTNOLL, R. (Eds) *AIDS, Drugs and Prevention: Perspectives on individual and community action*, London: Routledge.

HEALTH AND WELFARE CANADA (1992) *Canada's Drug Strategy*, Ottawa: Government of Canada.

HEATHER, N. and TEBUTT, J. (Eds) (1989) *The Effectiveness of Treatment for Drug and Alcohol Problems: An Overview*, National Campaign Against Drug Abuse, Monograph Series No. 11, Canberra: Australian Government Publishing Service.

HERKT, D. (1993) 'Peer-based user groups: the Australian experience', in HEATHER, N., WODAK, A., NADELMANN, E. and O'HARE, P. (Eds.) *Psychoactive Drugs and Harm: From Faith to Science*, London: Wurr Publishers.

HESTER, R.K. (1993) 'Psychological, behavioural and psychodynamic treatments for substance abuse', in WHO, *Approaches to Treatment of Substance Abuse*, Geneva: Programme on Substance Abuse, World Health Organization.

HUDELSON, P.M. (1994) *Qualitative Research for Health Programmes*, Geneva: Division of Mental Health, World Health Organization.

INTERNATIONAL NARCOTICS CONTROL BOARD (1996) *Report of the International Narcotics Control Board for 1995*, Vienna: United Nations.

JILEK, W.G. (1993) 'The role of traditional healing in the management of substance abuse', in WHO, *Approaches to Treatment of Substance Abuse*, Geneva: Programme on Substance Abuse, World Health Organization.

JOINT UNITED NATIONS PROGRAMME ON HIV/AIDS (1996) *UNAIDS: Fact Sheet*, Geneva: UNAIDS.

JOSE, B., FRIEDMAN, S.R., NEAIGUS, A. *et al.* (1992) ' "Frontloading" is associated with HIV infection among drug injectors in New York City', VIII International Conference on AIDS, Amsterdam.

JOSE, B., FRIEDMAN, S.R., NEAIGUS, A., CURTIS, R., SUFIAN, M., STEPHERSON, B. and DES JARLAIS, D.C. (1996) 'Collective organisation of injecting drug users and the struggle against AIDS', in RHODES, T. and HARTNOLL, R. (Eds) *AIDS, Drugs and Prevention: Perspectives on individual and community action*, London: Routledge.

KALANT, H. (1993) 'Pharmacological treatment of dependence on alcohol and other drugs: An overview', in WHO, *Approaches to Treatment of Substance Abuse*, Geneva: Programme on Substance Abuse, World Health Organization.

KANGA, K. (1996) 'Drug intervention/awareness among IDUs in the slum', Abstract Mo.D.242, XI International Conference on AIDS, Vancouver.

KOESTER, S. (1996) 'The process of drug injection: Applying ethnography to the study of HIV risk among IDUs', in RHODES, T. and HARTNOLL, R. (1995) *AIDS, Drugs and Prevention: Perspectives on individual and community action*, London: Routledge.

LASKI, G. (1991) 'A longitudinal analysis of needle sharing among San Francisco injection heroin users', Abstract MD4090, VII International Conference on AIDS, Florence.

LLOSA, T. (1994) 'The standard low dose of oral cocaine used for treatment of cocaine dependence', *Substance Abuse*, **15**, pp. 215–20.

LOXLEY, W. and OVENDEN, C. (1995) 'Friends and lovers: needle sharing in young people in Western Australia', *AIDS Care*, **7**, pp. 337–51.

LURIE, P. and DRUCKER, E. (1996) 'An opportunity lost: Estimating the number of HIV infections due to the US failure to adopt a national needle exchange policy', Abstract Tu.C.324, XI International Conference on AIDS, Vancouver.

LURIE, P. and REINGOLD, A.L. (1993) *The Public Health Impact of Needle Exchange Programs in the United States and Abroad: Summary, conclusions and recommendations*, San Franciso: University of California.

McCOY, A.W. (1991) *The Politics of Heroin: CIA Complicity in the Global Drug Trade*, Chicago: Lawrence Hill Books.

McGeorge, J., Crofts, N. and Burrows, C. (1996) *Injecting Drug Users and the Disinfection of Used Injecting Equipment*, 7th International Conference on the Reduction of Drug Related Harm, Hobart, Tasmania.

McKeganey, N.P. and Barnard, M.A. (1992) *AIDS, Drugs and Sexual Risk: Lives in the Balance*, Buckingham: Open University Press.

McKeganey, N.P., Barnard, M.A., Leyland, A.H. and Follet, E. (1992) 'Female streetworking prostitution and HIV infection in Glasgow', *British Medical Journal*, **305**, pp. 801–4.

Maharjan, S.H. and Singh, M. (1996) 'Street-based outreach program for injecting drug users', Abstract Mo.D.244, XI International Conference on AIDS, Vancouver.

Mattick, R. and Darke, S. (1995) 'Drug replacement treatments: is amphetamine substitution a horse of a different colour?', *Drug and Alcohol Review*, **14**, pp. 389–94.

Mattick, R. and Hall, W. (Eds) (1993) *A treatment outline for approaches to opioid dependence: quality assurance project*, National Campaign Against Drug Abuse, Monograph Series No. 21, Canberra: Australian Government Publishing Service.

Millar, A. (1996) 'The medical prescription of anabolic steroids', *The International Journal of Drug Policy*, **7**, pp. 15–18.

Miller, W.R. and Rollnick, S. (1991) *Motivational Interviewing*, New York: Guilford Press.

Mitcheson, M., Edwards, G., Hawks, D. and Ogborne, A. (1976) 'Treatment of methylamphetamine users during the 1968 epidemic', in Edwards, G., Russell, M., Hawks, D. and MacCafferty, M. (Eds), *Drug and Drug Dependence*, Farnborough: Saxon House.

Normand, J., Vlahov, D. and Moses, L.E. (Eds) (1995) *Preventing HIV Transmission: The Role of Sterile Needles and Bleach*, Washington: National Academy Press.

Pickens, R.W., Leukefeld, C.G. and Schuster, C.R. (Eds) (1991) *Improving Drug Abuse Treatment*, Research Monograph Series 106, Rockville: National Institute on Drug Abuse.

Porter, L., Argandoña, M. and Curran, W.J. (in press) *Drug and Alcohol Policies, Legislation and Programmes for Treatment and Rehabilitation*, Geneva: World Health Organization.

Power, R. (1996) 'Promoting risk management among drug injectors', in Rhodes, T. and Hartnoll, R. (Eds) *AIDS, Drugs and Prevention: Perspectives on individual and community action*, London: Routledge.

Rhodes, T. (1994) *Risk, Intervention and Change*, London: Health Education Authority.

Rhodes, T., Gallagher, M., Foy, C., *et al.* (1989) 'Prevention in practice: obstacles and opportunities', *AIDS Care*, **1**, pp. 257–68.

Rhodes, T.J., Bloor, M.J., Donoghoe, M.C., *et al.* (1993) 'HIV prevalence and HIV risk behaviour among injecting drug users in London and Glasgow', *AIDS Care*, **5**, pp. 413–25.

Rihs-Middel, M. (1995) 'La prescription de stupéfiants sous contrôle médical et la recherche en matière de drogues à l'Office fédéral de la santé publique (OFSP)', in *La Prescription de Stupéfiants sous Contrôle Médical*, pp. 9–16, Genève: Éditions Médicine et Hygiène.

Saunders, J.B. and Roche, A.M. (1991) 'Medical education in substance use disorders', *Drug and Alcohol Review*, **10**, pp. 263–75.

Saxon, A.J., Calsyn, D.A. and Jackson, T.R. (1994) 'Longitudinal changes in injection behaviours in a cohort of injection drug users', *Addiction*, **89**, pp. 191–202.

SHERMAN, J.P. (1990) 'Dexamphetamine for "speed" addiction', *Medical Journal of Australia*, **153**, p. 306.

SHRESTA, D.M., SHRESTA, N.M. and GAUTAM, K. (1995) 'Methadone treatment programme in Nepal: A one-year experience', *Journal of Nepalese Medical Association*, **33**, pp. 33–46.

THE SPIKE COLLECTIVE (1995) 'Lost the plot', *The Spike: News and Views for Injecting Drug Users*, Issue 17, Auckland.

STIMSON, G.V. (1994) 'Reconstruction of subregional diffusion of HIV infection among injecting drug users in south-east Asia: Implications for early intervention', *AIDS*, **8**, pp. 1630–2.

STIMSON, G.V. (1995) 'AIDS and injecting drug use in the United Kingdom, 1987–1993: The policy response and the prevention of the epidemic', *Social Science and Medicine*, **41**, pp. 699–716.

STIMSON. G.V. and DONOGHOE, M.C. (1996) 'Health promotion and facilitation of individual change: The case of syringe distribution and exchange', in RHODES, T. and HARTNOLL, R. (Eds) *AIDS, Drugs and Prevention: Perspectives on Individual and Community Action*, London: Routledge.

STIMSON, G.V. and HUNTER, G. (1996) 'Interventions with drug injectors in the UK: trends in risk behaviour and HIV prevalence', *International Journal of STD & AIDS*, **7**, suppl. 2, pp. 52–6.

STRANG, J., DES JARLAIS, D.C., GRIFFITHS, P. and GOSSOP, M. (1992) 'The study of transitions in the route of drug use: The route from one route to another', *British Journal of Addiction*, **87**, 3, pp. 473–83.

STRANG, J., RUBEN, S., FARRELL, M. and GOSSOP, M. (1994) 'Prescribing heroin and other injectable drugs', in STRANG, J. and GOSSOP, M. (Eds) *Heroin Addiction and Drug Policy: The British System*, pp. 193–206, Oxford: Oxford University Press.

UCHTENHAGEN, A., DOBLER-MIKOLA, A. and GUTZWILLER, F. (1996) 'Medically controlled prescription of narcotics: A Swiss National project', *The International Journal of Drug Policy*, **7**, pp. 31–6.

UNITED NATIONS (1995) *Basic Facts about the United Nations*, New York: United Nations.

VAN AMEIJDEN, E.J., VAN DEN HOEK, J.A., VAN HAASTRECHT, H.J. and COUTINHO, R. A. (1994a) 'Trends in sexual behaviour and the incidence of sexually transmitted diseases and HIV among drug-using prostitutes, Amsterdam 1986–1992', *AIDS*, **8**, pp. 213–21.

VAN AMEIJDEN, E.J., VAN DEN HOEK, J.A.R., HARTGERS, C. and COUTINHO, R.A. (1994b) 'Risk factors for the transition from noninjection to injection drug use and accompanying AIDS risk behavior in a cohort of drug users', *American Journal of Epidemiology*, **139**, pp. 67–77.

VAN DEN HOEK, J.A.R., VAN HAASTRECHT, H.J.A. and COUTINHO, R.A. (1990) 'Heterosexual behaviour of intravenous drug users in Amsterdam: implications for the AIDS epidemic', *AIDS*, **4**, 449–53.

VANICHSENI, S., WONGSUWAN, B., STAFF OF THE BMA NARCOTICS CLINIC NO. 6, CHOOPANYA, K. and WONGPANICH, K. (1991) 'A controlled trial of methadone maintenance in a population of intravenous drug users in Bangkok: Implications for prevention of HIV', *International Journal of Addictions*, **26**, pp. 1313–20.

VLAHOV, D. (1996) 'Backloading and HIV infection among injection drug users', *The International Journal of Drug Policy*, **7**, pp. 52–7.

WARD, J., MATTICK, R. and HALL, W. (1992) *Key Issues in Methadone Maintenance Treatment*, Sydney: New South Wales University Press.

WARD, J., MATTICK, R. and HALL, W. (1994) 'The effectiveness of methadone maintenance treatment: an overview', *Drug and Alcohol Review*, **13**, pp. 327–36.

WATTERS, J.K. (1996) 'Americans and syringe exchange: Roots and resistance', in RHODES, T. and HARTNOLL, R. (Eds) *AIDS, Drugs and Prevention: Perspectives on individual and community action*, London: Routledge.

WHO (1978) *Primary Health Care: Report of the International Conference on Primary Health Care*, Geneva: World Health Organization.

WHO (1981) *Global Strategy for Health for All by the Year 2000*, Geneva: World Health Organization

WHO (1986) *Health Promotion: Ottawa Charter*, WHO/HPR/HEP/95.1, Geneva: World Health Organization

WHO (1990) *Basic Documents*, 38th Edn., Geneva: World Health Organization

WHO (1993a) *National AIDS Programme Management: Prevention of HIV Transmission through Injecting Drug Use*, Geneva: Global Programme on AIDS, World Health Organization

WHO (1993b) *Tabular Information on Legal Instruments Dealing with HIV Infection and AIDS*, WHO/GPA/HLE/93.1, Geneva: Global Programme on AIDS, World Health Organization.

WHO (1993c) *Drug use and sport: Current issues and implications for public health*, WHO/PSA/ 93.3, Geneva: Programme on Substance Abuse, World Health Organization.

WHO (1993d) *Approaches to Treatment of Substance Abuse*, WHO/PSA/93.10, Geneva: Programme on Substance Abuse, World Health Organization.

WHO (1993e) *Community Based Approaches to Treatment and Care of Substance Dependence: Report on a WHO Consultation*, Geneva: Programme on Substance Abuse, World Health Organization.

WHO (1994a) World Health Organization International Collaborative Group. *Multi-City Study on Drug Injecting and Risk of HIV Infection*, WHO/PSA/94.4, Geneva: World Health Organization.

WHO (1994b) *Primary Health Care Concepts and Challenges in a Changing World: Alma-Ata Revisited*, WHO/SHS/CC/94.2, Geneva: Division of Strengthening of Health Services, World Health Organization.

WHO (1995a) *Renewing the Health-For-All Strategy: Elaboration of a Policy for Equity, Solidarity and Health: Consultation Document*, WHO/PAC/95.1, Geneva: World Health Organization.

WHO (1995b) *Street Children, Substance Use and Health: Training for Street Educators*, WHO/ PSA/95.12, Geneva: Programme on Substance Abuse, World Health Organization

WHO (1996a) *WHO Drug Injecting Study Phase II: Report of Planning Meeting*, WHO/PSA/ 96.4, Geneva: Programme on Substance Abuse, World Health Organization.

WHO (1996b) *Report on Indigenous Peoples and Substance Use Project: Phase II Planning Meeting*, Geneva: Programme on Substance Abuse, World Health Organization.

WHO (1996c) *Report on Consultation Meeting on WHO Drug Substitution Project*, WHO/PSA/ 96.3, Geneva: Programme on Substance Abuse. World Health Organization.

WHO (1996d) *The World Health Report 1996: Fighting Disease, Fostering Development*, Geneva: World Health Organization.

WIEBEL, W., JIMENEZ, A., JOHNSON, W. *et al.* (1993) 'Positive effect on HIV seroconversion of street outreach interventions with IDU in Chicago, 1988–1992', VIII International Conference on AIDS, Berlin.

WIEBEL, W. (1996) 'Ethnographic contributions to AIDS intervention strategies', in RHODES, T. and HARTNOLL, R. (Eds) *AIDS, Drugs and Prevention: Perspectives on Individual and Community Action*, London: Routledge.

Methodology of the World Health Organization Multi-City Study on Drug Injecting and Risk of HIV Infection

David Goldberg

Much of the material presented in this book draws upon data collected in the World Health Organization Multi-City Study on Drug Injecting and Risk of HIV Infection, and from related studies. This study represents the largest international project to date on drug injecting and its consequences.

Prior to this study there were no internationally comparable studies of HIV-related risk behaviour between countries; the ones that existed employed different methods of sampling, information gathering and analysis. Therefore one of the primary reasons for setting up the multi-centre study was to develop a sampling methodology and establish data collection practices common to a variety of centres in different countries, including both developed and developing nations.

The study was initiated by the World Health Organization in 1987, and the main fieldwork took place between October 1989 and March 1992. Material presented in this book comes from 12 of the cities in the study.

The Collaborative Group

In October 1987 the World Health Organization's Global Programme on AIDS brought together researchers from various cities to design a cross-national study to improve the understanding of HIV-related risk behaviours of injecting drug users across parts of North and South America, Europe, South-east Asia and Australasia. This group of researchers constituted the WHO Collaborative Group.

Coordination and Funding

The study was initially co-ordinated by the WHO Global Programme on AIDS (GPA) and then by an *ad hoc* committee of collaborators. In 1992 the co-ordination of the study at the World Health Organization became the responsibility of the Programme on Substance Abuse (PSA), and was undertaken by an Executive Committee of collaborators. Funding for WHO to analyze the data and prepare the report was provided by the United Nations International Drug Control Programme. Most centres obtained funding from national agencies or from the World Health Organization itself.

Aims, Objectives and Study Design

The WHO Collaborative Group identified the overall aim of the study, which was to facilitate the reduction of HIV transmission, through influencing injecting behaviour. The study would provide needed information on the precise nature, extent and implications of injecting behaviour, as well as help to understand the psychosocial, cultural and legal factors that help determine the propensity for risk taking and, hence, the opportunities for risk reduction.

Three main objectives were to quantify types of HIV risk behaviour among IDUs, to determine the prevalence of HIV-1 infection among this population, and to contextualize drug injecting in the cultural and political environments of the different cities in different countries.

The specific objectives were to:

- identify and describe the types of high risk drug injecting practices and sexual behaviours in given populations of drug injectors;
- identify and describe the social and behavioural factors influencing drug injecting behaviour and attitudes to risk reduction;
- identify and describe the background cultural, legal and political environment in which these behaviours occur, including the presence or absence of intervention programmes;
- describe and measure behavioural changes that occur over time among drug injectors;
- consider the possible interaction between selected socio-political, legal and other environmental factors with patterns of drug injecting behaviour; and
- measure the prevalence of HIV-1 infection among given populations of drug injectors in selected cities.

Study Protocol and Design

The study protocol was designed by a technical working group of collaborators, under the auspices of the World Health Organization's Global Programme on AIDS (GPA).

The study involved period prevalence studies in different cities throughout the world that could potentially be repeated periodically in order to provide information on changing patterns and trends in drug injecting and the associated risk of HIV-1 infection. By mid-1989 the researchers had developed a standardized study methodology, a core interview schedule and an interview instruction manual, and the protocol was finalized in 1990.

Sample Selection

Because of the nature of drug injecting behaviour and the difficulties often encountered in identifying drug injectors, it is not possible to obtain representative samples. Drug injectors are known to have different rates of contact with drug treatment services and programmes. Sometimes this may be a function of the social, political and legal environment in question. Studies that totally depend for their recruitment on samples that are solely drawn from drug treatment programmes are necessarily open to questions of bias and lack of generalizability.

Problems of bias can also result from the fact that many drug injectors attend drug treatment programmes on the referral of law enforcement agencies. In these circumstances, drug injectors may not be inclined either to participate in studies or to provide reliable answers to questions posed.

The study therefore recruited drug injectors both 'in-treatment' and 'out-of-treatment'; thus respondents were drawn not only from within service environments, but also from their day-to-day social environments including drug use venues (such as 'shooting galleries'), street locations and other places frequented for the purposes of drug injecting and social functions.

Although none of these sources is entirely free from bias, this procedure minimizes overselection from any one segment of the drug injecting population.

Criteria for Recruitment into Study

The criteria for selection of 'in-treatment' respondents were:

1 that they must have injected drugs at least once within the last two months;
2 that they began a new episode of treatment in the last month;
3 that they be recruited from within a treatment centre as defined in the country-specific field protocol and questionnaire; and
4 that they had not been previously recruited and studied within the same period of the study phase.

The criteria for selection of 'out-of-treatment' respondents were:

1 that they had injected drugs at least once within the last two months;
2 that they be recruited in the same city as the treatment sample, but not from

within a treatment centre as defined in the country-specific field protocol and questionnaire; and

3 that they had not been previously recruited and studied within the same period of the current study phase.

Drug injectors undergoing medical treatment for conditions related to drug use were considered 'out-of-treatment' for the purpose of sampling criteria unless they were in medical treatment as a part of a drug treatment programme or some other risk-reduction initiative.

These selection criteria aimed to ensure that the samples taken in different cities and at different time periods were consistent and permitted comparability of data both cross-culturally and at different time intervals. The criteria were not established in order to assess the impact of treatment on drug injecting behaviour and the risk of HIV infection.

Knowledge of HIV-1 status was not a criterion for recruitment. Drug injectors were to be recruited into the study irrespective of whether they had or had not been tested in the past, and whether or not they were aware of their HIV-1 status.

Ethical Procedures

All collaborating centres were responsible for ensuring that the study was conducted according to local and national ethical guidelines.

Site Selection

Factors influencing which cities were selected for participation in the study were the representation of a range of global sectors, and each city having the capacity to undertake the research, the ability to recruit the required numbers of 'in-treatment' and 'out-of-treatment' respondents, and the means to mobilize national and local support for the project, including financial contributions. Cities were also selected on the basis that prevalences of HIV-1 infection, ranging from low to high, might be detected reflecting different stages of the epidemic in different parts of the world. Thirteen cities were initially selected: Athens, Bangkok, Berlin, Glasgow, London, Madrid, Naples, New York, Rome, Rio de Janeiro, Santos, Sydney and Toronto. Information for Naples was not available and data therefore apply to 12 centres.

At the time of planning the study, injecting drug use was not recognized as a major problem in most developing countries. Therefore, developed country sites were the main focus of the study. During the course of the study it became evident that IDU was emerging as a critical public health issue in the developing world, particularly in Asia, but also in areas of Africa, Latin America, the eastern Mediterranean and eastern Europe.

Interview Procedure and Schedule

The interview procedure involved the administration of the interview schedule by a trained interviewer and a request for a blood and/or saliva sample. The schedule consisted of an eligibility check, and questions on: personal demographics; drug use; needle and syringe sharing; sexual behaviour; HIV and AIDS knowledge and behaviour change; travel history; and previous HIV-1 testing. The questionnaire therefore comprised a set of core questions which could then be supplemented with questions specific to certain centres.

It was agreed that such a cross-sectional design should not attempt to obtain lifetime behavioural details since investigators' prior experience was of interviewees having poor recollection of such events; thus most behavioural questions referred to 'current behaviour' which was defined as the six-month period prior to the interview. On average an interview would take 30 minutes to complete.

The schedule, which took almost two years to design, was piloted in most of the centres, an exercise which involved the interviewing of approximately 50 IDUs in each centre. The questionnaire was then translated from English into Portuguese, Thai, German, Spanish, Italian and Greek.

Interviewer Recruitment

It was decided, in the main, to use interviewers who had no prior close or ongoing professional relationships with the IDUs (such as through treatment programmes or law enforcement) as this could bias responses. For example, if an IDU wants to maintain good relations with someone providing treatment this may influence his or her response. Interviewers were, however, expected to be sensitive to the subculture of injecting drug use, and were selected on the basis of familiarity with the subject and previous experience in the area.

Some centres used interviewers with prior experience of injecting drug use, or with access to networks of users, as this was a relatively efficient way of recruiting injectors to the study and gaining information from them.

Saliva and Blood Specimen Collection

Saliva specimens were collected in Athens, Glasgow, London, Rome and Toronto. A salivette was used to collect the specimens — this involved the respondent chewing on a piece of cotton wool in the form of a cylinder. Forty-five to sixty seconds of gentle chewing would suffice and the saturated cotton wool would then be placed in a container to be sent for storage and then antibody testing. The collection of saliva specimens was particularly useful for some centres that recruited injectors from community sites.

Samples of blood were taken in Athens, Bangkok, Madrid, New York, Rio,

Santos, Sydney and Toronto. Venepuncture was performed in each of these centres (in Toronto only on the 'in-treatment' sample) except Sydney, where drops of blood were obtained using an autolet device, and then transferred onto filter paper. In Toronto the 'out-of-treatment' sample were asked for saliva specimens, and finger-prick samples. The resultant dried blood spot was then stored, eluted out into solution and tested for HIV-1 antibodies.

Saliva testing involved an Elisa, Radio-immunoassay, Omnisal (Gacelisa, Gacria, or Saliva Diagnostic Systems) test and all reactive were then tested for confirmation using a Western Blot assay. Standard blood samples were tested using an Elisa assay (for example Wellcozyme) while the elutes from dried blood spots were tested using a particle agglutination test (for example Serodia). For all blood samples, reactives were confirmed using Western Blot.

Interviewee Recruitment

The study guidelines recommended that each centre adopt a recruitment strategy designated to yield a sample as representative as possible, of approximately 500 current drug injectors, with respondents drawn from both 'in-treatment' and 'out-of-treatment' sites.

Out-of-treatment sites covered a wide range of settings including needle and syringe exchanges, pharmacies, street sites, drug use venues, nightclubs, health centres and personal contacts. Thus each centre implemented a strategy based on local conditions in order to achieve a multi-site sample of injectors. Respondents recruited out-of-treatment were not necessarily a non-treatment sample (see below).

Centres were asked to ensure that no more than 50 per cent of injectors be recruited from drug treatment settings. Compliance with this requirement was extremely high and, with the exception of Rome, at least 25 per cent of the sample from each centre included injectors who had never received treatment. The types of recruitment site in each city are listed in Table A1.1.

Injecting drug use is a problematic and difficult area of research, due to its illegal and covert nature. The researchers attempted to overcome any constraints by ensuring wide-ranging samples, by establishing good rapport with drug injectors and by developing an insight into the socio-cultural and political environment that influences the behaviour of drug injectors.

Environmental Questionnaire

It was important that the questionnaire data from each centre be placed in context of the cultural, legal, political and social environments in which injecting and HIV risk-related behaviours occurred. An Environmental Questionnaire was developed for this purpose and completed by investigators from each of the centres. The principal aim was to obtain information which related to the time

Table A1.1 Recruitment sites

Site	'In treatment'	'Out of treatment'
Athens	therapeutic community, out-patient programme	prisons, military sites, in-patient and out-patient departments of a general hospital
Bangkok	narcotics clinics	immediate vicinity of narcotics clinics
Berlin	therapeutic community (SYNANON), in-patient transitional care unit, residential rehabilitation unit	six street sites, one prostitution site
Glasgow	community drugs project, residential rehabilitation centres, hospital in-patients and hospital out-patients	pharmacy shops, needle/syringe exchanges, detached sites and a community centre
London	hospital-based drug dependence units, advice and counselling agencies, residential rehabilitation units, community drug teams, and drugs projects	social networks of drug injectors recruited by indigenous interviewers using network techniques in public and private drug venues
Madrid	private drug treatment centre, Madrid treatment centres for drug addicts	between 20 and 30 street sites and a city hostel for the homeless
New York	a hospital detoxification ward and a hospital out-patient methadone maintenance treatment programme	a store-front
Rio de Janeiro	out-patient and in-patient clinics for drug users, and community resources.	detached sites, drug selling points and nightclubs
Rome	methadone clinics and residential communities	pubs, cafés, restaurants, private homes, public parks, street sites, telephone help-line/drop-in centre, and hospital
Santos	private drug and alcohol treatment centre managed by the Church and health centres where drug treatment was available	health centres where drug treatment was not available and users recruited on the street in the vicinity, houses with rooms rented to injectors and prostitutes, and other street sites
Sydney	information not available	
Toronto	treatment centres including in- and out-patient programmes, methadone maintenance programmes, detoxification units and some programmes operated from community agencies/centres	needle-exchange sites, community centres/drop-ins, youth and community social service agencies, and word-of-mouth contact

period when the study was conducted, and note any changes that may have occurred before, during and after the study period, particularly relating to government policy on and public attitudes to the issues of drug injecting and HIV/AIDS.

The main areas of information that the Environmental Questionnaire yielded were:

- general descriptions of the city, for example population, government, economy, ethnic and class make-up;
- history of drug injecting, the development of HIV/AIDS;
- availability of sterile injecting equipment, condoms and bleach;
- type and amount of drug treatment available;
- legal environment and policy formation;
- public attitudes to drug use;
- education about drug use, HIV and AIDS;
- the HIV/AIDS and drug injecting situation in prisons — including availability of condoms, bleach and treatment; and
- the existence of drug user and advocacy groups (including those for sex workers) and their influence on HIV/AIDS policy.

Data Collection, Collation and Analysis

The main phase of data collection related to the period between October 1989 and March 1992. The timescale of recruitment for each centre varied — from three months in late 1989 for Bangkok to 19 months from January 1990 for New York. The number of interviews performed by each centre was variable, though only two centres (Athens and Santos) completed less than 380. A total of 6436 interviews were conducted (Table A1.2).

Table A1.2 Sample size in each city, and proportion of sample recruited in and out of treatment

Cities	Total number in sample	Percentage recruited in treatment %	Percentage recruited out of treatment %
Athens	400	44	56
Bangkok	601	56	44
Berlin	380	51	49
Glasgow	503	34	66
London	534	22	78
Madrid	472	49	51
New York	1478	54	46
Rio	479	56	44
Rome	487	52	48
Santos	220	38	62
Sydney	424	32	68
Toronto	458	27	73

Although each centre developed its own systems for data coding, entry and analysis, it was necessary to merge the data from each centre into one standard file to permit full analysis across centres. Accordingly, each centre sent their data in various formats to Glasgow where the merging process was carried out. The formats included SPSS PC, SPSS Mainframe and the more common PC Database packages such as D Base 3 and D Base 4. Although each centre, in the main, asked all the core questions in the exact style that was agreed upon, the coding of the responses to these questions varied. Therefore, a template was developed and a common file produced, which now holds approximately 300 variables on injectors from the study centres. This is the largest ever global study of drug injecting.

Due to the local alteration of some questions, variability in naming conventions and coding, and limitations of time and resources, it has only been possible to merge and make comparative analyses using 57 selected variables from 12 cities. Each centre has completed extensive analyses on its own data set and an extensive list of publications has resulted.

The difficulties experienced illustrate the importance of ensuring standardization across centres of the wording of core questionnaire items and coding conventions prior to data collection. It also supports the argument for a shorter and simple core questionnaire when undertaking a multi-centre study, with the potential for centres to include additional items.

International Co-ordination

Co-ordination was provided by the WHO GPA and PSA and site investigators. The precise mechanisms for this co-ordination changed over time. Difficulties were encountered in this co-ordination for a variety of reasons. It is clear that multi-centre studies require considerable resources to ensure that all stages of the research are organized efficiently.

Future Research

The study has provided a wealth of data which has been used to inform both international and national drug and HIV/AIDS policies and programmes. It has helped place drug injecting and HIV issues on the international agenda.

Apart from the extensive data collected in each of the participating cities, the study has contributed much to the development of research methods for investigating this hard-to-reach population. It helped establish international collaborative networks, and encouraged the exchange of research skills and ideas between collaborators.

A valuable product of the study has been the development of a study methodology and standardized instruments which have application across a range of countries. The instruments have now been adopted for use in many subsequent studies which were not part of the original initiative.

The study has also raised a wide range of questions which requires a further programme of research. In particular, a need has been identified for the collection of information from a range of developing countries. The study was conceived in 1986–7 before there was much awareness of the problem of HIV infection among IDUs in developing countries. Bangkok, Rio de Janeiro and

Santos were the only centres that participated from developing countries. Considering the changes in the extent of injecting behaviour and the rapid spread of HIV infection in many developing countries, sites in Africa, Eastern Europe, Latin America and Asia should be included in any future studies. It has also become clear that much more needs to be known about the dynamics of the diffusion of drug injecting practices, since the ability to understand the reasons why, and the contexts in which injecting is adopted, should lead to the development of more effectively targeted interventions. Sexual risk behaviour of IDUs is also an important area for investigation.

The limited resources and expertise available in some developing countries often preclude the use of quantitative methods requiring large samples; therefore consideration should be given to the development and utilization of more rapid methods of assessment which can inform cost-effective and culturally appropriate interventions. This would include the application of qualitative methods to examine the context of drug injecting.

The study has highlighted the different courses of HIV epidemics among injectors in different countries. There is now substantial evidence from this and other studies that IDUs do change their behaviour in response to information about HIV/AIDS and with access to the means for behaviour change. There is evidence that in some cities epidemics have been prevented.

Examining the context of drug injecting has helped to inform our understanding of factors which influence the spread of HIV-1 infection among this population. Work associated with this study and reported in this book shows the factors that are important for curtailing HIV epidemics. This has required the development of methods for comparative international research. Prior to this study, little such work had been conducted. Comparative analyses require creative utilization of multiple types of information, including quantitative data about epidemic trends and risk behaviours, descriptions of policies and programmes, and an understanding of the environmental context. The study has indicated that such comparative analyses are essential to understanding the epidemic and the effect of interventions, that they are difficult to undertake but are nevertheless feasible, and that they must be a key feature of future research.

City Epidemics and Contexts

Fabio Mesquita, Paulo Telles, Francisco Bastos, and Gerry V. Stimson

The World Health Organization Multi-City Study on Drug Injection and Risk of HIV Infection was conceived in 1986/7 before there was much understanding of the course of HIV-1 epidemics. Data presented at the First International Conference on AIDS in Atlanta in 1985 showed high prevalence rates in New York and New Jersey within the range of 50 to 72 per cent. Data presented at the 1986 Paris AIDS Conference showed similar high prevalence rates, of around 50 per cent, in cities in Austria, Italy, Spain, France and Switzerland. In the United Kingdom rates of between 39 and 51 per cent were reported in Edinburgh and Dundee for the period 1983 to 1986. In many of these cities (with the exception of New York, which was earlier), the virus probably first arrived between 1980 and 1983. By 1988 there was startling evidence from Bangkok that HIV-1 prevalence had risen from approximately zero at the beginning of the year, to nearly 40 per cent towards the end of that year amongst samples at a major treatment hospital and within methadone treatment programmes. The evidence seemed to support the hypothesis that soon after HIV-1 infection was introduced into injecting populations, there could be rapid spread of infection to prevalence rates of 40 per cent and above.

As is apparent in this book, such rapid spread to high prevalence rates has not occurred in every city. There is now evidence to show that prevalence rates differ between cities, and that these different levels may change over time.

This appendix describes the early development of the epidemic of HIV-1 infection among injecting drug users (IDUs) in the cities involved in the WHO Multi-City Study. Up to about 1990, institutions in these cities varied widely in their willingness and ability to respond in the context of an emerging awareness of a potential public health disaster. This appendix describes the context in which the epidemics occurred and the ways in which policy and responses were — or were not — initiated. The description of the cities up to the end of the 1980s forms a backdrop for understanding the emergence and control of the epidemics among IDUs in a number of cities, and the context for more focused analyses presented in other chapters in this book.

Athens

Athens is the capital of Greece and has a population of 4.1 million. There was rapid population expansion during the decades immediately following the First and Second World Wars, mainly due to the influx of refugees and the establishment of much of Greece's industrial production in Athens. In the 1980s there was a significant decline in population growth, both in Athens and elsewhere in Greece. The spread of psychoactive substance use in Athens seems to be linked to unco-ordinated, intense economic growth which has led to important recent alterations in the standard of living and has also been followed by an increase in criminal activity and political problems.

Prior to 1970, drug use was quite limited in Greece and mainly confined to certain sections of the working-class city population. Drug users were generally of Asian origin and smoked cannabis as part of an Eastern Mediterranean cultural tradition. After the mid-1970s illicit drug use, including the use of opioids, spread widely, crossing the barriers of class, sex and age. The increased public and political concern following the change in the pattern of drug use, and its spread to younger age groups led, in the beginning of the 1980s, to a series of nationwide epidemiological studies being undertaken by Athens University. These aimed to assess the magnitude and the nature of drug use in Greece. Although a substantial increase has been observed in lifetime illicit drug use in the general population between 1984 and 1993 (from 5.9 per cent to 9.5 per cent), the ratio between genders remained unchanged. The most important increase in illicit drug use between 1984 and 1993 was observed in the 18–24 and 25–35 age groups. Both genders in the 18–24 age group, but more so females, have almost doubled their use between 1984 and 1993 (from 13.9 per cent to 20.1 per cent for males, and from 3.6 per cent to 9 per cent for females). In the student population the ratio of illicit drug use between boys and girls is 2:1 for lifetime use, while for more recent use the differences become more pronounced. No significant increase was observed between 1984 and 1993 in lifetime use for both sexes (6.0 per cent and 6.1 per cent respectively), while a significant increase for more recent use has been observed only for boys (from 4.8 per cent to 6.4 per cent for last year and from 2.3 per cent to 3.9 per cent for last month). Cannabis was the main drug used. Higher rates of illicit drug use were found in urban areas. In 1983 there were 9689 registered drug addicts of which 91 per cent were male. The main substances of use were heroin and cannabis. Approximately one-third of this drug using population had been hospitalized for treatment, mainly for opiate or tranquillizer addiction. According to official estimates, there were about 40 000 opiate users in a population of about 10 million and of those, 50 per cent were injectors of heroin (Kokkevi and Stefanis, 1991).

Treatment services at the time of the WHO Multi-City Study were inadequate. Optimistic estimates suggest that around 5 per cent of drug users had access to drug treatment services. There were no services prescribing methadone or other substitute drugs. Methadone treatment became available later.

Before the WHO Multi-City Study, high risk drug use practices, such as needle and syringe sharing, were reported by the majority of IDUs, despite there being no legal restrictions on purchasing needles and syringes. These could be obtained at low prices in most pharmacies, although these are rarely open at night. There were no needle exchange programmes. An educational campaign for IDUs was launched in 1985, using counselling and leaflets for IDUs in prison and in treatment. Confidential, anonymous testing for HIV was made available free of charge. Greek authorities made no attempt to encourage IDUs to use bleach to sterilize equipment.

In a sample of 140 IDUs in contact with health services in Athens in 1988 and 1989, 76 per cent reported some sharing of injecting equipment. However, frequent sharing was only reported by 19 per cent (Kokkevi *et al.*, 1992) and 'shooting galleries' were almost non-existent (Papaevangelou *et al.*, 1991). An earlier study conducted by Malliori *et al.* (1992), with a sample of 330 IDUs, found 'frequent sharing' in both street recruited and treatment samples. In addition, the majority of IDUs rarely, or never, used condoms during sexual intercourse (Malliori *et al.*, 1993; Malliori *et al.*, 1992).

HIV-1 has been present among injectors in Athens since at least 1982 (Papaevangelou *et al.*, 1991). The first case of AIDS in Greece was reported in 1984. The prevalence of HIV-1 infection is very low among IDUs in Greece and it seems that HIV-1 had not been substantially introduced into the IDU community at the time of the WHO Multi-City Study. Reports from the Ministry of Health and Welfare show that there were 277 cases of HIV infection to January 1990, with only 9 (3.2 per cent) being attributed to injecting drug use (Kokkevi *et al.*, 1992). A series of studies found a low level of HIV-1 infection among IDUs. One study showed that 2 per cent of a sample of 288 imprisoned IDUs were HIV-1 positive (Romelioutou-Karayannis *et al.*, 1987), while of 215 IDUs hospitalized for infectious diseases, none was positive. In both these studies subjects comprised all IDUs in the service during the research period (Tassopoulos *et al.*, 1989). In another study 400 IDUs were tested for both HIV-1 and hepatitis C (Malliori *et al.*, 1993); 0.5 per cent were HIV-1 positive compared to 82 per cent HCV positivity. These different findings for HCV and HIV raise important questions about the relationship risk behaviours and epidemic histories.

Limited information is available about the sexual lives of the Greek population, but from a religious point of view there is a negative attitude towards the use of condoms. Since the AIDS epidemic, family planning centres and other authorities have encouraged the use of condoms. Condoms have been available since 1984 in family planning services, as well as in STD/AIDS clinics. Studies have revealed that these efforts have had little impact, as the use of condoms remains low among all age groups in the general population.

Severe penalties are imposed for drug traffickers, with sentences ranging from a minimum of 10 years to life-time imprisonment. Arrested drug users are separated into dependent and non-dependent users. Non-dependent users who have been arrested for the first time for personal use are obliged to follow a counselling programme. No penal record is kept and emphasis is placed upon de-stigmatization. Those arrested for drug trafficking are considered fully responsible. For dependent users arrested for personal use, there are two possibilities, either following a voluntary detoxification programme or compulsory confinement in the prison detoxification unit for therapy without penalty. Those arrested for drug trafficking are offered similar options.

Approximately 60 per cent of the prison population has been sentenced for drug-related offences. As the number of drug users in prisons is high, the spread of HIV must be considered a high risk. Despite this, no needles and syringes are provided nor materials to clean syringes. People with HIV or AIDS are isolated from other inmates and put in solitary confinement. There is no specific treatment for drug dependent prisoners, and methadone and condoms are not available in Greek prisons.

There had been only a few systematic training programmes on drug abuse for either health professionals or for teachers. A pilot Health Education Programme to prevent drug abuse was in operation in schools between 1986 and 1989. The evaluation showed increased knowledge and awareness of the issues about drug abuse among pupils, parents and teachers. Since 1989–90 a similar programme was introduced in 21 schools in Peristeri, an Athenian community of about 300 000 inhabitants.

There are few organizations for IDUs in Greece. They are not set up to influence HIV/AIDS policy and they do not provide needle and syringe exchange or outreach services. There is one organization for sex workers in Greece, whose main activity is to encourage sex workers to use condoms. Public attitudes to IDUs are still negative in Greece.

Bangkok

Bangkok is the capital of Thailand and has a population of approximately 6 million out of the country's total population of 55 million. Thailand is a rapidly developing country with associated improvements in per capita income, and modernization in transportation and communication. Rapid urbanization has led to major problems of unemployment, slum inhabitation, poor sanitation, insufficient places for recreation, traffic congestion and water and air pollution. Affluent commercial buildings contrast with the estimated one million slum dwellings in the city. Thailand is a constitutional democracy, but there is a strong military influence in government and in many areas of state and business activity. The majority of the population are ethnic Thais, but there are substantial Chinese and Indian minorities, and other minority ethnic groups from elsewhere in Thailand.

The Bangkok Metropolitan Administration (BMA) is the city's local governing body, responsible for law and order, supervising municipal by-laws and other regulations, and providing roads and waterways, the drainage system, public health and sanitation, the medical service, and generally ensuring the good working order of the city. It has responsibility for education, the promotion of employment, the prevention and alleviation of public disasters and the improvement of slums and housing conditions. The BMA Department of Health is responsible for promoting and controlling public health services, family health care programmes, environmental health care, community hospitals, and drug abuse prevention and treatment.

In 1959 heroin was first found in Thailand, imported from Hong Kong, and heroin use spread among the old opium addicts as well as among new ones. During the mid-1970s, there was a major diffusion of heroin dependence throughout Thailand including Bangkok. A second heroin epidemic extended well into the 1980s. Injecting drug use is commonly reported by more than 60 per cent of clients in treatment services, and around 80 per cent of clients in Bangkok. Within a period of 25 years the drug dependence situation in Thailand had changed from indigenous opium dependence into a complex pattern of dependence on many types of drugs, with heroin predominating. The period from about 1967 to 1975 was a critical time when dependence on heroin, opium, amphetamine and perhaps inhalants was beginning to spread. The indigenous drugs problem developed as Thailand and other neighbouring countries became major opium producers and heroin refiners for the world market.

The drug scene of Bangkok is mainly characterized by people who made the transition from more traditional use of opium and heroin through smoking or inhalation — 'chasing of the dragon' — to the injection of heroin. Cocaine injection is very uncommon. A capture–recapture study in 1991 produced an estimate of 36 600 opiate users in Bangkok. About 90 per cent of the opiate users are injectors and heroin is the main drug injected. Most injectors are male (Choopanya *et al.*, 1991). Thai IDUs are more socially integrated than in other societies, with an especially striking contrast to their North American counterparts. In comparison with other countries, they have a very high level of employment. They also belong, with a few exceptions to the majority ethnic group in Thailand (Des Jarlais *et al.*, 1992).

HIV-1 was introduced in South East Asia relatively late, via the Americas and Africa. Molecular epidemiology studies support this hypothesis as they demonstrate a low nucleotide divergence among people infected with the same subtype in Asia and diversity has been documented as a function of the years of epidemic evolution (Quinn, 1994; Weniger *et al.*, 1994). This high degree of genetic homogeneity contrasts profoundly with the substantial diversity of those subtypes in the countries affected earlier by HIV-1 infection, especially in the first epicentres located in sub-Saharan Africa (Weniger *et al.*, 1994).

The first cases of AIDS were reported in 1985 and it was only after 1988 that HIV-1 infection escalated to epidemic proportions (Quinn, 1994). Serosurveys taken between 1985 and 1987 revealed very low seroprevalence rates among different populations, including sex workers, clients attending STDs clinics and IDUs. However, by 1988 repeated serosurveys signalled an escalation of seroprevalence among IDUs. Seroprevalence in IDUs recruited at drug treatment facilities increased from 1 per cent in late 1987 to 15 per cent in March 1988 and to 43 per cent by the end of the same year (Choopanya *et al.*, 1991). Extremely high seroconversion rates were found amongst survey participants in Bangkok: 20 per cent of IDUs who were seronegative at the beginning of 1988 had converted by September 1988, an incidence of 3 per cent per month. It is unclear when the first case of AIDS occurred among IDUs, but by 1990 there had been only seven cases of AIDS amongst IDUs throughout Thailand.

This wave of HIV-1 epidemic was followed by another among sex workers, although molecular epidemiology studies reveal that the two waves have relatively independent dynamics, as shown by the pattern of different subtypes between the two population groups. Subtype E has mainly been transmitted by sexual interaction and subtype B by the common use of needles and syringes (Weniger *et al.*, 1994). Seroprevalence levels seem to have stabilized at a high plateau in the beginning of the 1990s (Choopanya *et al.*, 1991). Des Jarlais *et al.* (1992, 1994) suggested that this apparent stabilization is secondary to deliberate risk reduction by IDUs themselves, plus the effect of preventive programmes.

Syringe exchange programmes had not been initiated in the city at the time of the study. IDUs were, rather, encouraged to disinfect needles and syringes. The cost of sterile injection equipment was approximately 6 baht, or US $0.25. Sterile injection equipment is available from pharmacies and other stores. Bleach was not available before about 1988, and IDUs were unaware of this method of syringe sterilization. From October 1988 onwards, provision of free bleach in packets, and instructions on needle disinfection, were introduced at many drug clinics. In 1989, 8600 bottles of bleach were distributed.

There were no major cultural or religious obstacles to the use of condoms at the time of the study. Major efforts had been made to promote condom use by male and female sex workers with condom information provided through flip-charts, leaflets, posters, cassette tapes and other media. There were also projects to encourage 100 per cent condom compliance in brothels. In 1989 111 000 condoms were distributed to IDUs by the BMA.

At the time of the study, drug use treatment at the 17 drug clinics of the Bangkok Administration consisted of long-term (45-day) out-patient methadone assisted detoxification, followed by 180 days of additional counselling and aftercare. Patients in methadone treatment were prescribed methadone linctus with a fixed upper limit of 100–150 mg per day. Daily attendance was generally required. Treatment facilities registered around 6000 individuals under treatment in 1991. In July 1988 a pilot programme for methadone maintenance was introduced at one drug clinic but methodone maintenance was not available to most IDUs at the time of the study. Other treatment facilities include in-patient detoxification at Thanyarak Hospital, and some detoxification undertaken by Buddhist monasteries.

A national advisory committee on AIDS was established in 1985 and a national programme on prevention and control of AIDS commenced in the period 1988 to 1991, supported by WHO with a budget of 12.5 million bhat. The Ministry of Public Health Executive Committee on AIDS Prevention and Control is chaired by the Permanent Secretary for Public Health. Under the impact of AIDS, the 1989 AIDS Prevention and Control Programme objectives for IDUs were (a) to determine the extent and trends of transmission of HIV; (b) to provide medical and social services to IDUs and to strengthen rehabilitation services; (c) to provide intensive education and information to IDUs on HIV infection and prevention; and (d) to alert the general population and in particular adolescents to the risks attributed to injecting drug use.

From 1988 the BMA began to introduce harm reduction measures including bleach, condom distribution, outreach work in slum communities, and AIDS counselling. Since 1988 the transmission of HIV amongst IDUs has been discouraged by posters, videos and counselling at many drug treatment clinics, by home and community visits by volunteer health workers and ex-IDUs. HIV/AIDS awareness-raising campaigns targeting IDUs and their spouses were introduced from 1988, just before the start of the study period. Outreach activities included IDU outreach workers being trained to educate IDUs in the use of bleach. IDUs probably became aware of HIV and AIDS from 1988 and 1989 onwards, by which time accurate knowledge about AIDS had reached 90 per cent in one study.

It is not known how many IDUs there are in prison in Bangkok, but imprisonment is a major risk factor for HIV infection, and 80 per cent of HIV positive individuals had been incarcerated after they had begun injecting drugs. The large numbers of people formerly incarcerated and subsequently released from prisons also seems to have had a crucial role in the 'efficient mixing' pattern of diffusion necessary for this rapid increase in HIV-1 levels, as reported by a number of studies (Choopanya *et al.*, 1991; Wright *et al.*, 1994).

No drug user or advocacy groups were in existence during the WHO Study period. Organizations for sex workers had not been established in the city before or during data collection.

Berlin

The years 1989 and 1990 were characterized as a period of major historical and political change for Berlin and the whole of Germany. On 9 November the Berlin Wall fell and one year later, on 3 October, Germany was formally reunited. The administrative unity of former East and West Berlin was accomplished in 1991. Berlin is now the capital of Germany with (in 1990) a total population of 3.4 million (West: 2.1 million; East: 1.3 million). The Islamic community (mainly from Turkey) is the largest minority with about 150 000 members. All other ethnic or religious minorities are of negligible size. Within the Federal Republic of Germany, Berlin has the status of a Federal State (Bundesland). In 1990 the State elections resulted in a coalition government of the two major political parties in Germany, the Social Democrats and the Christian Democrats. Despite the unification of Germany, stark socio-economic differences prevail between east and west.

The most widely used illicit drug in Berlin is cannabis: surveys among young adults (12–24 years) showed a lifetime prevalence of 3–4 per cent for East Berlin and of more than 20 per cent for West Berlin in 1990. Heroin injecting developed during the late 1960s, and in 1979 the number of heroin users was estimated to be 6000, and 8000 in 1990. More than 75 per cent of heroin users are thought to inject. Until 1990 no significant illicit drug use 'scene' had emerged in the former East Berlin. Heroin is the most commonly injected drug, but cocaine use, as well as speedballing, has increased (Kappeler *et al.*, 1993). In 1990, around 5 per cent of all drug users in treatment were treated for cocaine addiction.

The first AIDS cases registered in the former Federal Republic of Germany in 1982 were among homosexual men. These cases were reported in Berlin and Frankfurt. In 1983 the first cases among IDUs were reported. Since then the HIV epidemic in Germany, despite the profound socio-economic and political reformation following the reunification of the country, remains stable among all exposure categories (Stark and Kleiber, 1991). In 1986 IDUs accounted for around 3.3 per cent of AIDS cases: this increased to 14 per cent in 1990. This proportion declined to around 10 per cent of the total AIDS cases at the beginning of the 1990s when the WHO Multi-City Study commenced. The AIDS epidemic is mainly restricted to major metropolitan regions of the unified Germany: these have around 61 per cent of all AIDS cases registered up to 1993.

The number of newly registered HIV infections increased from 482 to 1576 in 1985 and decreased to 975 HIV infections in 1990. The proportion of HIV infected IDUs has declined from 10 per cent in 1985 to 5.3 per cent in 1990. However, these data have to be treated with caution as there were high rates of missing data.

Low levels of HIV-1 seroprevalence and few AIDS cases have been reported in the former Eastern Germany (including Eastern Berlin) — less than 1 per cent in contrast to 21 per cent in the unified Germany in the beginning of the 1990s (Hamouda *et al.*, 1993). One explanation for this is the almost complete absence of an injecting drug scene in the former Eastern territories, including the absence of homemade injecting preparations as observed in Poland (Kappeler *et al.*, 1993; EIGDU, 1993).

Drug laws do not restrict the purchase, or possession, of sterile needles and syringes. Since the mid-1980s, health authorities and non-governmental organizations have developed prevention strategies for HIV infection. These have improved the availability of sterile equipment, complemented by expanding sales in drugstores and vending machines. In 1988 syringe vending machines were established as part of AIDS prevention. Since 1989 sterile equipment has been distributed and exchanged at an increasing rate in storefront units and by streetworkers. Eight vending machines distributed more than 30 000 sets a month, accompanied by about 40 000 exchanged sets of injecting equipment in syringe exchange schemes. Low-threshold drug counselling facilities encouraged IDUs to use sterile injection equipment during the study period. Bleach bottles or packets for IDUs were neither promoted nor available in Germany.

Drug treatment in Berlin comprised two low-threshold facilities (accessible to everyone regardless of his or her actual intoxication status), 11 drug counselling agencies, three out-patient therapeutic services and 17 drug-free in-patient therapeutic communities. There was one drug emergency facility with a 24-hour service. There were minor changes in drug treatment services in response to the changing demands of HIV. Some agencies established special HIV wards, and drug counselling facilities were increased. Nevertheless there was a strong tendency for IDUs to avoid drug-free treatment. In 1991 about 1900 IDUs received either out-patient or in-patient treatment, which corresponds to about 20 per cent of all Berlin IDUs. Methadone substitution is regulated by the Federal Law on Narcotics, and mostly restricted to long-term drug users not showing a pattern of polydrug addiction, those who are HIV seropositive or suffering other persistent and severe health problems, or female drug users during pregnancy. By 1991, 171 drug users were participating in the methadone programme. Dosages varied from an initial 15 mg to a maximum maintenance dosage of 60 mg per day (Stöver and Schuller, 1992; Raschke and Kalke, 1993).

The period also saw the establishment of liberal coalitions of health professionals, social workers and educators (for example the 'Bundesverbandes fur akzeptierende Drogenarbeit und humane Drogenpolitik' — AKZEPT); the beginning of active self-help and advocacy groups (JES bringing together *J*unkies, *E*x-users and drug users under methadone treatment — *S*ubstituierte); and the participation of those organizations under the umbrella of the large non-governmental organization Deutsche AIDS-Hilfe (Stöver and Schuller, 1992; Hermann, 1993; EIGDU, 1993). There were four organization for commercial sex workers. HYDRA, established in 1979, is the oldest organization for sex workers in Germany. These organizations have attempted to change the law in favour of the legal acceptance of commercial sex work as a profession. Beyond that they have developed a programme of financial assistance to allow sex workers to cease their work.

There were no major cultural, religious or any other obstacles for the use of condoms. There was a satisfactory availability of condoms distributed free, and on sale through pharmacies and vending machines. Health authorities and non-governmental organizations have implemented efforts to improve the use of condoms.

According to surveys, the majority of the German population regards drug users as victims of dealers, and drug addiction as an illness. Beyond that, drug addiction is seen as a symptom of a weak personality. Nevertheless there are negative attitudes regarding IDUs, especially concerning the unsafe disposal of used syringes in public areas causing neighbourhood resentment.

Since 1985 there have been various HIV/AIDS awareness campaigns. AIDS-related information booklets were sent to each German household; film-spots were shown in cinemas and on television; posters and advertisements were displayed in public places; and peer education programmes were conducted in schools. No government-implemented HIV/AIDS awareness campaigns specifi-cally targeted IDUs.

The Federal Law of Narcotics was revised in 1982 and a distinction is made between possession of small and larger quantities of drugs. The sentence for possessing less than 1.5 g of pure heroin ranges from one day to one year. There were no HIV/AIDS education programmes in prisons. Every drug dependent prisoner had the choice of drug-free therapy as an alternative to imprisonment. At the time of the study there were no methadone substitution programmes in prison, and condoms and bleach were not available.

Glasgow

Glasgow, Scotland, is an industrial city with a population of approximately 700 000, and it has a wide social class mix. There are some small well-integrated ethnic groups including Asians and Chinese, but in the main the population is a homogeneous one with the great majority of people being white. There is a two-to-one ratio of Protestants to Catholics. Although Glasgow had made a concerted effort to tackle its 'inner-city' problems, there remains considerable poverty and deprivation.

Drug injecting was introduced into Glasgow in the late 1970s and early 1980s, though this did not escalate to any significant proportions until approximately 1983. The culture of drug use has always been predominantly based around injecting. Injecting has been mainly confined to deprived areas of the city, particularly areas with large municipal housing estates. In 1985 it was estimated that there were approximately 5000 injectors in Glasgow, a figure which had risen to approximately 8500 in 1990. Heroin, benzodiazepines and buprenorphine (Temgesic) constitute the main types of drug that have been injected in the last 10 years.

When reports began to emerge in 1986 that an estimated 50 per cent of IDUs in Edinburgh might be HIV postive (Robertson, Bucknall and Wiggins, 1986), questions began to be asked about the situation in Glasgow — a city no more than 70 kilometres from Edinburgh with a much larger drug injecting population. The first published reports on the situation within Glasgow came from staff at the Regional Virus Laboratory who, in 1985, found that out of 606 blood samples analyzed, there were only three HIV positive tests from IDUs living within the city (Follett et al., 1986). The same team tested a further 309 blood samples between October to December 1986 and identified 20 HIV positive samples (Follett, Wallace and McCruden, 1987). The possibility remained that either Glasgow was at an early stage of the epidemic spread, or that the rapid infection that had occurred in Edinburgh had not been carried over into Glasgow. One possible reason for the difference between Glasgow and Edinburgh was that IDUs within Glasgow were not sharing needles and syringes as frequently as their counterparts in Edinburgh (Robertson, Bucknall and Wiggins, 1986). To clarify the situation within Glasgow there was a clear need for a large-scale survey of IDUs.

This research, which formed part of the WHO Study, indicated that the level of HIV-1 infection amongst IDUs within Glasgow was between 1 and 2 per cent. The risk behaviour data also showed that injectors were attempting to reduce their risk of HIV infection by reducing the extent of their needle and syringe sharing (Frischer *et al.*, 1992; Rhodes *et al.*, 1993; Taylor *et al.*, 1994). Other research identified a close link between female street sex work within the city and injecting drug use. Of 206 sex workers surveyed, 71 per cent were injecting drugs — a higher proportion that that reported in any other UK city. Despite the high overlap between sex work and injecting drug use only very low levels of HIV-1 infection amongst street working women were found, with a prevalence rate of 2.5 per cent (McKeganey *et al.*, 1992).

Before March 1987 IDUs had difficulty purchasing needles and syringes. The first pilot needle exchange opened in June 1987 (Gruer, Cameron and Elliott, 1993). By December 1988, it was attracting 20 to 30 clients per week. By January 1989, a second needle exchange was opened and within a few weeks around 50 clients were attending each evening. At the time of the study there were four needle and syringe exchange schemes and approximately ten retail pharmacies which were the main outlets for the provision of sterile equipment. At needle and syringe exchange schemes, injection equipment is free of charge, and from a pharmacy the usual price of a needle and syringe was £0.40. In 1988, 2600 syringes were issued on the basis of 880 attendances, and by 1992, 238 500 syringes were issued on the basis of 27 990 attendances (ibid.). Prior to the establishment of needle and syringe exchange schemes, injectors were encouraged to use bleach to clean their equipment. By the time of the study, this policy had been dropped and replaced by the single unequivocal message of 'never share needles and syringes'.

There has been increasing availability of condoms for purchase, especially since the late 1980s and early 1990s, when messages promoting safer sex came to be increasingly important. Condoms have always been freely available through Family Planning Centres. Originally condoms could only be bought from pharmacies and vending machines, but they are now available from numerous outlets. There is opposition to their use by the Catholic Church, but it is not clear whether this has had any influence. Condoms are given free to injectors at needle and syringe exchanges and there is a health care drop-in for street sex workers which constitutes a major source of condoms.

There was little change in drug treatment and during the study period. Treatment consisted of a few hospital-based detoxification centres, one or two drug-free rehabilitation centres and a variety of self-help groups and voluntary organizations. Probably about 6 to 7 per cent of IDUs at any one time were in treatment during the study period. Almost no IDUs were on methadone treatment. Only later was a city-wide methadone programme established.

It was difficult to assess public attitudes to IDUs. If any attitude did prevail, it was one of slight compassion as part of an underlying feeling that factors such as unemployment, deprivation and the highly manipulative skills of drug barons were ultimately responsible for drug-using behaviour.

Drugs policy was markedly influenced by the report of the Advisory Council of the Misuse of Drugs in 1988, *AIDS and Drugs Misuse* (see under London).

This emphasized the importance of making contact with a greater proportion of the drug injecting population, and stressed that AIDS was a more important threat to public and individual health than drug misuse. The importance of working with the population of continuing injectors was also emphasized. There was a major development of harm reduction centred on syringe exchanges, and community drug and outreach teams. On a governmental level, Britain has stressed both its adherence to international conventions and the importance of police and customs work in reducing drug supply and demand. In 1988 a document 'HIV Infection and AIDS — towards an inter-agency strategy in Strathclyde' was published jointly by the Health Boards and Social Work Department. The aim of the document was to provide an integrated approach for the planning of drug and AIDS policies in the Glasgow area.

The greater Glasgow Health Board and the Social Work Department had implemented HIV/AIDS awareness-raising campaigns for the general public prior to the period of the data collection. At a national level there have been several advertising campaigns using television, radio and newspapers. Local campaigns were targeted at IDUs. Some were linked to drug treatment and needle and syringe exchange schemes while others were linked to pharmacies and general practitioners. Billboards highlighting the dangers of sharing needles and syringes were present in high-risk areas in the city.

Organizations for IDUs were not in existence before or during data collection. No organization for sex workers existed, though a centre for street workers was established in 1988. This is a social drop-in centre and is run by doctors, nurses and social workers.

UK legislation distinguishes drugs according to their perceived harmfulness and according to whether the offence involves trafficking/supply or only possession. Many prisoners have a history of drug injecting. *Ad hoc* HIV/AIDS education programmes for prisoners began in 1988/9. However, the turnover for persons committing drug related offences is usually high and education programmes for prisoners were never comprehensive, ongoing or well structured. Bleach was not officially available for the decontamination of injecting equipment in Scottish prisons. In some prisons, it was sometimes possible to obtain bleach, but it would have been necessary to disguise the purpose for which the bleach was intended. Treatment for drug dependent prisoners was virtually non-existent. Methadone maintenance was not available for drug dependent prisoners. Condoms were not available.

The focus of research in Glasgow has switched from identifying whether an epidemic of HIV was to occur to explain why low levels of infection have been maintained over a number of years (Bloor *et al.*, 1994; Taylor *et al.*, 1994). Explaining why something *did not* happen is more difficult than explaining why something *did* happen. However, it is likely that the speedy response to developing a network of needle exchanges, along with the development of outreach interventions and high levels of media coverage of HIV in Edinburgh, all played a part in limiting the spread of infection within Glasgow. The city's network of needle and syringe exchanges has now been complemented by the development of a city-wide methadone substitute prescribing service.

London

London is the capital of the United Kingdom. In 1990, the Greater London population was 6.8 million, about 11.8 per cent of the total population of the UK (including Northern Ireland). Greater London comprises 13 inner and 20 outer London boroughs. Local boroughs are responsible for social, educational and other services (apart from health or police in their area). There are significant demographic, cultural and economic differences between inner and outer areas. Socio-economic deprivation is generally higher in inner London (even though inner London contains pockets of extreme affluence). About 20 per cent of the population are black or from other ethnic minorities. There is no single health or metropolitan authority for London. At the time of the study, London health services were covered by four health regions, serving populations of around 3.5 million each. Smaller District Health Authorities were responsible for purchasing health and medical services from a variety of organizations, both within and outside the National Health Service.

IDUs have existed in significant numbers in London since the 1960s, and most injectors use heroin and other drugs. The most noticeable trend in the early 1980s was a continuing rise in the availability and use of heroin. The early 1980s saw the diffusion of drug injecting into new population groups, which in turn was part of a Europe-wide increase in heroin use. A particular features was the spread of heroin use and injecting among people living in deprived areas of inner cities. The size of the injecting population was, and remains, unknown, but in the mid-1980s estimates suggested that there were approximately 20 000 injectors living in London.

In 1986 there was an awareness of the potential for an epidemic of HIV-1 infection to occur among IDUs. The first case of AIDS in an IDU occurred in 1984. Following the introduction of the HIV antibody test in 1985, HIV-1 was discovered among IDUs in several parts of the country, including London. The first reported study in 1986 found a prevalence among IDUs of 0.7 per cent (Webb *et al.*, 1986). Subsequent studies in 1987 and 1988 found prevalences ranging between 3.7 per cent (Hart *et al.*, 1989) and 7.0 per cent (Hart *et al.*, 1991). Studies conducted between 1983 and 1987 showed that syringe sharing was common: in London between 60 and 80 per cent of drug injectors regularly shared syringes (Stimson, 1995).

Between 1986 and 1989 there was a growing national AIDS awareness, and intense media interest in HIV and AIDS. Reports of high HIV spread among IDUs in Edinburgh brought a new dimension to governmental and public concern. Drug injectors were thought to be a particularly important focal group, being viewed, in the language of the time, as a 'bridge' for the spread of HIV infection to others. They were also considered a difficult group in which to encourage changes in behaviour.

The HIV-1 outbreaks in Edinburgh (see under Glasgow) and Dundee were unique in the UK. But similar rapid epidemic spread was known to have occurred in cities elsewhere. A Scottish investigation into HIV infection among IDUs heard that the rapid spread of infection in Edinburgh was helped by police activity to discourage sale and possession of syringes, medical opposition to maintenance prescribing and the low level of investment in services for drug users (Scottish Home and Health Department, 1986). It suggested that making sterile needles and syringes available to people who inject drugs, along with improved treatment services and substitute prescribing would help to reduce sharing levels and the spread of HIV infection. The report is the first government document to refer to 'safer drug taking'.

In England the sale of syringes to IDUs was never illegal, but pharmacists operated a voluntary sales ban from 1982. This was rescinded in 1986. During 1986 a few drug agencies began distributing syringes — the earliest in April in Peterborough (70 km from London), and later at the Kaleidoscope Project in a suburb of London. By late 1986, an exchange had been established in central London.

In late 1986 the Department of Health and Social Security and the Scottish Home and Health Department initiated a pilot syringe exchange programme in England (including sites in London) and three in Scotland. It was the first government funded response to AIDS among IDUs. The years from 1987 to 1990 saw the development of major changes in working philosophy and practices in drug services, as the ideas of harm minimization, accessibility, flexibility and multiple and intermediate goals were developed (Advisory Council on the Misuse of Drugs, 1988; Stimson, 1995). Recognizing that many people who inject drugs are unable and unwilling to stop injecting, services tried to find ways of helping them to change their behaviour to reduce the risks of HIV infection. Early harm minimization projects focused on syringe exchange, with nearly 200 exchanges in the UK by 1990 (Lart and Stimson, 1990). Needles and syringes became increasingly available during the study period and IDUs were directly encouraged to use sterile injection equipment, distributed free and exchanged at syringe exchange schemes, together with information and advice leaflets and condoms. It is estimated that there were approximately 35 syringe exchanges within London at the time of the study. Approximately 25 per cent of pharmacies were willing to sell syringes, which were generally purchased for £0.10 each. Some helping agencies have promoted bleach as an alternative option when sterile syringes are unavailable, but bleach has not been a popular risk reduction method in London. Also important was the literature on harm minimization with posters, leaflets and comics including advice on safer drug use.

Overall there are no major cultural or religious obstacles to the use of condoms (though their use is opposed by some religious groups). There was an increase in the promotion of condom use, but data so far do not suggest major changes in sexual behaviour in the general population. Most drug agencies promote condom use through the display of safer sex posters, and condoms are often available free to clients of syringe exchanges and drug agencies. Condoms are also available free of charge from Family Planning Centres.

Most districts in London have access to a range of drug treatment services including drug dependency clinics, residential communities, advice and information agencies, crisis centres, self-help groups, community drug teams, Narcotics Anonymous and private rehabilitation units based on the Minnesota Model. General medical practitioners and probation officers are also important sources of help. Given the fragmented nature of the drug treatment services, estimating the proportion of IDUs in treatment is extremely difficult. However, on the basis of (now outdated) studies, it is possible that about 10 per cent of IDUs injecting mainly opiates were in treatment contact. The proportion of stimulant injectors in treatment contact is probably much less. From 1988 there was an expansion of outreach activities (Rhodes, Hartnoll and Johnson, 1991).

Drug treatment centres attempted to increase their attractiveness and accessibility to patients. The drug of choice in treatment is methadone, but this is prescribed in a rather arbitrary and *ad hoc* fashion. At the time of the study there were no methadone maintenance programmes within the NHS system. The predominant methadone prescribing regime by NHS doctors was a low-dose reducing regime. A variety of methadone preparations are prescribed including oral, tablets and injectables; however, the majority of NHS prescribing is of oral methadone. Any medical practitioner may prescribe methadone for the treatment of addiction.

Across London, the majority of the population is probably indifferent to drug injectors, with the exception of a few areas where drug using and dealing have caused localized problems.

IDUs were not involved in the process of HIV prevention policy development in any major way. However, there were attempts to involve IDUs as volunteers within drug agencies, for example in the distribution and collection of needles and syringes. The organizations for sex workers that existed did not have a major influence on HIV and AIDS policy.

About 10 per cent of the prison population in England has a recent history of drug injecting. HIV and AIDS education programmes for prisoners began in 1986, in the form of general education packages. They were not specifically aimed at IDUs. Treatment for drug dependent prisoners was rudimentary. There was no formal provision of methadone detoxification or maintenance for opiate dependent prisoners. Methadone maintenance programmes were available for pregnant women prisoners until the births of their babies. Bleach and sterile syringes were not available. Condoms were not available to prisoners, and there was considerable resistance to condom distribution in prisons, both at governmental and prison officer level.

Madrid

Madrid is the capital of Spain and has a population of 3.9 million. Madrid City is located in the Comunidad Autonoma de Madrid (CAM), which contains nearly 5 million people, out of the total Spanish population of 40 million. The Government of CAM, and Spain itself, is Socialist (Party Socialists Obrero Espanol), but the Government of the City of Madrid is Conservative (Partido Popular). The official language Castellano (Spanish) was the language used for the WHO questionnaire. The principal ethnic group is white (Caucasian), with Gypsies, Latin-Americans and North Africans in the minority.

Drug use in Madrid began to increase between 1970 and 1975, first with the use of LSD, cannabis and amphetamines. Around 1977 heroin use started to spread and it is now the most commonly injected drug in the city, followed by cocaine. Between 1981 and 1985 a comparative study of drug treatment centres in five Spanish cities showed 92 per cent of patients were injecting heroin. Levels reduced to 85 per cent in 1986/7 and to 58 per cent in 1991 (Escohotado, 1994). Although heroin use appeared to decline up to the beginning of the WHO Study, there still appeared to be an extremely high prevalence of heroin injecting. Health authorities estimated that there were around 24 000 IDUs in Madrid.

The first case of AIDS in Spain was reported in 1981; the first case in Madrid, in 1982. The first case related to IDU in Madrid was reported in 1983. Since reporting began, the biggest group of AIDS cases has been IDUs, both in the country as a whole and in the city of Madrid. In 1989 IDUs accounted for 64 per cent of all AIDS cases in Spain; about one quarter of all cases were in Madrid, and at the time of the study, 72 per cent of AIDS cases were associated with injecting drug use.

Syringes and needles have always been available. Spanish legislation has never restricted their sale at pharmacies. All of the 1800 pharmacies in Madrid were selling syringes when the study began, but few were open at night or on public holidays. The cost of syringes, in relation to average salaries and general cost of living, was not high at about 50 ptas. In 1990 and 1991 it was reported that almost half the IDUs in the city always used sterile injection equipment. The first needle exchange opened in 1991.

There is opposition to the use of contraception by the Catholic Church, which is the principal church in Spain. Men are culturally accustomed to rejecting the use of condoms, partly due to 'machismo' and partly due to the lack of information about their use. Condom use has increased, but is still not very widespread. Campaigns by authorities and family planning centres, encouraging people (particularly adolescents and other young adults) to use condoms have been implemented, but these have been subject to a counter-campaign launched by the Catholic Church.

In 1990, more than 25 100 drug treatment episodes at official treatment centres were notified to the State System of Information on Drug Abuse in Spain: 97 per cent were related to heroin use; 2 per cent to cocaine and 2 per cent to other opioids. Over 3250 cases were from treatment services in Madrid. Between

1989 and 1990 15 drug treatment centres were established in Madrid. All were public and treatment was free of charge. Only one centre ran a methadone maintenance programme, available to 200 people in advanced stages of AIDS. Dosage ranged from 20 to 50 mg per day. There were also some other drug treatment services in the city, most of which were therapeutic communities. There were no harm reduction programmes or prevention activities to reduce the spread of AIDS within the drug treatment programmes. The increase of AIDS cases among IDUs, at the time of the WHO Study, did not lead to a greater interest in drug treatment. Estimates indicated that between 10 and 20 per cent of IDUs in Madrid were in treatment on an average day.

The public's attitude towards IDUs is negative, because of the perceived threat to citizen safety and traditional values, and the fear that children will adopt behaviour related to drug consumption. The mass media mainly focus on this latter subject, and in a sensationalist way; that is, most of the time news about IDUs is transmitted in reports covering AIDS or issues related to crime, the family and the social order.

A national plan on AIDS was established in 1984 to collect data on AIDS. In 1987 the analysis of blood samples was started by law. The national prevention policy was based on mass media advertising campaigns, addressed to adolescents and to the general population. There was a national campaign on AIDS prevention in 1988, but no national campaign addressed to IDUs before the period of the study. Several campaigns were aimed at drug abstinence, and the number of drug treatment centres with that goal were increased. Between 1985 and 1987 IDUs became aware of HIV/AIDS through mass media, and from the staff of drug treatment centres. Prevention programmes based on harm reduction did not start in Madrid until 1990, with the small methadone maintenance programme mentioned above, operated by Médicin du Monde. Both were financed by the government.

Changes in politics have influenced the legal environment in Spain. The severe penalties for possession, use or traffic in the dictatorship period (Franco) were replaced by liberal legislation from 1983 to 1987 with the beginning of the Socialist Government. A new change occurred in 1988, bringing back strong legislation against possession and trafficking. The consumption of drugs is not penalized, but possession of small amounts is often considered indicative of drug dealing. This is a subjective decision, often dependent on the IDU or the views of the arresting officer or judge. Punishment for possession of drugs can be more severe than that for murder. Eighty per cent of prisoners in Madrid are in prison for a drug related offence. HIV/AIDS education programmes for prisoners started in 1987. From 1989, on entering jail, prisoners were given a kit which contains condoms, bleach, toothbrush, soap and so on. They also receive condoms when they have contact with their partners. Syringes are not available. Prisoners are given treatment in jail, but the range and type is limited. Methadone programmes are not provided.

There are few advocacy groups in Spain; they are relatively small and have little influence on HIV/AIDS policy. There are a few organizations which work with sex workers in Spain, and some of these are government-funded. Institutes which work with sex workers are The Institute for Women (set up by the Minister for Social Affairs) and two programmes run by Medicos del Mundo (an NGO) and Caritas — a Catholic organization.

New York

New York City has a population of slightly over 7 million. The greater New York–northern New Jersey–southern Connecticut consolidated metropolitan area has a population of approximately 20 million. There is a diverse economic base, with strengths in communications, financial services and manufacturing. The political system is a two-party representative democracy. City, state and federal laws all apply to the city, and there is often conflict between the city, state and federal governments. There is great ethnic diversity in the city, which has traditionally been the leading immigrant city in a 'nation of immigrants'. The most common racial/ethnic groups are 'Whites', 'Blacks' (African-Americans) and 'Hispanics' (Latinos). It should be emphasized, however, that there are very important ethnic differences within each of these broad groups, for example Jews, Irish and Italians within Whites, 'US' and Afro-Caribbean within Blacks, and Puerto Rican, Dominican and Mexican within Hispanics.

For many years New York was considered the capital of narcotic movement and usage in the world. The injection of drugs started from the nineteenth century and then spread in the first decades of the twentieth century. There was an 'epidemic' of increased heroin use in the late 1960s–early 1970s, and a great increase in cocaine use during the 1980s, including the 'crack' cocaine epidemic in the mid-1980s. In New York there are an estimated 200 000 injectors, distributed among many different socio-economic and racial/ethnic groups. Heroin and cocaine (and often the mixture of both — 'speedball') are the drugs most commonly injected.

HIV entered New York City sometime in the early to mid-1970s among homosexual/bisexual men. The virus then spread to homosexual/bisexual men who injected drugs and then to heterosexual IDUs. The first cases of AIDS were identified among gay men in New York in 1981 (among the first in the world), and the first cases in heterosexual drug users were also identified in 1981. Initially, the few cases of AIDS among IDUs did not generate a great deal of public health concern. However, after the availability of HIV-1 antibody tests in 1985, this concern radically intensified. These tests revealed that approximately half of the IDUs in New York had been infected with HIV-1 (Des Jarlais and Friedman, 1993).

The spread of HIV-1 within the IDU population may have occurred in the 1970s, long before AIDS was well known. This certainly would account for the relatively high rates of HIV-1 infection among IDUs. The first IDUs were probably infected around 1975 and there may have been a rapid spread of HIV-1 between 1978 and 1983. Unfortunately, in such a high seroprevalence area even relatively low levels of risk may lead to high rates of new HIV-1 infection. Many factors, such as injecting in 'shooting galleries' (where syringes can be rented by many different drug users), drug dealers that lend injection equipment to customers and the group purchasing of drugs, could possibly have contributed to the rapid spreading of HIV-1 in New York (Des Jarlais and Friedman, 1993; Des Jarlais and Friedman, 1990).

Possession and purchase of injection equipment were illegal at the beginning of the WHO Multi-City Study. During the period of data collection, underground AIDS activist syringe exchanges were set up, and some outreach programmes made syringes available on a small scale, but these did not reach a large proportion of active IDUs. Cleaning with bleach as an official method of sterilizing injection equipment was not encouraged in New York as it was in other places in North America, except in a very small number of unofficial programmes. Outreach programmes provided HIV/AIDS education and encouraged IDUs not to share injection equipment. The illicit market in sterile injection equipment expanded in response to increased demand. Small-scale, unofficial programmes have distributed bleach since 1986. These programmes involved approximately 50 to 75 outreach workers. An official outreach strategy was in place since 1987. During the period of data collection, this involved more the promotion of bleach as a method of syringe sterilization, rather than actual bleach distribution. Since then bleach distribution has become more widespread.

There are approximately 40 000 to 50 000 treatment slots for IDUs in New York. The most common form of drug treatment is methadone, although detoxification and drug-free residential services also exist. Both the capacity and attractiveness of drug treatment services have increased little since the advent of HIV and AIDS. HIV/AIDS education was added to existing drug treatment programmes and these programmes also developed some capacity for providing additional medical services to persons with HIV infection. Persons with AIDS were generally given priority for drug treatment. There were waiting lists of around 1000 persons during the time of the data collection, and it is estimated that during this period around 15 to 20 per cent of IDUs were in treatment on an average day.

The majority of methadone patients were on 'high dose, long-term' methadone treatment. Methadone maintenance was developed in New York, and the city has the world's largest system of methadone treatment programmes, with over 30 000 methadone treatment slots in the city. The Dole-Nyswander approach of high dosage of indefinite treatment is the official policy of most programmes, although a substantial percentage of staff encourages patients who are doing well to try to detoxify and remain abstinent.

Illicit drug use, particularly heroin and cocaine use, is generally highly stigmatized, and considered a crime and a moral failure of the individual. Attitudes towards illicit drug use also reflect racial/ethnic conflicts, with minority groups stigmatized for their drug use; this goes as far back as Chinese opium smoking around the turn of the century. Negative attitudes towards illicit drug use are also reinforced by the connections between drug use and violent crime.

The primary drug policy in the USA was supply reduction. The great majority of persons arrested on drug charges were low-level street dealers. At the time of the study harm reduction approaches to drug use had little influence. However, from around 1992 this changed and harm reduction is now the official policy response within New York.

Government-implemented AIDS awareness media campaigns began around 1985, before the data collection period. AIDS awareness campaigns specifically targeted at IDUs began in 1986. Data show that IDUs were aware of the risks of HIV/AIDS around 1984, prior to specific health education strategies and seven years after the epidemic began (1977).

Possession of small amounts of drugs for personal use is a criminal offence. However, the criminal justice system is so overloaded that possession of small amounts of illicit substances would only rarely lead to a prison sentence. There is, however, considerable police harassment of drug users on the street. It is estimated that around 60 per cent of the prison population have drug misuse problems and that 40 per cent of that total are IDUs. During the time of the study there were AIDS education programmes in jails and prisons. Condoms were available to prisoners, but by request only, so they were not frequently used. To date, bleach is not available in prisons.

The Association of Drug Abuse Prevention and Treatment (ADAPT) was formed in 1985 to represent IDUs. Although not specifically a users group, ADAPT has had some degree of influence on related policy and has organized outreach programmes, bleach distribution, and more recently syringe exchange schemes. In the period since data collection, drug users' organizations have begun to be developed in New York City, and these are affiliated to the North American Users' Network formed in March 1994. There were no formal organizations of sex workers at the time of the study.

The increase in incidence and increased severity of non-AIDS illnesses associated with HIV-1 among IDUs are noteworthy, especially the increased incidence of tuberculosis and its multidrug-resistant strains. It is estimated that a high percentage of tuberculosis patients in New York City are infected with HIV-1. Afro-Americans and Latinos (ethnic minority groups) are at disproportionate risk of HIV-1 infection as well as of tuberculosis (Curtis *et al.*, 1993; Friedman *et al.*, 1993; Friedman *et al.*, 1987).

Rio de Janeiro

Rio de Janeiro is the second city of Brazil (after São Paulo). The city is divided into 30 administrative regions and the population registered by the 1991 census was 5.5 million (excluding the surrounding Grande Rio area). Fifty-two per cent of the total population are female and just over a third are under 19 years of age. Ethnic variability is inaccurately registered as no precise definition of ethnicity exists. However, the population is mainly comprised of 'mulattos' (black/white Mestizos), whites (mainly of Portuguese heritage) and blacks. Brazil is a federal state, and since the mid-1980s, the country has been a democracy ruled by an elected president.

For more than a hundred years the drug of preference in Brazil was marijuana, mostly used by blacks and mulattos. In the 1960s marijuana use spread to the white middle-class population during the counter-culture movement. However, some fictional Brazilian literature refers to the use of cocaine during the 1920s. The diffusion of cocaine use in Brazil is very clearly related to the recent North American political 'War on Drugs'. In the last 15 years Brazil has gradually become a cocaine trafficking route. In this time international drug traffickers have developed a local market in order to guarantee consumption of the surplus. The relationship between cocaine trafficking routes and the AIDS epidemic is evident in Brazil and has been verified in recent years (Mesquita, 1992; Bastos, 1995). Cocaine is the most commonly injected drug. Very little was known about cocaine injection prior to the registration of the first AIDS cases among IDUs. Most IDUs inject cocaine. At the time of the WHO study, heroin use was uncommon in Brazil and was generally restricted to non-Brazilians or wealthier Brazilians who have lived abroad.

The HIV/AIDS epidemic appears to have begun in Brazil in the late 1970s. The first AIDS case in Brazil occurred in São Paulo, the largest city in Brazil, in 1982. The first AIDS case related to IDU occurred in Rio de Janeiro, in 1983.

The prevalence of HIV-1 infection among IDUs is around 30 per cent. When HIV/AIDS among IDUs first came to public awareness, in the late 1980s, HIV-1 probably already had a relatively high prevalence in this population. In the period between 1982 and 1986 IDUs represented only 3 per cent of the national registered AIDS cases. In 1992 this figure had increased to around 24 per cent. An important trend, observed in Rio de Janeiro city and state and also elsewhere in Brazil, is the significant increase of AIDS cases among women through heterosexual transmission, both from IDUs and bisexual partners. Data from two studies among IDUs suggest that the prevalence of HIV-1 infection among IDUs is around 30 per cent. Despite this, the significance of IDUs in the overall AIDS cases in Rio de Janeiro was not as important as it was in other cities in Brazil, such as in the state of Saõ Paulo.

Drug policies have been based on demand and supply reduction. Few preventive efforts directed to IDUs are based on 'harm reduction' strategies. Since the beginning of the 1990s a few interventions have been tried, such as outreach work, distribution of condoms and the training of health personnel. At the time of the WHO study there were no drug user advocacy groups.

Needles and syringes can generally be purchased in pharmacies without prescription and they are not expensive. However, considering that the salaries in Brazil are low for the majority of the population, they are expensive. Although bleach is both cheap and widely available, it is not commonly used by IDUs to clean injecting equipment.

Aside from the commonly reported negative feelings surrounding condom use (such as shame, prejudice, nuisance and uneasiness) there are two main obstacles against use of condoms. The first is the strong influence of the Catholic Church, and the other is for many people the high price of condoms. However, the National AIDS Program is attempting to reduce the price of condoms. Family planning centres in Brazil, generally funded by external sources (mainly USA), take a major role in the free distribution of condoms. There is a significant lack of condom distribution programmes targeted at IDUs compared with the reasonable availability of free condoms and educational programmes for other 'at risk' groups such as male and female sex workers, homosexual or bisexual men, or sexual partners of infected persons.

Rio de Janeiro has only one free public treatment facility for drug users, which is NEPAD, an out-patient service operated by the State University of Rio de Janeiro since 1986. Other provision includes self-help groups such as Drug Addiction Anonymous and religious groups. There is a major shortage of treatment facilities and there are long waiting lists. There are also private treatment institutions, but they are too expensive for most potential clients.

The main obstacle to providing adequate treatment services in Brazil is a lack of public funding. What is available is out of reach for many drug users as they are unable to afford private clinics. There was no reliable estimate of how many IDUs there were in Rio at the time of the WHO Study or how many are receiving drug treatment. An informed estimate would suggest 6 to 10 per cent. There were no methadone programmes.

The laws on drug use and the drug policy in Brazil are seen as anachronistic and there is an intense debate in the Brazilian society about changes in the law, including the decriminalization of marijuana. Impediments to change in policies and legislation include the strong influence of their North American neighbours.

Public attitudes to IDUs are generally unsymphathetic. Discussions about new treatment options or public policies emphasizing a harm reduction approach were, in general, not welcomed in Brazil. Traditionally, Brazilian drug policies are strongly dependent on and similar to USA policies, so supply reduction was the primary and dominant approach of the National Drug Policy at the time of survey. NGOs tend to have a greater tolerance and openness to deal with controversial issues though, due to limited resources, they have a restricted coverage.

Since the middle of the 1980s there have been national government HIV/AIDS awareness campaigns, although none specifically targeting IDUs. The only local initiative that included information about less hazardous injection practices took place in Santos, São Paulo, at the beginning of the decade. Generally government campaigns are cautious in handling sensitive issues, for example drug use and men-to-men relationships.

There are no reliable data on the percentage of the prison population that are IDUs. There had been no educational programmes targeting incarcerated IDUs, and no programmes of bleach or condom distribution in Rio de Janeiro's prisons. No specific treatment programme is available for incarcerated drug users. Brazil has very few known cases of heroin injectors so there is little demand for methadone maintenance programmes for drug users in prisons.

There are, to date, no drug user and advocacy groups and the role and influence of current IDUs is negligible. Since the middle of the 1980s Rio de Janeiro has had sex workers' associations, mainly supported by international agencies active in Rio.

Rome

The involvement of Italy in the WHO Multi-City Study commenced in recognition of the heterogeneity of Italian city epidemics in a country with marked cultural and socio-economic differences. Italy was one of the countries where the concept of regional sub-epidemics proved at an early stage to be fruitful for epidemiological analyses and the establishment of preventive strategies (Cantoni *et al.*, 1995).

The cities initially enrolled in the study were Rome, Naples, Milan, Verona and Cagliari, although only data from Rome are included in this book. They vary in geographical location — Verona and Milan in the north; Rome, the capital, in the middle; Naples in the south and Cagliari on the island of Sardinia. Rome, Naples and Milan are big cities with over 3 million inhabitants, whereas Verona and Cagliari are middle-size cities with around 800 000 inhabitants. One common feature is that, despite regional differences, the overall AIDS epidemic in Italy is strongly influenced by high levels of infection among IDUs. The patterns of HIV infection and AIDS is similar to that in Spain (around 65 per cent of all the AIDS cases in both countries are among IDUs).

The Italian political system is a liberal democracy, and more than 10 parties have representatives in the parliament. At the time of the study, the national government was run by a coalition of five parties. Regional government has a certain degree of autonomy, particularly regions like Sardinia (Cagliari). Coalitions running regional governments may differ from those running the national government. Ethnic variation in Italy is limited.

The prevalence of injecting drug use increased significantly in Italy during the second half of the 1970s/1980s, as demonstrated both by the increase of death by overdose and by an increase of drug users attending drug treatment services. Heroin was the most commonly injected drug, being initially injected by largely young middle-class people in specific urban areas. This pattern was subsequently replaced by a more diffused one, crossing social classes in most urban centres and proving to be particularly common among the unemployed. The yearly average number of IDUs in Rome, during 1980–8 was estimated around 12 000 (out of a population of 3 million) (Perucci *et al.*, 1992). This rose to approximately 20 000 in 1992.

The first AIDS case in Italy was reported in 1982 and the first case related to IDU was reported in 1984. The analyses of frozen blood samples suggest that in 1979 HIV-1 infection was present among IDUs in the Milan area (Tempesta and Giamantomo, 1990). HIV spread rapidly in the first half of the 1980s in cities like Milan and Cagliari. However, large geographical variations were observed in 1985/6 with the highest rates of HIV among IDUs in the northern provinces. Cross-sectional surveys showed seroprevalence of HIV-1 ranging from 5 per cent in Naples, to 30 per cent in Rome, to approximately 50 to 60 per cent in Milan. Up to 1990, 5236 subjects with HIV infection and 848 cases of AIDS were reported to the HIV and AIDS Surveillance System of the Epidemiology Unit of the Lazio Region. IDUs accounted for 59 per cent of the HIV infected subjects and 57 per cent of the AIDS cases.

The purchase or possession of sterile needles and syringes has not been restricted and injecting equipment is sold in pharmacies at low prices. Despite this, high rates of syringe sharing were reported in the 1980s. This suggested that deeply embedded social habits were involved in the genesis and dynamic of the Italian epidemic among IDUs. There were also particular settings where syringes and needles were not always available.

Treatment services have been available free of charge since 1980. They offer mainly methadone treatment and a low dose detoxification regime. There are no waiting lists for treatment. During the 1980s the number of drug users attending drug treatment increased. Methadone maintenance is available, although it was not officially endorsed. No efforts were made to make drug treatment services more attractive during the study period. It is estimated that approximately 30 per cent of IDUs in Italy were in treatment during the study period. No harm reduction programme was set up before 1994.

Possession of small quantities of drugs was, and is, tolerated in Italy. Public attitudes regarding drug use range from compassion to hostility. At the time of the study, drug users were not involved in the formation of strategies for prevention or assistance to their peers. The direction of public campaigns related to HIV/AIDS was always general, without any specific focus on IDUs, despite their epidemiological significance.

Until 1989 the Catholic Church had a considerable influence over the Italian Government policy regarding condom use. However, after this period there have been no real obstacles to the use of condoms. Family planning centres were not really implementing strategies to promote the use of condoms. No convincing effort was made to promote condom use among IDUs.

Public attitudes towards drug users in Italy vary between hostility and pity. Attempts to introduce harm reduction approaches met obstacles at both political and public opinion levels. Demand reduction has received more emphasis as a national policy for dealing with drug problems. The harm reduction approach has been more broadly accepted since the beginning of the 1990s, including distribution of syringes in vending machines (after 1992), although the use of bleach has never been promoted.

Mass media HIV/AIDS awareness-raising campaigns were implemented at a national level in 1988. The campaigns were not specifically targeted at IDUs, but focused instead on general HIV/AIDS information. Studies of behavioural change and HIV incidence data indicate that IDUs became alerted to the risk of HIV infection through injecting practices around 1986/7.

No regional or national policy focused specifically on prison populations. Only the occasional HIV/AIDS education programmes have been directed towards prisoners. Bleach was not available for cleaning injecting equipment. The only treatment available for drug users was drug-free treatment, that is detoxification. Methadone treatment was not available for incarcerated prisoners, and condoms were not provided.

There were no organizations for IDUs. Before the study period, organizations for sex workers had been established. However, very few sex workers were actively involved. These organizations have been unable to influence HIV/AIDS policy nationally.

Santos

Santos is situated in the south-east of the State of São Paulo, and is the largest port in South America. The city has 428 526 inhabitants (53 per cent females, and 33 per cent of the population under 19 years of age). The health services are localized and extend to smaller surrounding towns such as Bertioga, São Vicente, Guaruja, Praia Grande and Cubatao. Ethnic variability is inaccurately registered, as no precise definition of ethnicity exists. However, the population is comprised of 'mulattos', white (mainly of Portuguese heritage) and blacks. Brazil is a federal state and, since the mid-1980s, the country has been a democracy ruled by an elected president.

In Santos the first AIDS cases were reported in 1984 and, since then, drug injection has appeared as the transmission route in one in four of the AIDS cases reported each year. Injecting drug use has become a growing problem in the HIV epidemic. Since 1988 Santos has had the highest incidence of AIDS cases in Brazil. About half of the AIDS cases in the city have been directly related to injecting drug use.

Cocaine is the main drug that is injected. The social and economic conditions in Brazil make dealing in small quantitities of cocaine a means of subsistence for many people in Santos, as elsewhere in the country.

The Brazilian law on drugs permits the purchase and possession of syringes. Legislation dating from 1976 makes the implementation of needle exchange programmes, or any other preventive programmes, difficult. It is possible to buy and possess needles and syringes without a prescription. Sterile injecting equipment can be bought in most pharmacies at low cost (approx US $0.20), although, as observed by our fieldworkers, IDUs did not like to spend money on injecting equipment. At the time of the WHO Study there was no system of syringe exchange in Santos, but, given the increasing incidence of AIDS cases among IDUs, there has been some political pressure to make such a programme available. There is a vociferous debate in Brazilian society about these programmes, but at the time of the WHO Study no needle exchange programme, or any other strategy to reduce the harm caused by the injection of drugs, had been implemented in Santos. During the latter part of the study period (1992) the municipal government initiated a programme to promote the sterilization of needles and syringes. The use of bleach was encouraged through posters, leaflets, counselling and by outreach workers and municipal health professionals. Since the study period, these promotional activities are being supplemented by the distribution of bleach kits.

The importance of the Catholic Church in Brazil has proved an obstacle to the use of condoms in the country. Despite this influence, national health authorities have emphasized the need for the use of condoms for prevention of HIV/AIDS. People in Brazil rarely use condoms. Condoms are very expensive in Santos (US $0.50 per unit), and distribution programmes are few and far between. A programme of condom distribution was implemented through the STD/AIDS Control Program in Santos in 1989. Initially, health professionals found it difficult to discuss issues concerning HIV and AIDS.

There are few drug treatment places and most are private and very expensive. Few government-funded centres offer drug treatment, and access to government-funded programmes is difficult. Public drug treatment was not available in Santos at the time of the WHO Study. Some religious NGOs offered drug treatment, but without any quality control by the health authorities. Patients who are HIV-1 positive, in particular female patients, would have the greatest difficulty in obtaining treatment. In Brazil most drug users are cocaine dependent and unlike the use of methadone for heroin misusers, there is no substitute drug for cocaine.

Although drug use was common among prisoners, injecting drug use was not. Condoms were available for prisoners. However, it is important to note that the prison population is more resistant to condom use than the rest of the community. One education project in São Paulo was aimed specifically at prisoners. The project is based on a harm reduction philosphy and organizes the distribution of condoms and educational materials, but not bleach or syringes as this is a proscribed activity in Brazilian prisons.

There was no organized group for drug users in Santos and no organizations for sex workers. It is estimated that very few sex workers inject drugs. Since 1989, STD/AIDS prevention programmes for sex workers have distributed condoms, provided safe-sex education and offered free treatment and medicines.

Sydney

The make-up of Sydney's 3.9 million population is reasonably representative of the general Australian population. Approximately a third are born to Australian parents, a third are born overseas, and a third are born in Australia to parents from overseas. The local government holds no responsiblity for health matters: local health services are administered through the State Government of New South Wales.

Injecting drug use was very limited until the late 1960s when during the Vietnam war, visiting US servicemen facilitated the growth of drug injecting populations in both rural and urban areas in Australia. Eastern parts of Sydney have always been the major focus because of proximity to the major airport and seaport. Heroin is the most commonly injected drug; however, the injection of amphetamine has increased in popularity since the mid-1980s and large numbers of other drugs are also injected. A conservative estimate suggests there are between 8000 and 10 000 injectors in Sydney.

The first cases of HIV and AIDS involving IDUs were reported in 1986.

At the early stages of the HIV epidemic, injecting equipment could not be lawfully obtained and this legislation was strengthened in 1985. In November 1986 a pilot needle and syringe exchange scheme was established and began distributing free injecting equipment to IDUs. In December 1986 the NSW Government encouraged pharmacies to sell needles and syringes to IDUs and by the time of the WHO Study implemented a series of measures designed to make sterile injection equipment readily available to IDUs. Bleach distribution began in 1988. Government attempts to encourage IDUs to modify their risk behaviour started in 1987, as well as specific attempts to increase utilization of pharmacies and exchange schemes. These education campaigns used pamphlets and posters, and a variety of media including television and cinema advertisements. The cost of injecting equipment is generally very low, ranging from nothing to US \$0.50 depending on where the equipment is acquired. Bleach distribution began in 1988.

Condoms have been readily available for decades. Availability improved during the 1980s in response to the HIV/AIDS epidemic. Some groups in the community are opposed to barrier methods of contraception, but their views are not given much prominence and community attitudes to condoms have been fairly liberal for many years. Condoms were available from a wide variety of outlets including pharmacies, needle and syringe exchanges, family planning centres and community groups established in response to the HIV/AIDS epidemic. IDUs have been encouraged to use condoms by official government campaigns since the late 1980s.

Efforts to improve treatment for IDUs began in the mid-1980s in response to concerns about the level of illicit drug use in the community. The most common forms of treatment, at the time of the study, were detoxification, residential rehabilitation, methadone maintenance and out-patient counselling. Capacity of methadone prescribing increased by about 15 per cent per year during the late 1980s, but still never met demand. Those groups specifically targeted for drug treatment were women, prisoners, aborigines, non-English speakers and young people. Methadone programmes vary, although there was increasing emphasis on higher dose long-term maintenance and a decrease in emphasis on low dose short-term treatment with the aim of abstinence. It is difficult to estimate the proportion of Sydney's IDUs engaged in treatment. However, at the time of data collection, it was unlikely that more than 25 per cent were enrolled in a treatment programme. It is presumed that there has been an increase in this proportion as the demand for treatment has continued to increase.

Attitudes to IDUs have changed over time. Following the National Campaign Against Drug Abuse, people became more understanding. Media portrayals of drug users are much more likely to indicate the complexity of drug issues, rather than portraying IDUs as deviants. In 1985 harm reduction was accepted as the national objective of drug policy. The recognition in the mid-1980s that contentious steps needed to be taken quickly, enabled the rapid adoption and implementation of HIV prevention measures. Major HIV/AIDS awareness-raising campaigns were conducted nationally from the early 1980s, including a shock campaign which received considerable criticism, but which was remarkably successful in putting the subject high on the national agenda. Campaigns targeting IDUs were developed from 1987. A government-funded IDU group in NSW was established in 1988 and was functioning actively by the time of data collection.

Possession of a narcotic, without necessarily intention to supply, results in a charge and often a conviction. Police say unofficially that action may not be taken if the quantity is small and there are no previous convictions. HIV/AIDS education is provided in the prison system, and bleach has been sporadically provided since 1990. Treatment for drug problems has been available in the prison system in a number of years, but availability of drug treatment does not meet demand. Methadone maintenance was available for about 500 of the 6000 prisoners. Condoms have not been made available despite numerous recommendations from health professionals. Prison officers remain adamant in their opposition to the introduction of condoms.

IDUs have been involved in the development and implementation of responses to HIV/AIDS from the mid-1980s. This usually means ensuring that they are included on committees which have responsibility for developing and implementing policy. An organization to represent sex workers was successful in influencing policy regarding sex work and also gained support for HIV prevention policies for IDUs.

Toronto

Metropolitan Toronto is the capital and financial hub of Ontario, includes several urban municipalities, and has a total population of 3.9 million. Within Metropolitan Toronto, the City of Toronto in the downtown core has a population of 635 395 and has its own city council and public health department. The official language is English, although Toronto is considered to be a multi-lingual, multi-cultural city, with many different cultures co-existing within its boundaries. The population has changed with a large immigrant population choosing to settle in the area.

The Government in Canada has a three-tiered system. The Federal Government consists of an elected House of Commons and a Senate which is appointed. Provincial governments are elected within each of ten Canadian provinces with major powers in areas such as health and education. In Metropolitan Toronto there is a municipal government for each constituent municipality as well as a Metro Toronto Council, with representation from each of these municipalities. Each level of government has its own designated areas of authority and responsibility.

There is low lifetime heroin usage in the Toronto population – about 1 to 2 per cent among students, and lifetime use among adults is less than 1 per cent. There was a decline in use among street youth between 1990 and 1992. Lifetime cocaine use among adults was estimated at around 2 per cent in 1991. Cocaine use among students shows a continuing decline since its peak of 6 per cent in 1985. Marijuana use increased during the 1960s, but declined during the 1980s and 1990s. In the late 1980s and early 1990s crack use was evident in Toronto. Use among the population is estimated to be 1 per cent.

The first case of AIDS involving an IDU was recorded in 1984. Injecting drug use accounts for 1 per cent of all AIDS cases and is the second most commonly reported risk behaviour among those testing HIV-1 positive in Canada. HIV-1 prevalence rates among IDUs range from less than 1 per cent to around 17 per cent. The highest rates of HIV-1 among IDUs have been found in Montreal, Quebec.

Possession of injecting equipment is not illegal in Canada. Until 1989 Ontario's College of Pharmacists' policy stated that provision of needles and syringes to non-diabetics was not professionally ethical. In 1989, the policy was changed, indicating that providing needles and syringes to IDUs might be appropriate in the light of HIV/AIDS. However, sales were still subject to the personal discretion of the pharmacists. At the time of the study needles and syringes were available through syringe exchange schemes and through a number of pharmacies. In 1989 there was one syringe exchange scheme in Toronto, and by 1993 the number had risen to nine. A recent survey showed that 88 per cent of pharmacies in the Toronto area were willing to sell injecting equipment to non-diabetics in at least some cases. Distribution of bleach began in 1987/8. The DPH sponsored a bleach kit programme with distribution at syringe exchange sites and other centres. It includes bleach, water for rinsing, an alcohol swab, a cotton ball, condoms, standardized instructions for syringe cleaning and condom use.

The willingness to use condoms varies, reflecting the multicultural and multireligious nature of the population. Contraception in Canada became legal in 1969. Condoms are available through pharmacies, sex shops, community agencies, family planning centres, condom shops and by mail order. Condom distribution by the City of Toronto, Department of Public Health began in 1983. By 1988, free condoms were available in city-funded birth control and STD clinics.

Drug treatment was available at seven treatment centres before and during the study period. All programmes had waiting lists. The most common forms of treatment were detoxification, rehabilitation, out-patient counselling and methadone maintenance and reduction. Only a small number of methadone treatment slots were available (about 200 to 300) during the study period. Although it is difficult to estimate figures, less than 5 per cent of IDUs would be in treatment on an average day. Ten per cent of IDUs in methadone programmes were on low dose/short-term treatment and the remaining on high dose long-term treatment.

Media portrayals of IDUs are generally negative, and there is public concern about drug-related violence. In some areas residents' groups have attempted to rid the neighbourhood of drug users and sex workers. Some people believe that drug users do not deserve service provision, and prefer to emphasize legal sanctions.

Harm reduction is gaining a foothold in drug services but was not the dominant strategy at the time of the study. Initial harm reduction orientated programmes received funding as experimental projects. During the study period, current IDUs did not have direct involvement with policy development or implementation, although there was indirect involvement through community agencies working with drug users.

All forms of media were used to help increase the awareness of HIV/AIDS, including forums in schools and local malls. A major information campaign was conducted in 1988, containing basic AIDS information and the telephone number of the AIDS hotline. Campaigns specifically targeting drug users were more on a community level, with agencies serving the clientele doing most of the educating. The risks associated with sharing injection equipment were incorporated into national and local campaigns directed at the general public, although issues such as syringe exchange and other harm reduction practices were left to the local campaigns. IDUs became aware of HIV/AIDS around 1987, mainly through HIV/AIDS health education.

The Narcotic Control Act (NCA) specifies which drugs are illegal and all of those are defined as narcotics for legal purposes. The Food and Drug Act (FDA) deals with ensuring that foods, cosmetics, medicine and medical devices are safe for human consumption and use. At mid-point in the data-collection period, convictions for possession of narcotics resulted in sentences ranging from discharge or parole to 3.5 years' imprisonment. There are two prison systems. A provincial prison is for those sentenced for two years or less, and those sentenced for over two years are committed to a federal prison. A recent study of HIV prevalence in Ontario correctional facilities found that 12.5 per cent of males and 20 per cent of females had a history of injecting drug use. HIV/AIDS education programmes have been conducted within federal prisons since the 1980s. In the provincial system, there is some access to drug treatment and initial withdrawal is generally monitored by health-care staff. In the federal system, a variety of treatment services are available, although methadone maintenance for prisoners is not generally available. If users are on a programme prior to incarceration the treatment may be continued. Condoms have been available in all federal prisons since early 1992, and in the provincial system since late 1993. Bleach is not officially provided in Ontario correctional facilities, though some IDUs, have managed to get access to bleach whilst in prison.

Drug policy is primarily under federal jurisdiction. However, municipal Boards of Health will often initiate local policies on treatment for drug use and HIV. For example, the Board of Health for the city of Toronto approved the introduction of syringe exchange in the city.

Organizations for IDUs did not exist in Toronto prior to the study period. Organizations for sex workers were established before 1989/90. Sex workers organized at both local and national levels and attempted to have their voices heard in discussions about syringe exchange services in the city. The sex worker organizations ran their own HIV/AIDS awareness programme for sex workers, although these groups did not have a substantial influence in HIV/AIDS policy.

References

ADVISORY COUNCIL ON THE MISUSE OF DRUGS (1988) *AIDS and Drug Misuse: Part 1*, London: HMSO.

BASTOS, F. (1995) 'Ruina & Reconstruçào — AIDS e drogas injectávceis na cena contemporänea', Rio de Janeiro: Relume Dumará & ABIA.

BLOOR, M., FRISCHER, M., TAYLOR, A. *et al.* (1994) 'Tideline and turn? Possible reasons for the continuing low HIV prevalence among Glasgow's injecting drug users', *Sociological Review*, **2**, pp. 738–57.

CANTONI, M., LEPRI, A.C., GROSSI, P. *et al.* (1995) 'Use of AIDS surveillance data to describe subepidemic dynamics', *International Journal of Epidemiology*, **24**, 4, pp. 804–12.

CHOOPANYA, K., VANICHSENI, S., DES JARLAIS, D.C. *et al.* (1991) 'Risk factors and HIV seropositivity among injecting drug users in Bangkok', *AIDS*, **5**, 12, pp. 1509–13.

CURTIS, R., FRIEDMAN, S.R., NEAIGUS, A. *et al.* (1993) 'TB among injecting drug users: Current strategies may be counterproductive', Abstract, American Public Health Association, Annual Meeting, San Francisco.

DES JARLAIS, D.C. (1994) 'Cross-national studies of AIDS among injecting users', *Addiction*, **89**, pp. 383–92.

DES JARLAIS, D.C. and FRIEDMAN, S.R. (1990) 'Shooting galleries and AIDS: Infection probabilities and "tough" policies', *American Journal of Public Health*, **80**, pp. 142–4.

DES JARLAIS, D.C. and FRIEDMAN, S.R. (1993) 'Harm reduction: A public health response to the AIDS epidemic among injecting drug users', *Annual Review Public Health*, **14**, 41, pp. 3–50.

DES JARLAIS, D.C., CHOOPANYA, K., WENSTON, J. *et al.* (1992) 'Risk reduction and stabilization of HIV seroprevalence among drug injectors in New York City and Bangkok, Thailand', in ROSSI, G.B. *et al.* (Eds) *Science Challenging AIDS*, Basel: Karger.

DES JARLAIS, D.C., CHOOPANYA, K., VANICHSENI, S. *et al.* (1994) 'AIDS risk reduction and reduced HIV seroconversion among injection drug users in Bangkok', *American Journal of Public Health*, **84**, 3, pp. 452–5.

EIGDU (EUROPEAN INTEREST GROUP OF DRUG USERS) (1993) *The situation of the drug using population in Europe*, Memorandum, Berlin: Deutsche AIDS-Hilfe.

Escohotado, A. (1994) 'La situación en Europa: el caso espanhol', *História de las Drogas*, **3**, pp. 336–42.

Follet, E.A.C., McIntyre, A., O'Donnell, B. *et al.* (1986) 'Antibody in drug abusers in the West of Scotland: The Edinburgh connection', *Lancet*, **i**, pp. 446–7.

Follet, E.A.C., Wallace, L.A., McCruden, E.A.B. (1987) 'HIV and HBV infection in drug abusers in Glasgow', *Lancet*, 18 April.

Friedman, S.R., Sotheran, J.L., Abdul-Quader, A. *et al.* (1987) 'The AIDS epidemic among blacks and hispanics', *The Milbank Quarterly*, **65**, suppl 2.

Friedman, S.R., Jose, B., Neaigus, A. *et al.* (1993) 'Multiple minority status as a risk factor among drug injectors', IX International Conference on AIDS, Berlin.

Frischer, M., Bloor, M., Finlay, A., Goldberg, G. *et al.* (1991) 'A new method for estimating prevalence of injecting drug use in an urban population', *International Journal of Epidemiology*, **20**, pp. 21–6.

Frischer, M., Green, S.T., Goldberg, D.J., Haw, S., Bloor, M., McKeganey, N. *et al.* (1992) 'Estimates of HIV infection among injecting drug users in Glasgow, 1985–1990', *AIDS*, **6**, pp. 1371–5.

Gruer, L., Cameron, J. and Elliott, L. (1993) 'Building a city wide service for exchanging needles and syringes', *British Medical Journal*, **306**, pp. 1394–7.

Hamouda, O., Schwartländer, B., Koch, M.A. *et al.* (1993) *AIDS/HIV 1992 — Bericht zur epidemiologischen Situation in der Bundesrepublik Deutschland zum 31.12.1992*, Berlin: AIDS-Zentrum in Bundesgesundheitsamt.

Hart, G.J., Carvell, A.L.M., Woodward, N., Johnson, A.M., Williams, P. and Parry, J.V. (1989) 'Evaluation of needle exchanges in Central London: Behaviour changes in anti-HIV status over one year', *AIDS*, **3**, pp. 261–5.

Hart, G. M., Woodward, N., Johnson, A. M., Tighe, J., Parry, J. V. and Adler, M. W. (1991) 'Prevalence of HIV, hepatitis B and associated risk behaviours in clients of a needle exchange in Central London', *AIDS*, **5**, pp. 543–7.

Hermann, W. (1993) 'JES — History, demands and future', in *Aspects of AIDS and AIDS-Hilfe in Germany*, Berlin: Deutsche AIDS-Hilfe.

Kappeler, M., Barsch, G., Gaffron, K. *et al.* (1993) 'Die Entwicklung des legalisierten und ilegalisierten Drogenkonsums unter Schuterinnen der Sekundarstufe im Ostteil der Stadt Berlin — Ergebnisse der zweiten Wiederholungsuntersuchung im Jahr 1992', *Forschungsbericht* (Research report, p. 65), Berlin: Institut fur Sozialpädagogik der Wilhelm-Griesinger Krankenhauses.

Koch, U. and Ehrenberg, S. (1992) 'Akzeptanz AIDS-präventiver Botschaften: Evaluation der Autklärungs- und Beratungsarbeit bei i.v. Drogenabhägigen in Bundesrepublik Deutschland', in *AIDS und Drogen II — Evaluation AIDS-Präventiver Botschaften*, Berlin: Deutsche AIDS-Hilfe.

Kokkevi, A. and Stefanis, C. (1991) 'The epidemiology of licit and illicit substance use among high school students in Greece', *American Journal of Pubic Health*, **81**, pp. 48–52.

Kokkevi, A., Alevizou, S., Arvanikis, Y. *et al.* (1992) 'AIDS related behaviour and attitudes among IV drug users in Greece', *International Journal of Addictions*, **27** (1), pp. 37–50.

Lart, R.A. and Stimson, G.V. (1990) 'National survey of syringe exchange schemes in England', *British Journal of Addictions*, **85**, pp. 1433–43.

McKeganey, N., Barnard, M., Leyland, A., Coote, I. and Follet, E. (1992) 'Female streetworking prostitution and HIV infection in Glasgow', *British Medical Journal*, **305**, pp. 801–4.

Malliori, M., Kokkevi, A., Hatzakis, A. *et al.* (1992) 'Behavioural changes in IV drug users in Greece: personal perception and self reported practices', VIII International Conference on AIDS, Amsterdam.

MALLIORI, M., HATZAKIS, A., KATSOULIDOU, A. *et al.* (1993) 'Hepatitis C virus (HCV) seroepidemiology provides important insight in the understanding of the spread of HIV epidemic in intravenous drug users', IX International Conference on AIDS. Berlin.

MESQUITA, F. (1992) 'Capitulo VI, Março de 1989', in *AIDS na Rota da Cocaina*, São Paulo: Anita Garibaldi.

PAPAEVANGELOU, G., ROUMELIOTOU, A., STERGIOU, G. *et al.* (1991) 'HIV infection in Greek intravenous drug users', *European Journal of Epidemiology*, **7** (1), pp. 88–90.

PERUCCI, C.A., FORASTIERE, F., RAPITI, E., DAVOLI, M. and ABENI, D. (1992) 'The impact of intravenous drug use on mortality of young adults in Rome, Italy', *British Journal of Addictions*, **87**, pp. 1637–41.

QUINN, T.C. (1994) 'Population migration and the spread of types 1 and 2 human deficiency viruses', *Proceedings of the National Academy of Sciences*, **91**, pp. 2407–14.

RASCHKE, P. and KALKE, J. (1993) 'Substituitionstherapie in der Bundesrepublik Deutschland', *Neue Praxis*, **3**, pp. 207–18.

RHODES, T.J., HARTNOLL, R. and JOHNSON, A. (1991) *Out of the Agency and on to the Streets: A review of HIV Outreach Education in Europe and the United States*, London: Institute for the Study of Drug Dependence.

RHODES, T.J., BLOOR, M., DONOGHOE, M.C. *et al.* (1993) 'HIV prevalence and HIV risk behaviour among injecting drug users in London and Glasgow', *AIDS Care*, **4** (5), pp. 413–25.

ROBERTSON, J.R., BUCKNALL, A.B.V. and WIGGINS, P. (1986) 'Regional variations in HIV antibody seropositivity in British intravenous drug users', *Lancet*, **i**, pp. 1435–6.

ROUMELIOTOU-KARAYANNIS, A., TASSOPOULOS, N., KARFODINI, E., TRICHOPOULOU, E., KOTSIANOPOULOU, M. and PAPAEVANGELOU, G. (1987), 'Prevalence of HBV, HDV and HIV infections among intravenous drug addicts in Greece', *European Journal of Epidemiology*, **3**, pp. 143–6.

SCOTTISH HOME AND HEALTH DEPARTMENT (1986) *HIV Infection in Scotland*, Edinburgh: Scottish Committee on HIV Infection and Intravenous Drug Misuse.

STARK, K. and KLEIBER, D. (1991) 'AIDS und HIV-infektion bei intravenös Drogenabhängigen in der Bundesrepublik Deutschland', *Deutsche Medizin Wochenschrift*, **116**, pp. 863–9.

STIMSON, G.V. (1995) 'AIDS and injecting drug use in the United Kingdom, 1987–1993: The policy response and the prevention of the epidemic', *Social Science and Medicine*, **41**, 5, pp. 699–716.

STÖVER, H. and SCHULLER, K. (1992) 'AIDS prevention with injecting drug users in the former West Germany: A user-friendly approach on a municipal level', in O'HARE, P. *et al.* (Eds) *The Reduction of Drug-related Harm*, London: Routledge.

TASSOPOULOS, N., KALAFATAS, P., NIKOLAKAKIS, P., GIOTSAS, Z., MELA, H. and HATZAKIS, A. (1989) 'Prevalance of antibodies against human immunodeficiency virus-1 in Greek homosexuals and intravenous drug abusers', *Latriki*, **55**, pp. 77–80.

TAYLOR, A., FRISCHER, M., GREEN, S.T., GOLDBERG, D., McKEGANEY, N. (1994) 'Low and stable prevalence of HIV among drug injectors in Glasgow', *International Journal of STD and AIDS*, **5**, pp. 105–7.

TEMPESTA, E. and GIANNANTONIO, M. DI (1990) 'The Italian epidemic: a case study', in STRANG, J. and STIMSON, G.V. (Eds) *AIDS and Drug Misuse*, London: Routledge.

WEBB, G., WELLS, B., MORGAN, J.R. and McMANUS, T.J. (1986) 'Epidemic of AIDS-related virus infection among intravenous drug abusers', *British Medical Journal*, **292**, p. 1202.

WENIGER, B.G., LIMPAKARNJANARAT, K., UNGCHUSAK, K. *et al.* (1991) 'The epidemiology of HIV infection and AIDS in Thailand', *AIDS*, **5**, 2, pp. 571–85.

WENIGER, B.G., TAKEBE, Y., OU, C.Y. and YAMAZAKI, S. (1994) 'The molecular epidemiology of HIV in Asia', *AIDS*, **8**, suppl. 2, S13–S28.

WHO (1994) WHO International Collaborative Group, *Multi-City Study on Drug Injecting and Risk of HIV Infection*, Geneva: World Health Organization.

WRIGHT, N., VANICHSENI, S., AKARASEWI, P. *et al.* (1994) 'Was the 1988 HIV epidemic among Bangkok's injecting drug users a common source outbreak', *AIDS*, **8**, pp. 529–32.

Contributors and Collaborating Agencies in the World Health Organization Multi-City Study on Drug Injecting and Risk of HIV Infection

AUSTRALIA (Sydney)

Dr Alex Wodak

St Vincent's Hospital
Rankin Court
866 Victoria Street
Darlinghurst
New South Wales 2010
Australia

Dr Michael Ross
Aaron Stowe
Margaret Kellaher

National Centre in HIV Social
   Research
University of New South Wales
354 Crown Street
Surrey Hills
New South Wales 2010
Australia

BRAZIL (Rio de Janeiro)

Dr Francisco Bastos
Dr Elson Lima
Dr Paulo Roberto Telles
Dr Maria Thereza de Aquino
Dr Saul Bogea (deceased)

NEPAD/UERJ
Rua Fonseca Teles 121, 4 andar
CEP29940–200 São Cristovao
Rio de Janeiro
Brazil

BRAZIL (Santos)

Dr Fábio C. Mesquita
Dr Regina De Carvalho Bueno
Dr Giselda L. Turienzo
Dr Milton A. Ruiz
Dr Heraclito Carvalho
Dr Eduardo Massad

IEPAS (Instituto de Estudos e
   Pesquisas em AIDS de Santos)
Av Almirante Cochrane 130
Santos, S-P
CEP 11040.000
Brazil

CANADA (Toronto)

Dr Randall Coates (deceased)
Dr Peggy Millson
Dr Ted Myers

Dr Margaret Fearon
Ms Carol Major
Dr James Rankin

Department of Preventive Medicine
  and Biostatistics
University of Toronto
12 Queens Park Crescent West
Toronto, Ontario M5 1A8
Canada

GERMANY (Berlin)

Dr Wolfgang Heckmann

AIDS Research Unit
Willibald-Alexis-Str 39
W-1000 Berlin 61
Germany

Dr Dieter Kleiber
Dr Anand Pant

Freie Universitaet Berlin
Psychological Department
Habelschwerdter Alee 45
14195 Berlin
Germany

GREECE (Athens)

Dr Meni Malliori
Professor C. Stefanis
Dr D. Mitsikostas
Dr M. Economou

Department of Psychiatry
Eginition Hospital
Athens University Medical School
Vas Sofias 74
11528 Athens
Greece

Dr A. Hatzakis

Department of Hygiene and
  Epidemiology

Athens University Medical School
M Asias 75
11527 Athens
Greece

Dr F. Zafiridis

Therapy Centre for Dependent
  Individuals
Sorvolou 24
11636 Athens
Greece

ITALY (Rome)

Dr Giovanni Rezza
Dr Carlo Perucci
Dr Marina Davoli
Stefano Salmaso
Dr Damiano Abeni
Alessandra Anemona

Osservatorio Epidemiologica Regione
  Lazio
Via Santa Costanza
Rome
Italy

Dr A. Saracco

Hospital Sacco
Infectious Diseases Unit
Via GB Grassi
Milan
Italy

SPAIN (Madrid)

M. Angeles Rodriguez-Arenas
M. Victoria Zunzunegui Pastor
J. Carlos Romero Bellido

Centro Universitario de Salud
  Publica
General Oraa 39

28006 Madrid
Spain

THAILAND (Bangkok)

Dr Kachit Choopanya
Dr Suphak Vanichseni
Dr Suwanee Raktham
Dr Wandee Sonchai

Department of Health
Bangkok Metropolitan
  Administration
173 Dinsoa Road
Bangkok 10200
Thailand

UNITED KINGDOM (Glasgow)

Dr David Goldberg
Dr Sally Haw
Dr Martin Frischer
Dr Stephen Green
Dr Neil McKeganey
Dr Avril Taylor

AIDS Surveillance Programme
  Scotland
Communicable Diseases (Scotland)
  Unit
Ruchill Hospital
Glasgow G20 9NB
Scotland

UNITED KINGDOM (London)

Professor Gerry V. Stimson
Martin Donoghoe
Gillian Hunter
Tim Rhodes
Dr Betsy Ettore
Adam Crosier

The Centre for Research on Drugs
  and Health Behaviour
Charing Cross and Westminster
  Medical School
200 Seagrave Road
London SW6 1RQ
UK

UNITED STATES OF AMERICA (New York)

Dr Don Des Jarlais
Patricia Friedmann

Beth Israel Medical Centre
215 Park Avenue South, 15th Floor
New York
NY 10003
USA

Dr Samuel R. Friedman
Jo Sotheran

National Research and Development
  Institutes Inc.
11 Beach Street
New York
NY 10013
USA

WORLD HEALTH ORGANIZATION

Dr Andrew L. Ball
Programme on Substance Abuse

Dr Manuel Carballo
Global Programme on AIDS (until
  1990)
Programme on Substance Abuse
  (until 1992)

World Health Organization
1211 Geneva 27
Switzerland

Contributors

Damiano Abeni
Laboratorio di Epidemiologia
Instituto Dermopatico
  dell'Immacolata – Istituto di
  Ricovero e Cura a Carattere
  Scientifico
Rome
ITALY

Massimo Arcà
Epidemiology Unit
Lazio Regional Health Authority
Rome
ITALY

Andrew Ball
Programme on Substance Abuse
World Health Organization
Geneva
SWITZERLAND

Christovam Barcellos
Department of Health Information
Oswaldo Cruz Foundation
Rio de Janeiro
BRAZIL

Francisco Bastos
Department of Health Information
Oswaldo Cruz Foundation
Rio de Janeiro
BRAZIL

Regina Bueno
Instituto de Estudios e Pesquisas em
  AIDS de Santos

and Secretaria Municipal de Higiene
  e Saude de Santos
Santos
São Paulo
BRAZIL

Kachit Choopanya
Office of the Permanent Secretary
Bangkok Metropolitan
  Administration
Bangkok
THAILAND

Marina Davoli
Epidemiology Unit
Lazio Regional Health Authority
Rome
ITALY

Don C. Des Jarlais
Chemical Dependency Institute
Beth Israel Medical Center
New York
UNITED STATES OF AMERICA

Kate Dolan
National Drug and Alcohol Research
  Centre
University of New South Wales
Kensington
AUSTRALIA

Martin Donoghoe
Programme on Substance Abuse
World Health Organization
Geneva
SWITZERLAND

Samuel R. Friedman
National Development and Research
  Institutes, Inc.
New York
UNITED STATES OF AMERICA

Patricia Friedmann
Chemical Dependency Institute
Beth Israel Medical Center
New York
UNITED STATES OF AMERICA

Martin Frischer
Department of Medicines
  Management
Keele University
Staffordshire
UNITED KINGDOM

David Goldberg
Scottish Centre for Infection and
  Environmental Health
Ruchill Hospital
Glasgow
SCOTLAND

Steven Green
Scottish Centre for Infection and
  Environmental Health
Ruchill Hospital
Glasgow
SCOTLAND

Holly Hagan
Seattle-King County Department of
  Public Health
Seattle
Washington
UNITED STATES OF AMERICA

Gillian Hunter
Centre for Research on Drugs and
  Health Behaviour
London
UNITED KINGDOM

Bengt Ljunberg
Department of Infectious Diseases
University Hospital
University of Lund
Lund
SWEDEN

Neil McKeganey
Centre for Drug Misuse Research
University of Glasgow
Glasgow
SCOTLAND

Meni Malliori
Greek Organization for Combatting
  Drugs (OKANA)
Athens
GREECE

Fabio Mesquita
Nucleo de Pesquisas Epidemiologicas
  em AIDS da Universidade de São
  Paulo
and Instituto de Estudios e Pesquisas
  em AIDS de Santos
Santos
São Paulo
BRAZIL

Peggy Millson
Department of Preventive Medicine
University of Toronto
Toronto
CANADA

Ted Myers
Department of Health
  Administration
University of Toronto
Toronto
CANADA

Carlo A. Perucci
Epidemiology Unit
Lazio Regional Health Authority
Rome
ITALY

Andrea Pugliese
Department of Mathematics
Universita di Trento
Povo
ITALY

David Purchase
Point Defiance AIDS Prevention
    Project
Tacoma
Washington
UNITED STATES OF AMERICA

Tim Rhodes
Centre for Research on Drugs and
    Health Behaviour
London
UNITED KINGDOM

M. Angeles Rodriquez-Arenas
Centro Universitario de Salud Publica
Universidad Autonoma de Madrid
Madrid
SPAIN

Michael Ross
University of Texas
Houston
Texas
UNITED STATES OF AMERICA

Massimo Sangalli
Epidemiology Unit
Lazio Regional Health Authority
Rome
ITALY

Gerry V. Stimson
Centre for Research on Drugs and
    Health Behaviour
London
UNITED KINGDOM

Paulo Telles
Treatment and Research Centre on
    Drug Abuse
and State University of Rio De
    Janeiro
São Cristovao
Rio de Janeiro
BRAZIL

Kerstin Tunving
Department of Psychiatry and
    Neurochemistry
University of Lund
Lund
SWEDEN

Alex Wodak
St Vincent's Hospital
Darlinghurst
New South Wales
AUSTRALIA

Maria Victoria Zunzunegui
Escuela Andaluza de Salud Publica
Campus Universitario de Cartuja
Granada
SPAIN

Index